HEALING WITH YOGA

Yamini Muthanna

Om Books International

First Published in 2025 by

Om Books International

Corporate & Editorial Office
A-12, Sector 64, Noida 201 301
Uttar Pradesh, India
Phone: +91 120 477 4100
Email: editorial@ombooks.com
Website: www.ombooksinternational.com

Sales Office
107, Ansari Road, Darya Ganj
New Delhi 110 002, India
Phone: +91 11 4000 9000
Email: sales@ombooks.com

Photographer: Sudeep Gurtu and Arjunjith

Interior Design & Layout: Sheena Agarwal Sharma

ISBN: 978-93-63956-12-4

Printed in India

10 9 8 7 6 5 4 3 2 1

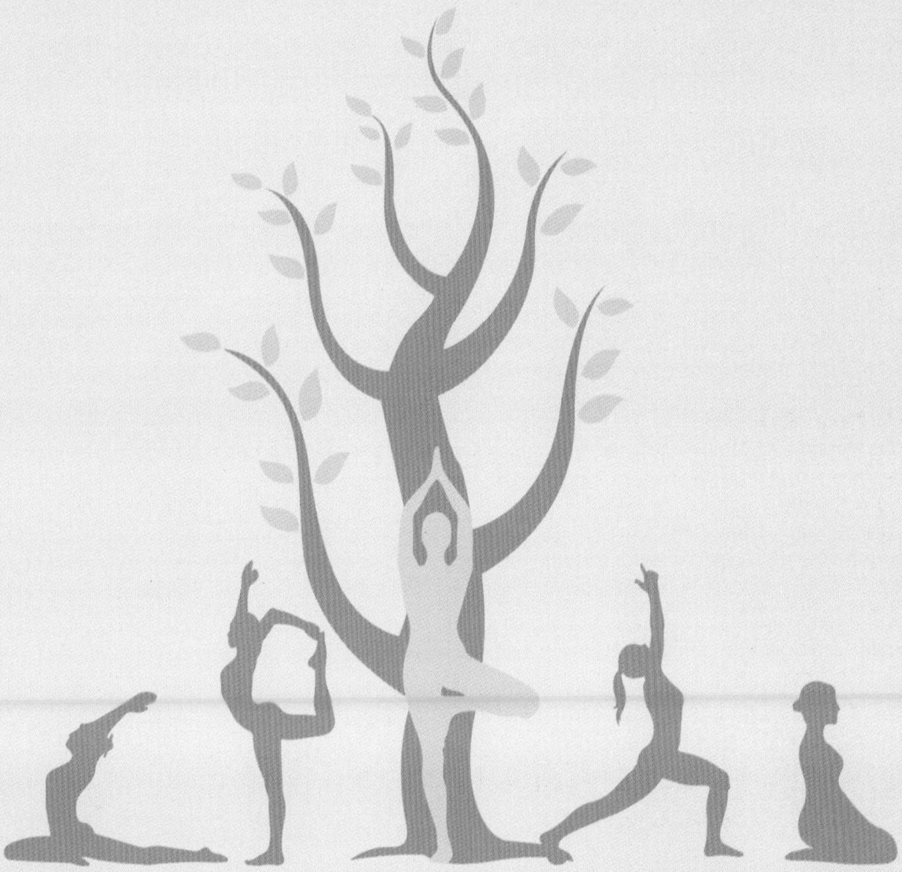

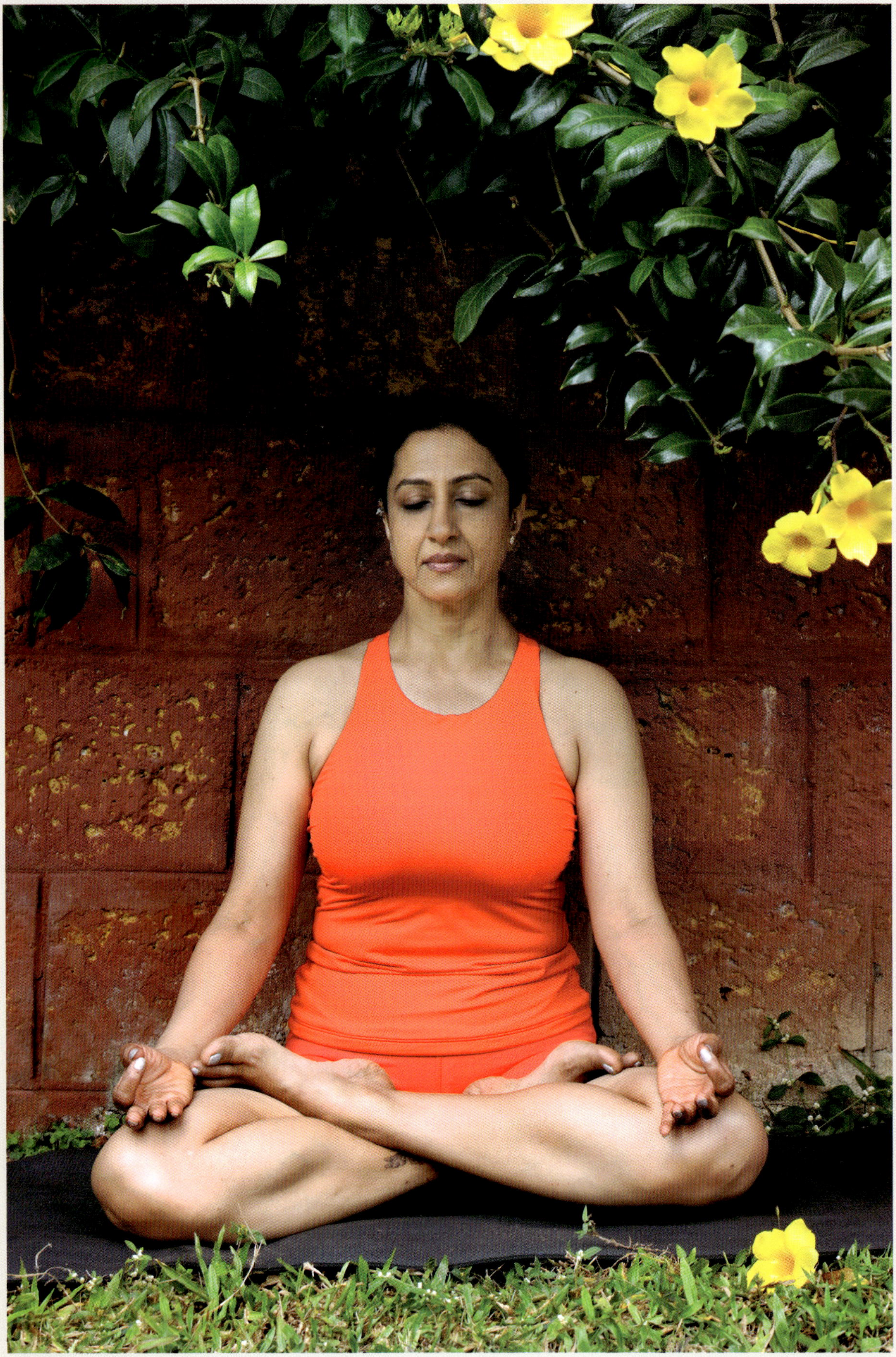

CONTENTS

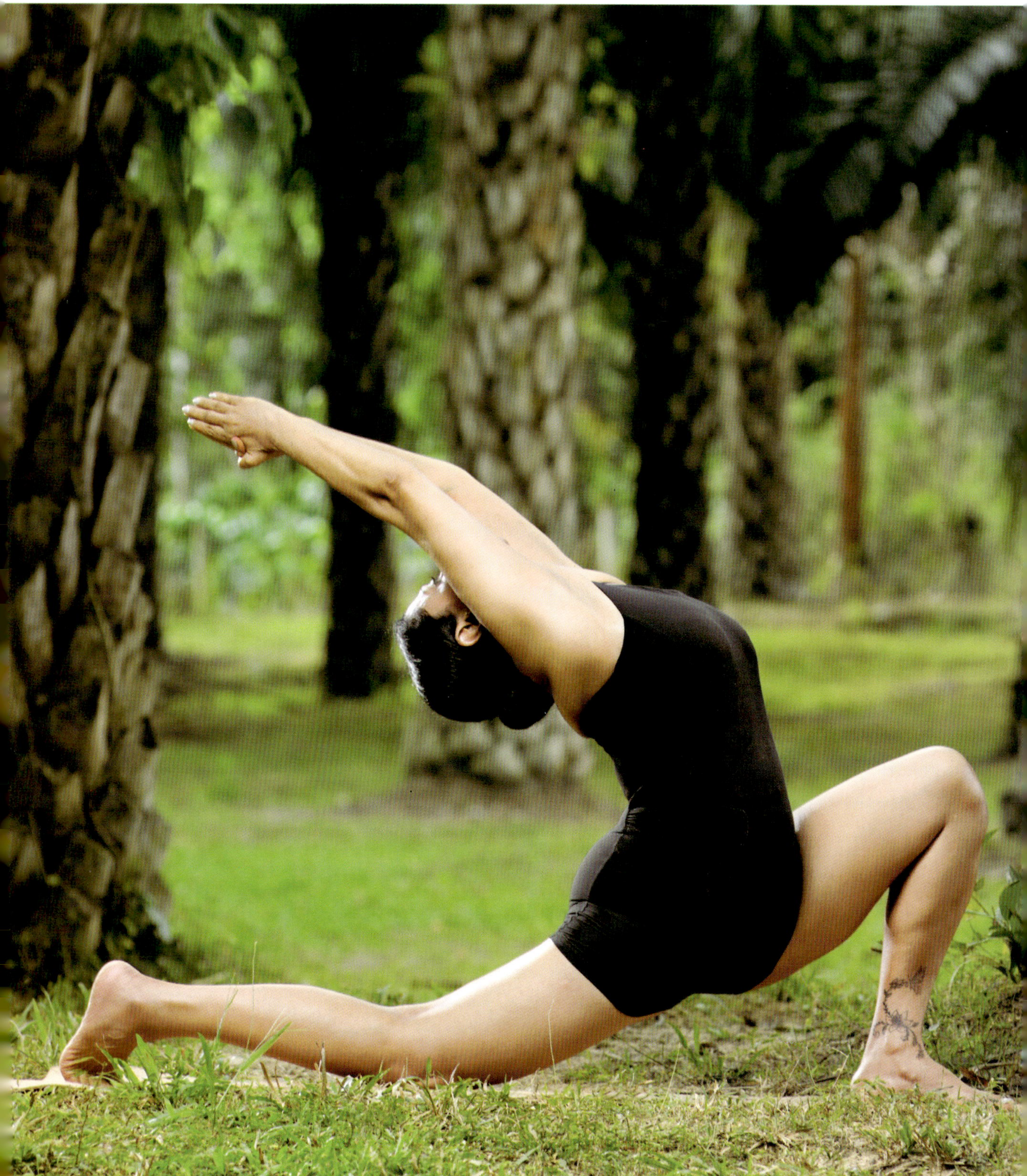

ACKNOWLEDGEMENTS

This book is a personal compilation of my learning, practice, teaching and research spread across over three decades. I am grateful to all the sacred books and documents with regard to yoga and Ayurveda. I have integrated this knowledge system into my lifestyle and have immensely benefited from it. This book is all about sharing my valuable study. I have tried my best to make sure of the accuracy of the contents shared. I humbly hope that I have remained true to the ever-evolving knowledge. I have worked on this book on my own for more than four years, compiling research and documenting from various sources and teachers.

My deepest gratitude is to my revered yoga guru, Shri B.N.S. Iyengar of Mysuru, whose knowledge and passion inspired me to keep the study going. I am not a qualified Ayurvedic doctor but a practitioner who has been following Guruji's tips and instructions through various stages of my life. His teachings were not confined to a structured syllabus or a traditional classroom setting. Instead, they were shared organically, offered only when a student was truly ready to receive them. The knowledge shared in this book is the result of 12 years of dedicated study under his guidance, coupled with 20 years of self-practice—seamlessly woven into my contemporary life as a city-dwelling mother of two grown-up children, a yoga *acharya*, a *natya* acharya, and the author of exclusive, practical yoga books tailored for the modern lifestyle.

I would like to convey my admiration and respect to my revered Bharatanatyam guru, 'Amma' Dr Vasundhara Doraswamy, who has always inspired me with her discipline and strength to keep the challenges of life going. An ardent practitioner of yoga herself, she has blessed my work in classical dance and yoga as always.

I have been blessed with some wonderful students from across the globe at my school of yoga, Yogastala, in Bengaluru which has completed 24 years now. My students have always encouraged and supported me with all the means to make this book come to life. I would like to especially thank Mr Shankar Maruwada for the support during the photoshoots and research tours. I would like to thank all those students who helped me financially to make this book. My special thanks to my dear friends Late Ramki Srinivasan (may his soul rest in peace) and Swarna Srinivasan for introducing me to Om Books International who have been the publishers of my work ever since.

A heartfelt acknowledgement to my friend and photographer Mr Sudeep Gurtu for the fabulous pictures that were not easy to take in the beautiful location of Kodagu. Thanks to photographer Arjunjit for the beautiful mudra photographs. Thanks to my dear cousin Karan Subbaiah for taking us to the most beautiful locations for the photoshoot. I am also thankful to our gracious hosts Prashanth Chinnappa and his gorgeous

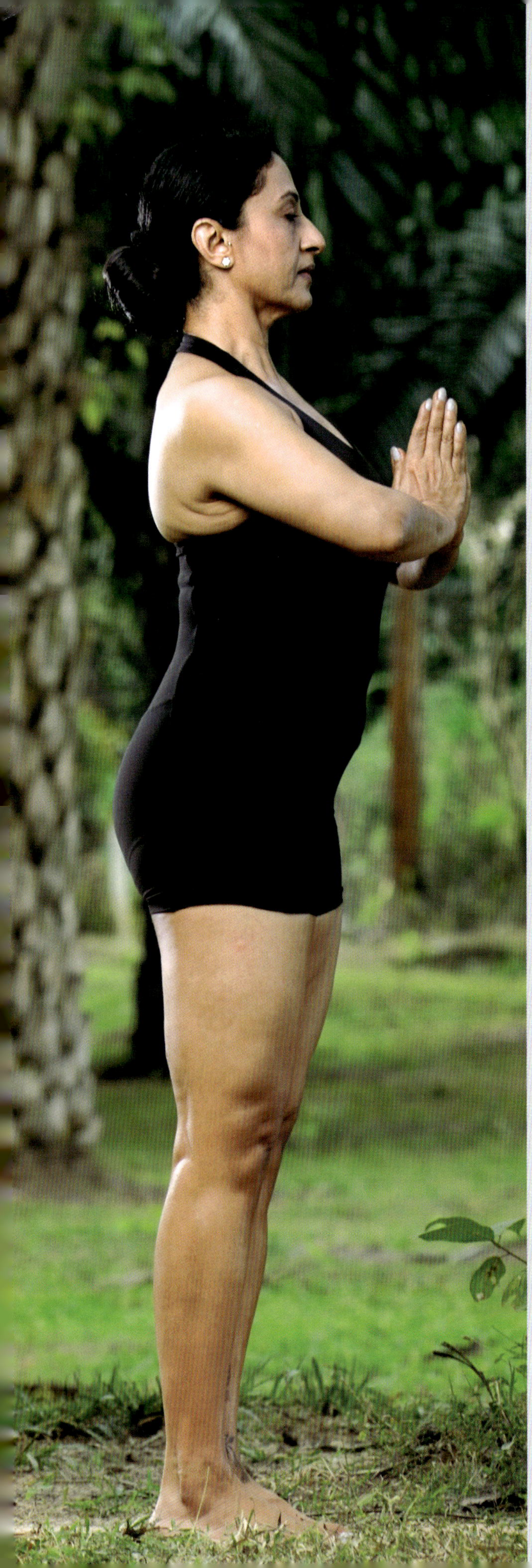

wife Disha Chinnappa for opening their estate for the photoshoot and serving us the most delicious food.

A special thanks to my family for their constant support and help in all my undertakings. My late parents have been a source of encouragement in everything I do. My daughter Manya Muthanna who has done the first proofreading of this book; my son who has been an assistant during the photoshoots; my husband whose silent support has been most valuable. My work is always blessed by my parents-in-law Mr Kotera Chengappa and Mrs Radha Chengappa. My dear brother Vachan Chinnappa has been my constant critic and support.

My sincere thanks to Mr Ajay Mago, publisher at Om Books International, for always bringing out the most beautiful designs and print of the book. Grateful to the editor of the book Ms Sakschi Verma for the accuracy and thorough editing of the contents. Thanks Sheena Agarwal Sharma for the fabulous design of the book and arranging the contents such that it makes for a very informative and enjoyable read. The books published by Om Books have inspired many to adopt yoga into their lifestyle.

INTRODUCTION

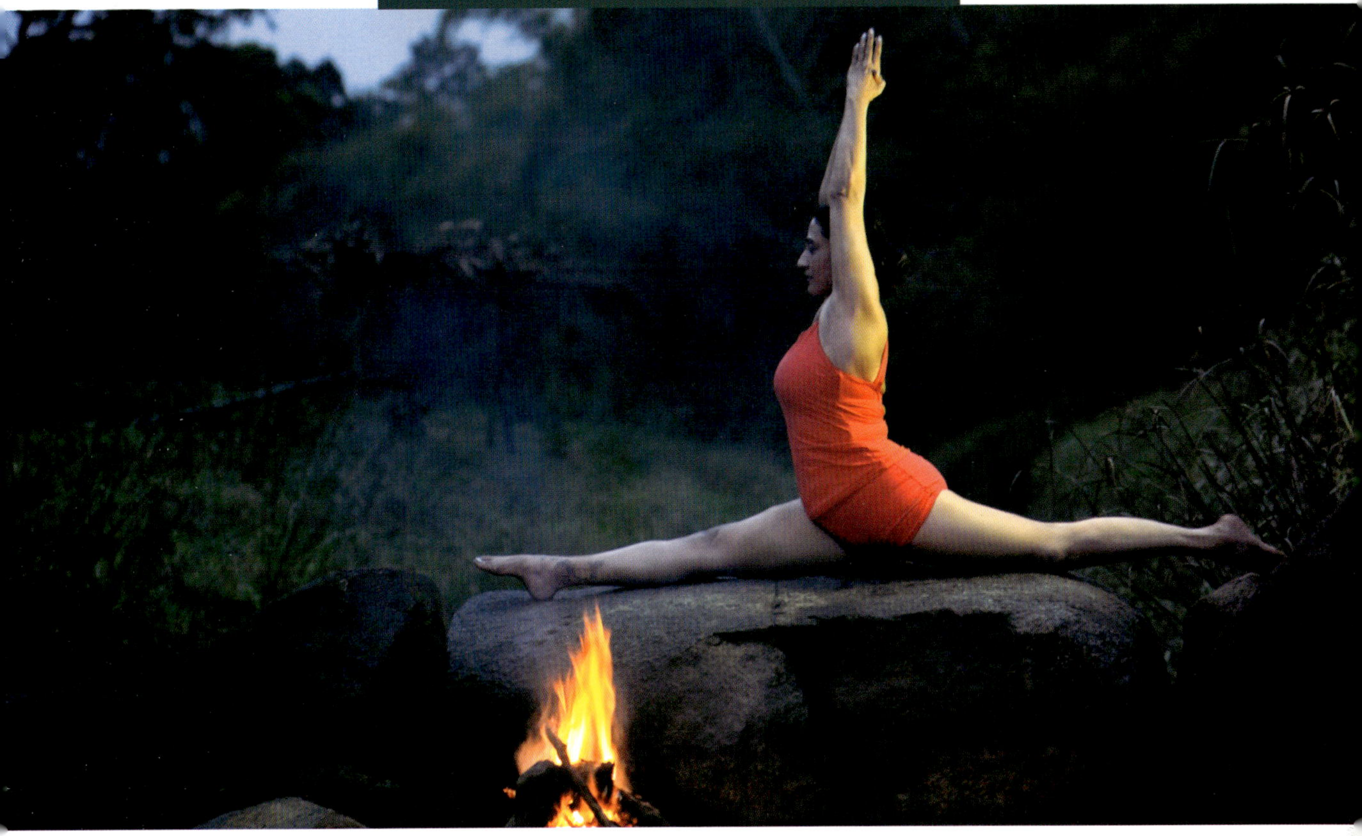

Yoga is a lifestyle. It is an ancient practice that helps align and connect the *sharira*, *prana*, *manas* and *atma*. Good health is not about the absence of disease, it is the alignment of these four aspects. It can be seen in modern times that psychological well-being is becoming vital for maintaining physical health. The lifestyle we choose forms an important factor in determining our health and happiness.

With more than three decades of practice and teaching asanas, pranayama and *pratyahara*, I was faced with a very potent question: 'What lies beyond the mat?' I started seeking for the value and essence of my yoga practice. Yoga is defined as the 'union of the Self with the Divine'. This looked like a simple definition but it was very difficult for me to understand, thus sending me on a journey of exploration. It took a lot of time and questioning to understand this definition. Most of the points that helped me find some answers are explained in this book, and I hope it helps you dive deeper into what yoga means as a practice.

A peek into how the ancient practices of yoga evolved and the changes it went through during the course of many centuries makes the study fascinating to read. The practice of yoga stems from the timeless wisdom of enlightened sages and rishis, who thoughtfully gathered their valuable insights, ensuring that future generations could embrace its benefits. Each of their findings was tried and tested and then documented. The essence of yoga is referred to in Vedas, Upanishads, *Yoga Sutra*s, the Bhagavad Gita, and many more valuable texts that serve as treasure house of knowledge.

While this knowledgeis timeless and extremely insightful, it is not simple to understand. I have embarked upon this journey with the honesty and innocence of a child who is very keen to understand the same. This book is a compilation of my simple notes from various texts and my own thoughts and experimentations, trying to understand these teachings. It will serve as an all-encompassing guide for a contemporary yogi, one who desires

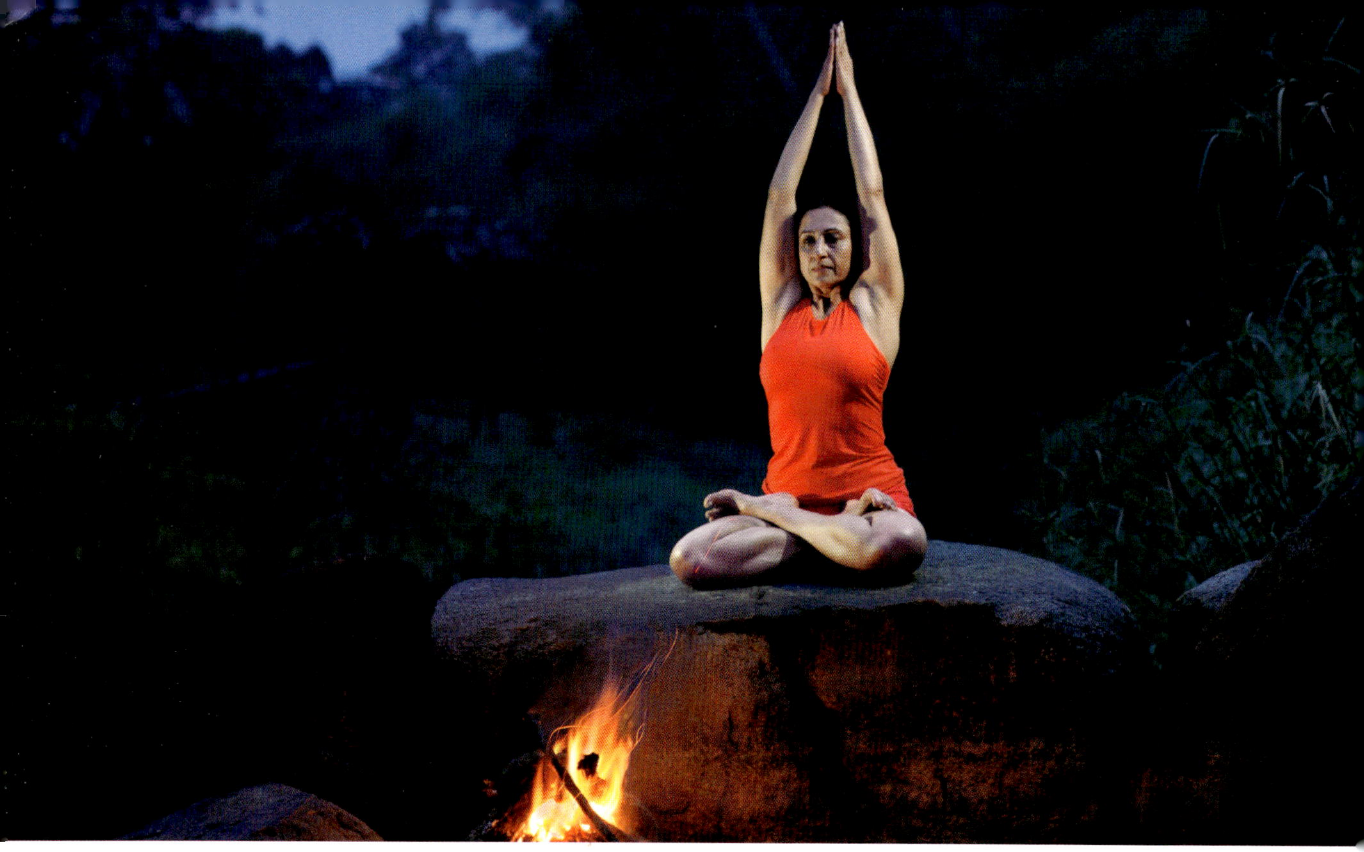

a transformation towards a more yogic lifestyle that is beyond practising asanas and pranayama. The information provided in this book has been collected from a vast treasury of ancient texts, which are profound and deep.

However, this book does not replace the depth of original Sanskrit texts or the invaluable guidance of a guru. It is a compilation of my insights and notes to encourage further exploration. The interpretations of scriptures may vary among gurus, and their wisdom remains essential in understanding this vast subject.

In modern times, yoga is interpreted in diverse ways—meditation, sport, healing and spiritual exploration, to name a few. The abundance of several approaches can feel overwhelming. Yet, most practitioners begin their journey with asana practice. While asanas build discipline, health, mental clarity and well-being, they alone do not chart the path to the deeper quality of life explained in yogic texts. To grasp this, it is important to explore how the ancient understood the body, mind and spirit. Ultimately, yoga guides the practitioner towards moksha or *kaivalya*—the state of complete freedom.

Just as the body requires physical exercise for maintenance, its other faculties also need care. The body is far more complex than a combination of bones, flesh, blood and muscles—it consists of multiple layers that influence overall well-being. This book offers insights into these layers, providing guidance on how to recognize and understand them. It includes practical suggestions, lifestyle tips, and their relevance in everyday life. For many practitioners, the therapeutic sequencing of asanas will be a key highlight, while others may find the philosophical yet practical explanations of yogic concepts both intriguing and transformative.

Additionally, the book introduces accessible yet powerful knowledge from Ayurveda, such as how to manage *dosha*s, using mudras to balance the body's five elements or *pancha bhoota*s, and planning a diet tailored to individual needs. It also outlines step-by-step meditation techniques. This book also delves into the importance of the right use of *jnanedriya*s and *karmendriya*s.

I hope *Healing with Yoga* helps bridge the gap between asana practice and a holistic yoga lifestyle, offering a concise yet essential understanding of yogic scriptures and philosophy.

HOW TO READ THIS BOOK

SECTION A: PHYSICAL LANDSCAPE OF THE BODY

The first section contains a simple explanation to a panoramic perspective of the energy body, the mind and the spirit. It also covers valuable information that has the potential to equip us with the philosophical equilibrium and the skills that are useful in abandoning attachments and uncertainties from life's circumstances. The easy-to-understand and practical tips will help you take a step towards a healthier lifestyle.

SECTION B: PRANIC LANDSCAPE OF THE BODY

The second section covers the functions of the prana. The prana, or the life force moving in and out of the body, is responsible for balancing the various patterns of energy in the mind and body. The book suggests simple guideline to identify these patterns and understand them.

Yogic texts describe the universe as a complete organism. As per this philosophy, the universe is not made up of discrete particles like building blocks of atoms and molecules—they are streams of information and energy. And this section is a brief introduction to such an energy system.

SECTION C: KARMIC LANDSCAPE OF THE BODY

This final section is a combination of yogic and Vedantic principles to provide a comprehensive understanding of yoga as a philosophy. It covers the four major pillars, or *purusharthas*, on which the success of a human life depends. It also covers the eight limbs of *Ashtanga Yoga* in *Yoga Sutras*. Simple meditation techniques to understand the concepts better and heal the mind from the general state of confusion are the highlights of the chapters within this section.

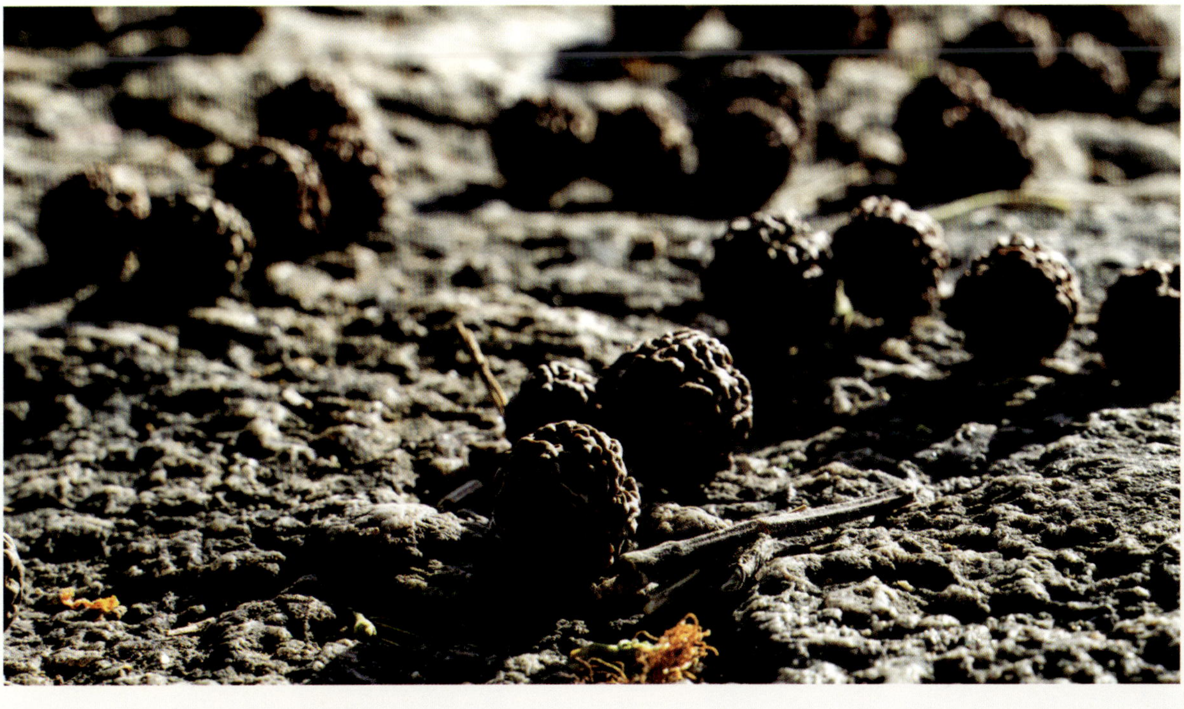

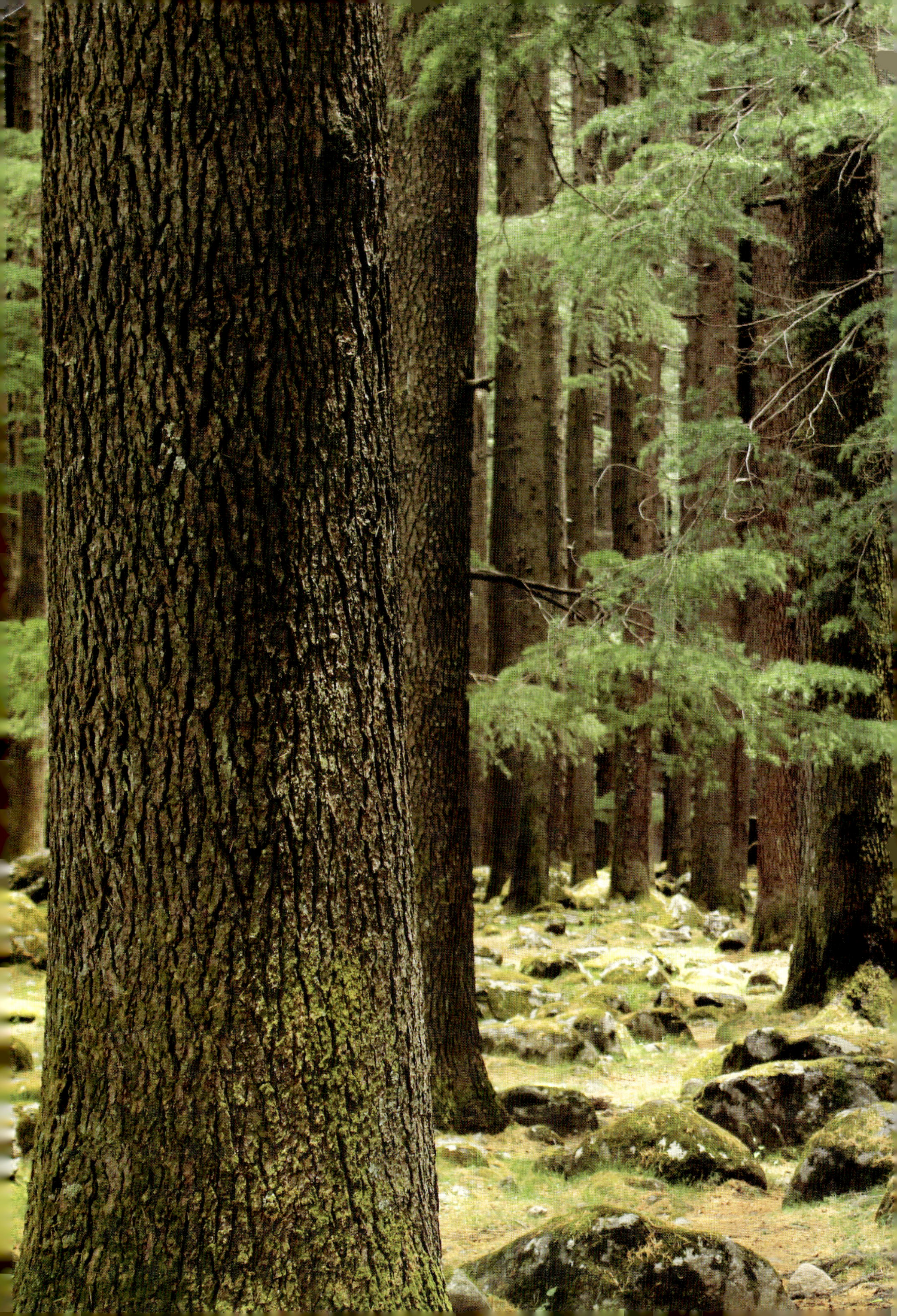

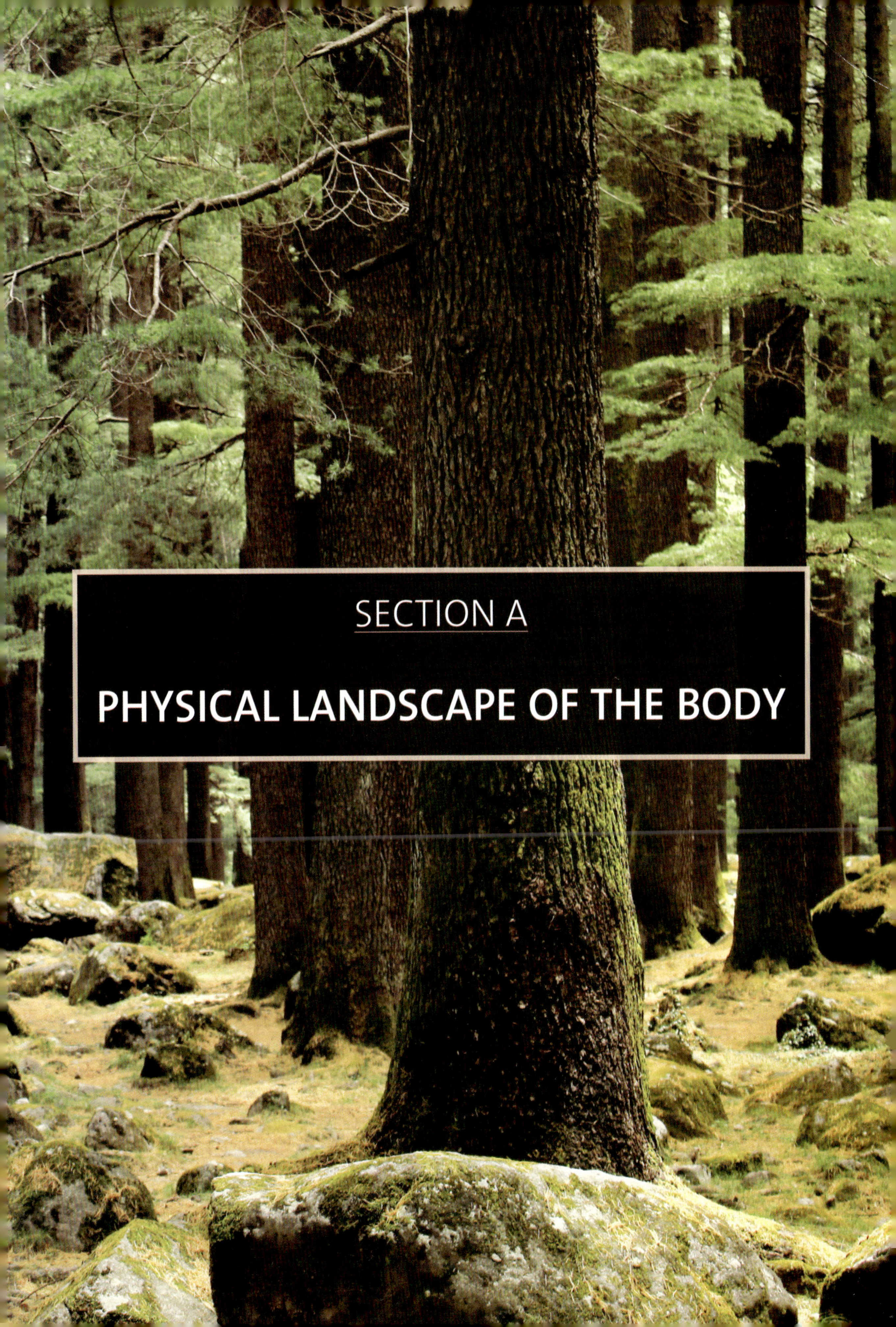

SECTION A

PHYSICAL LANDSCAPE OF THE BODY

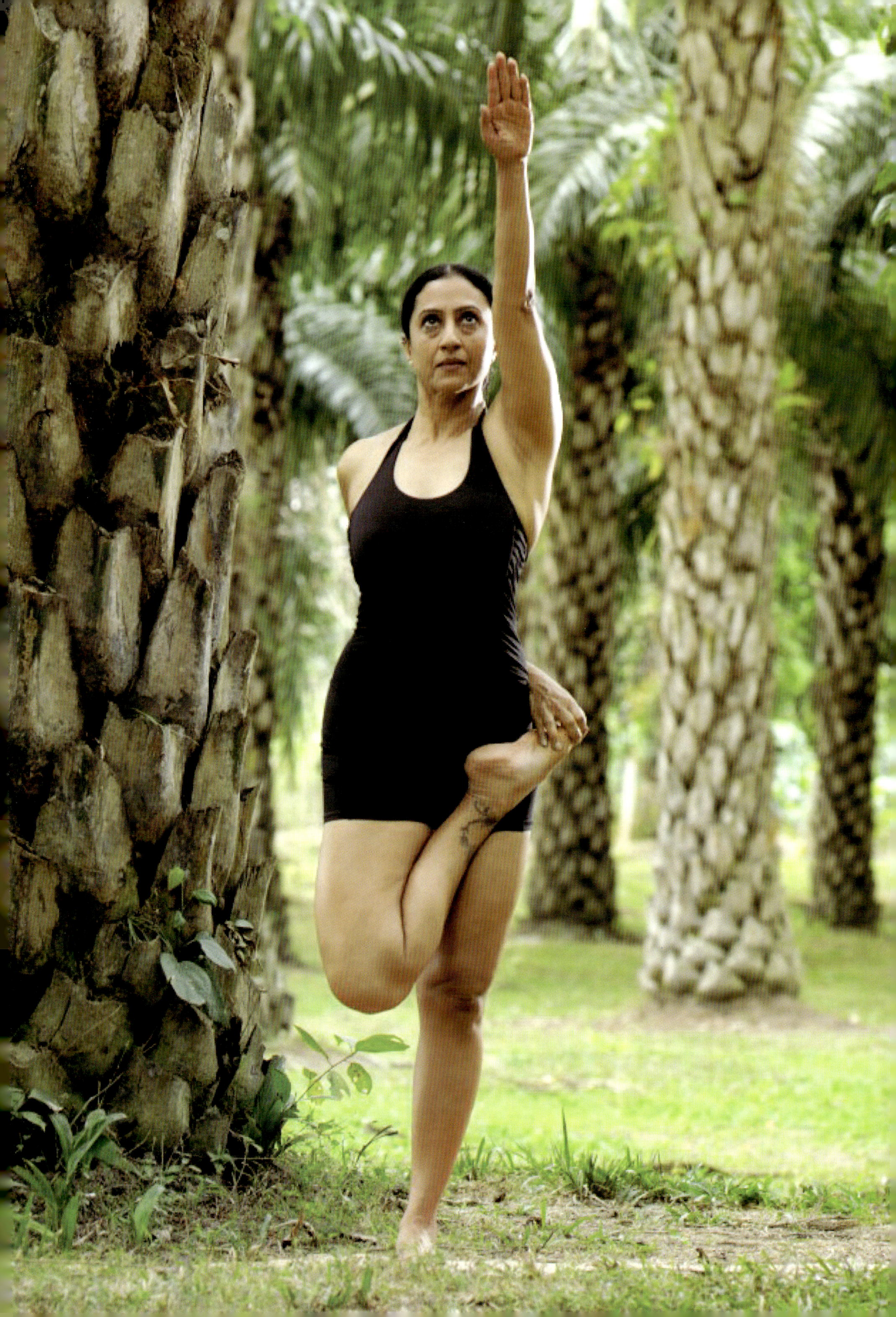

CHAPTER 1
SHARIRA TRAYA

The Sanskrit definition of sharira translates to 'that which decays', highlighting the impermanent nature of physical existence. *Sharira traya* refers to the three primary layers of energy bodies present in all living beings. When these layers are aligned and connected, they create harmony between the body, mind and spirit. This interconnectedness leads to a balanced and integrated state of being.

STHULA SHARIRA

This is the physical body comprising heads, legs, torso and sense organs. Each part of *sthula sharira* has two essential aspects: the physical structure and the energy that enables its function. Sthula sharira is the locus of all experiences. It is where the five fundamental elements of the body which are *prithvi* (earth), *agni* (fire), *vayu* (wind), *jal* (water) and *akasha* (space) exist. These are called Pancha Bhootas.

Sthula Sharira, created at birth, is subject to ageing and death. It is forever changing, thus requiring food to sustain.

SUKSHMA SHARIRA

This is the power driving the physical body, keeping it alive with life energy. *Sukshma sharira* is the Sanskrit word for 'subtle body'. It comprises prana or the vital energy. Physiological functions, like inhalation, digestion, reproduction, etc., along with the functions of the brain, form the sukshma sharira. It is housed within the sthula sharira, and is therefore the invisible body.

The sukshma sharira houses the sensory body, which includes manas and *buddhi*. Manas governs unintentional mental activities, such as emotions and spontaneous thoughts, while buddhi oversees intentional mental activities, involving conscious choices, such as reasoning and decision making.

The subtle body is most vividly experienced in the dream state, where the physical body rests, but the mind and intellect remain active. It departs or perishes along with the physical body upon death.

KARANA SHARIRA

This is referred to as the causal body, as this is the cause for the body to exist. Within the practice of spiritual yoga, *karana sharira* is referred to as 'atma' in the texts. This is considered to be the most complex knowledge in the yoga syllabus. The causal body has no beginning or end; it exists in all forms of life as a potential state of being and takes shape upon creation. (Just imagine the idea of a seed already carrying the tree it will grow into).

In Sanskrit, the word *karana* means 'causing' or 'making'. It is believed that this sharira connects the individual and the cosmic consciousness. It is also believed to be the storehouse of information from past lives. Karana sharira continues to exist even after the body perishes. It simply moves to another body and life continues. This sharira is most active in deep dreamless sleep.

KEYWORDS

- Atma is the essence of life and existence of a person. It is the power behind existence of every living thing in the universe. Atma is seen as eternal and unchanging.
- Moksha refers to the release from the cycle of rebirth, and attainment of the final state of liberation.
- Karma is an individual's residual past from which the present destiny is determined according to the past actions in many previous lives.

REFERENCE FOR SURYA NAMASKARA (A)

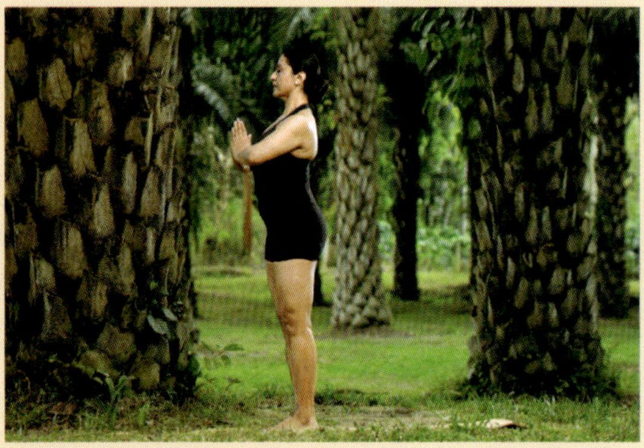

1.

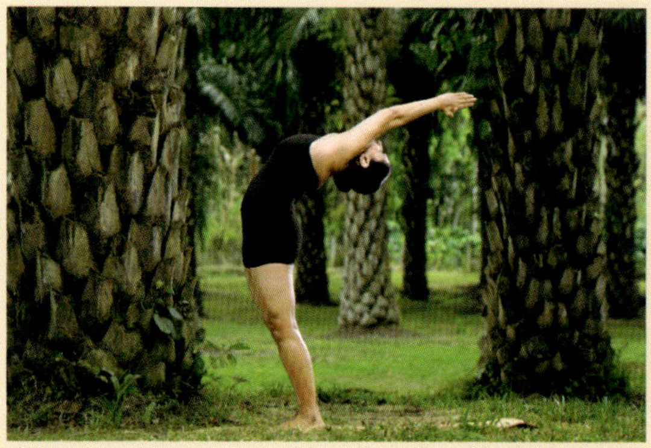

2.

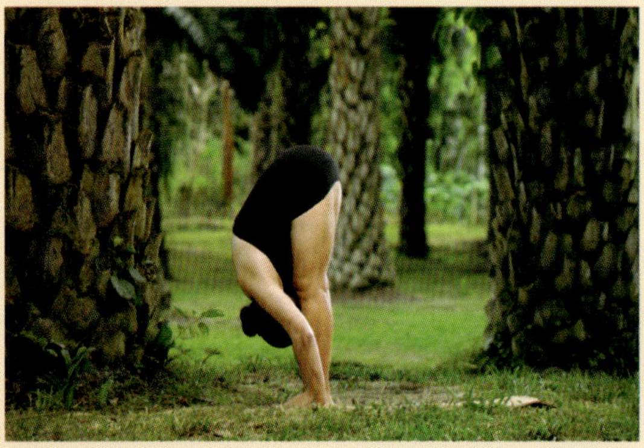

3.

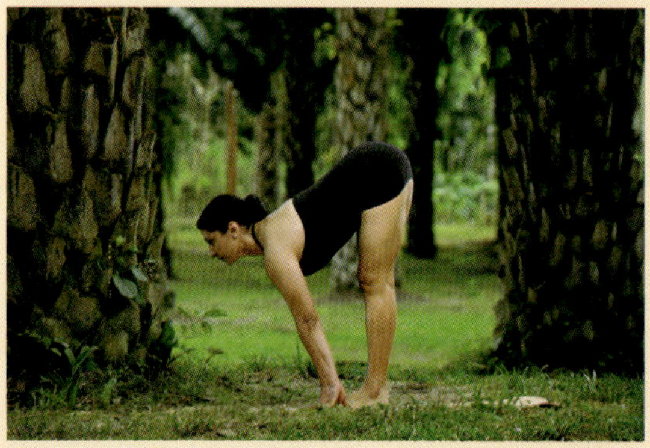

4.

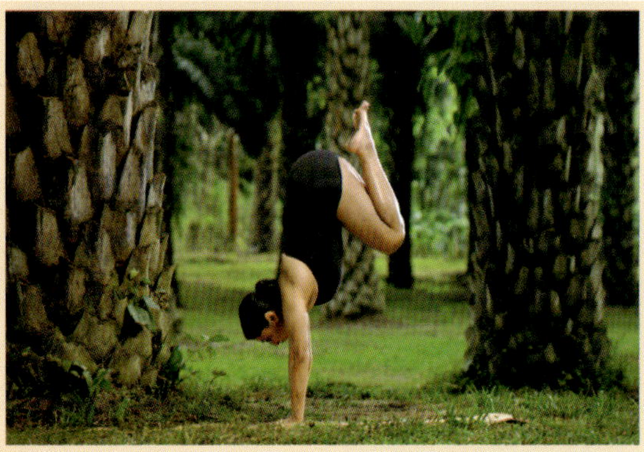

5.

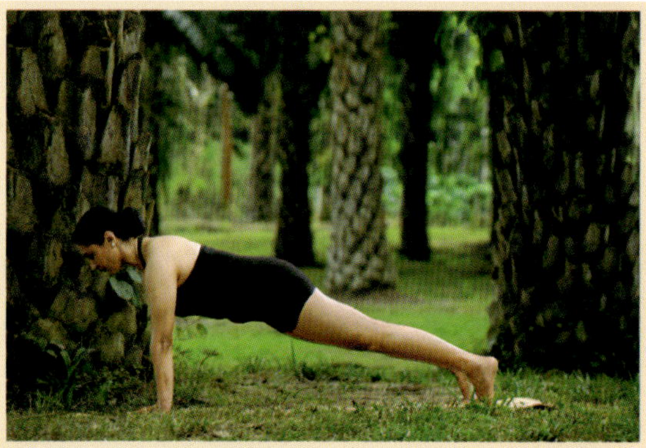

6.

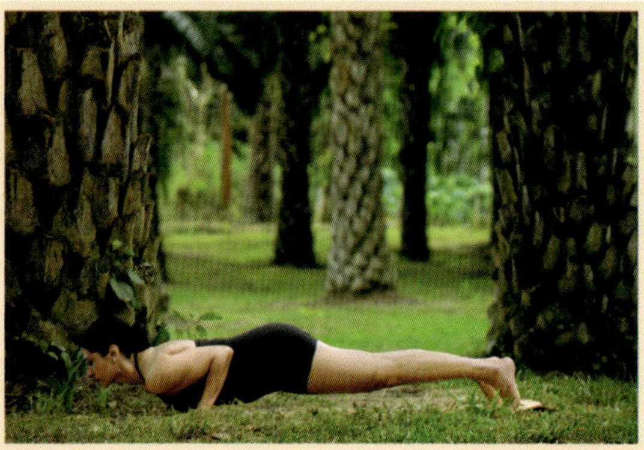

7.

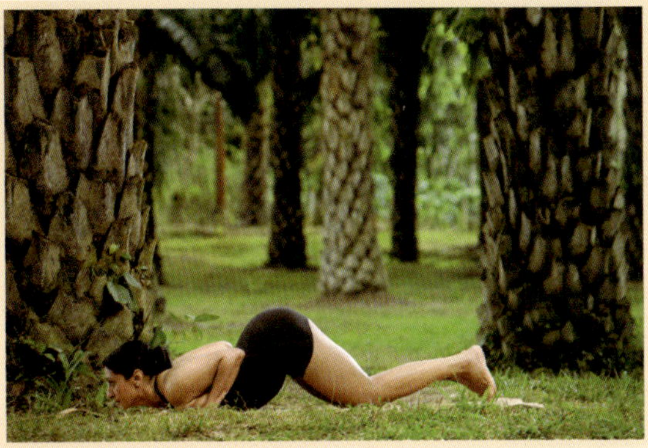
8.

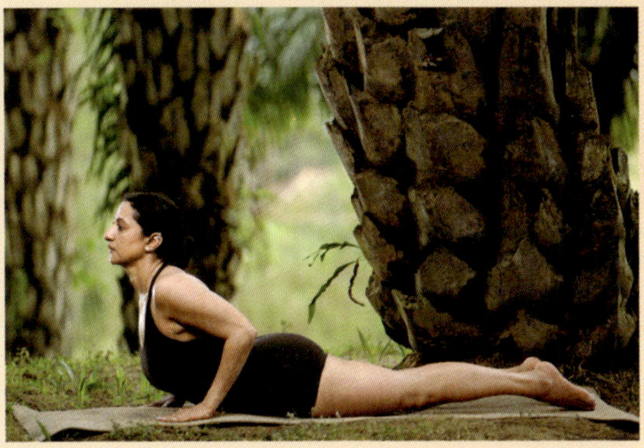
9.

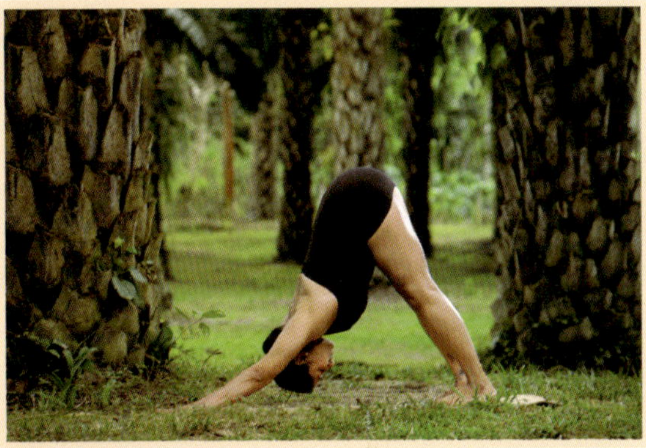
10.

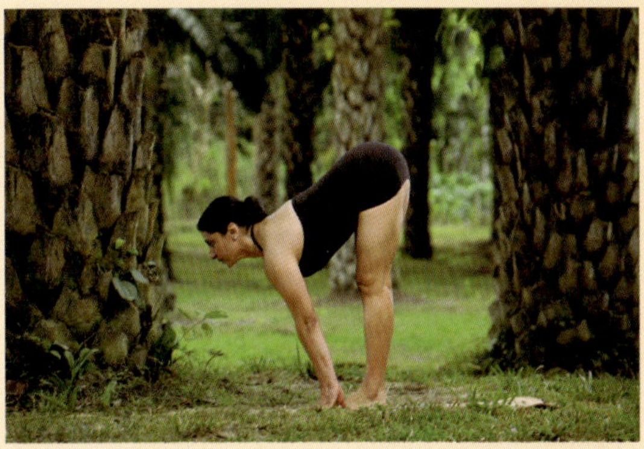
11.

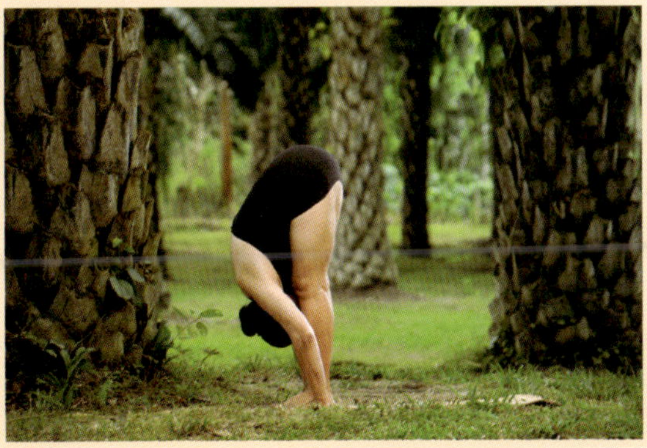
12.

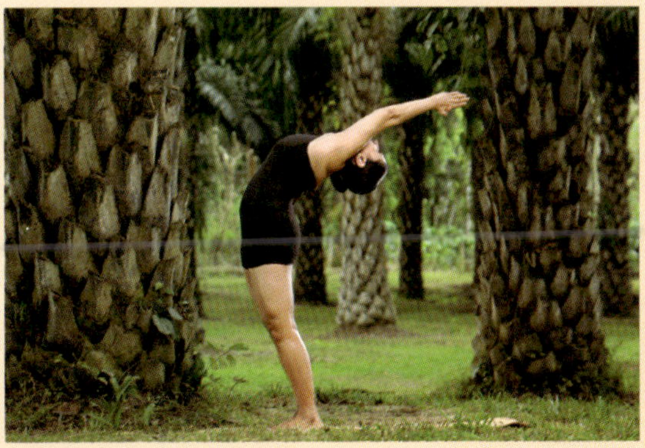
13.

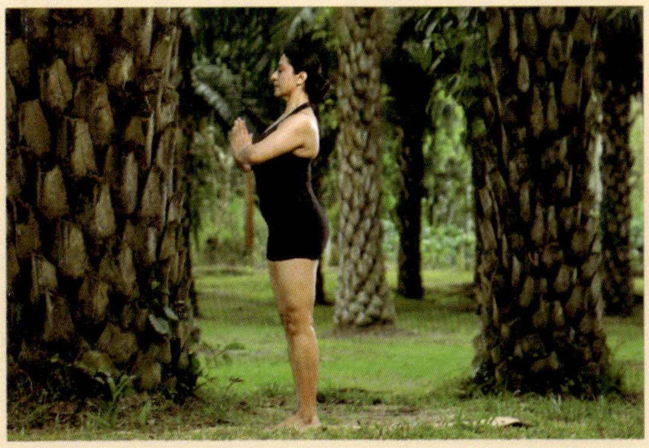
14.

REFERENCE FOR SURYA NAMASKARA (B)

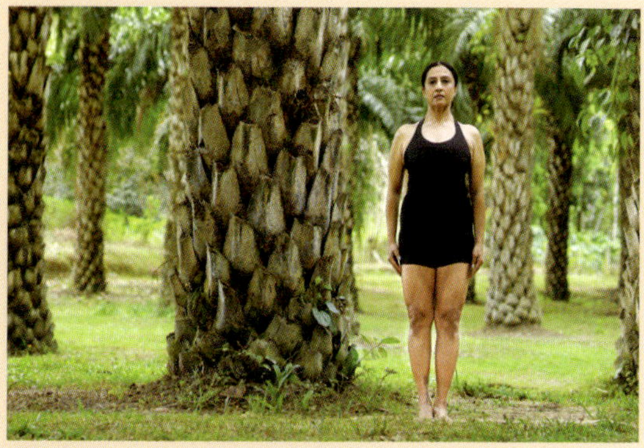
1.

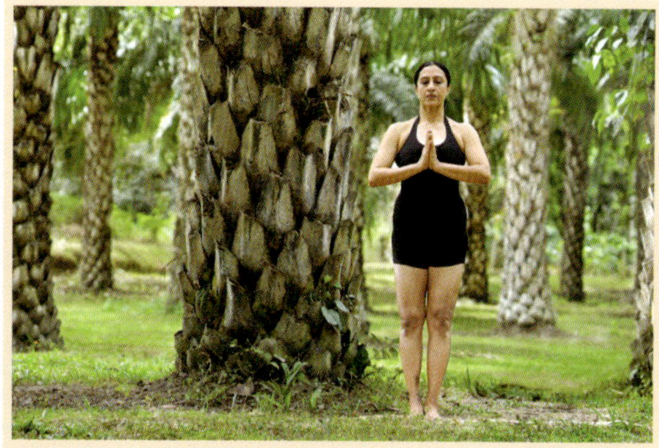
2.

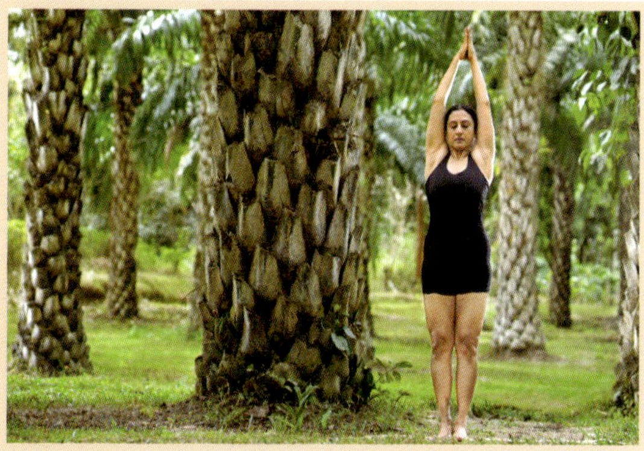
3.

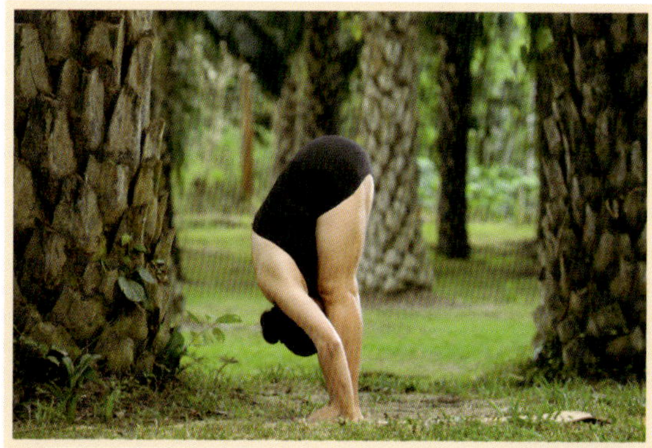
4.

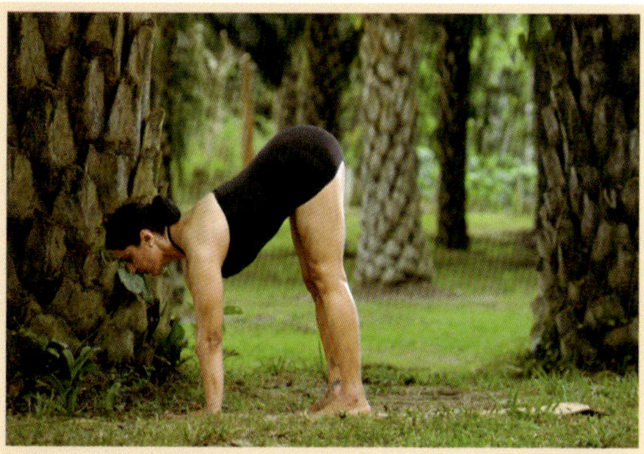
5.

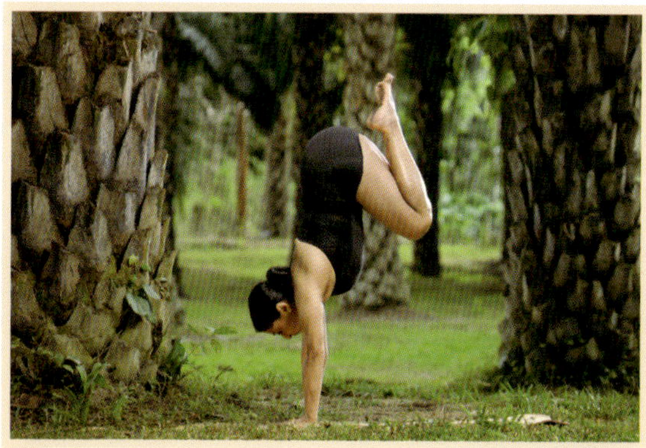
6.

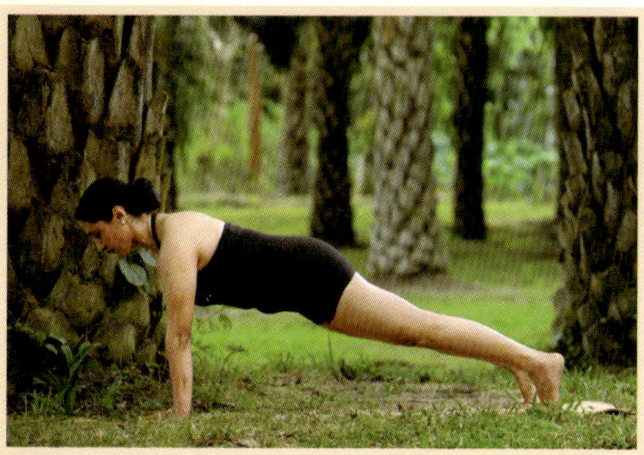
7.

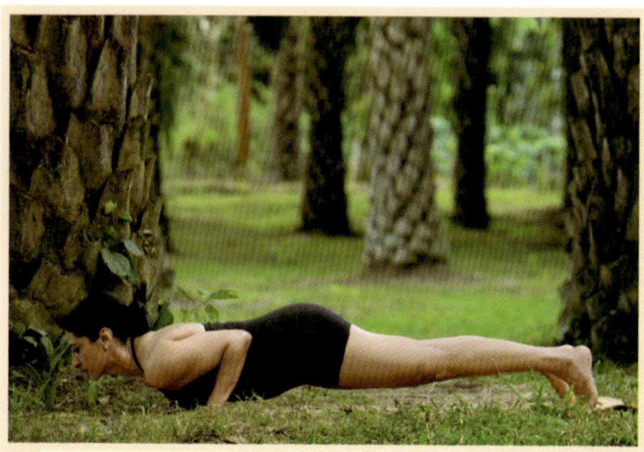
8.

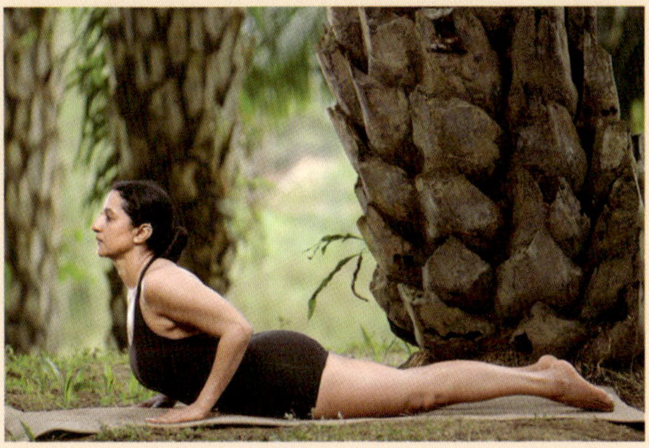

9.

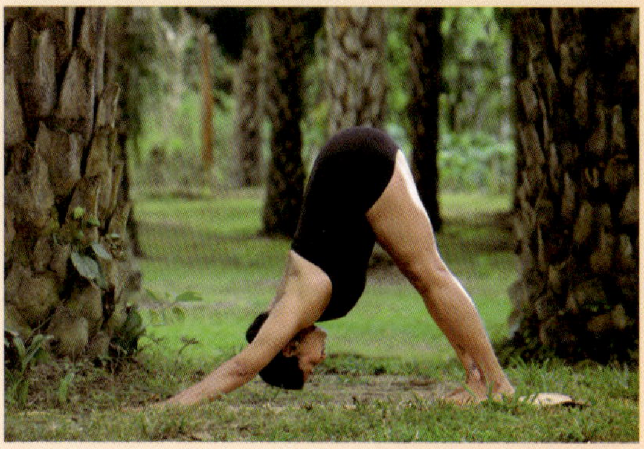

10.

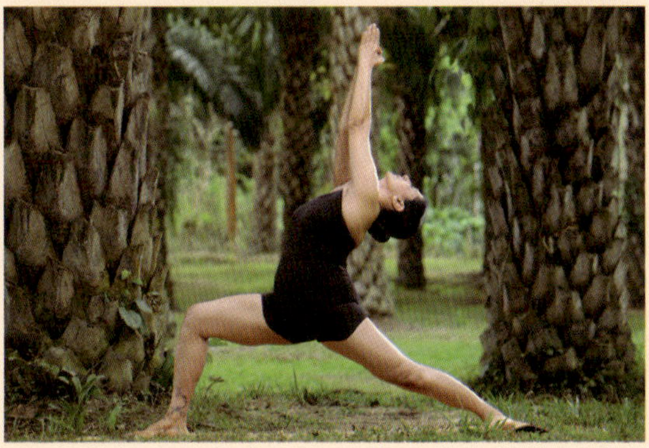

11.

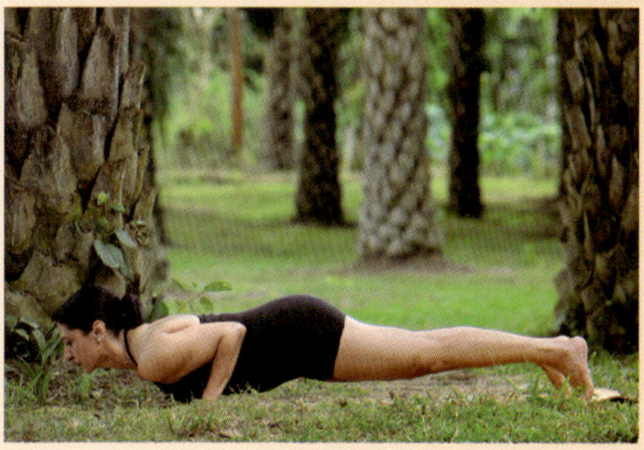

12.

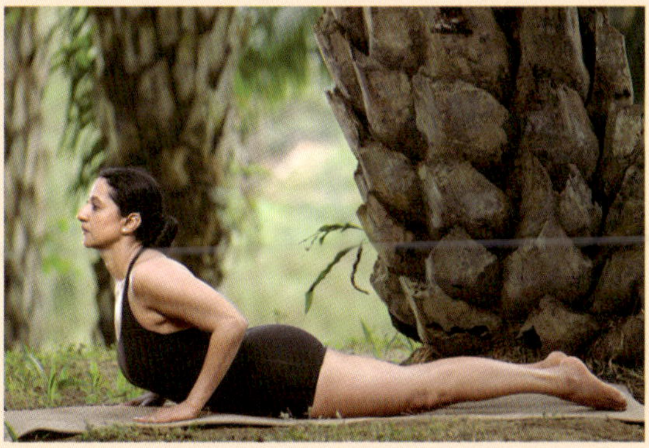

13.

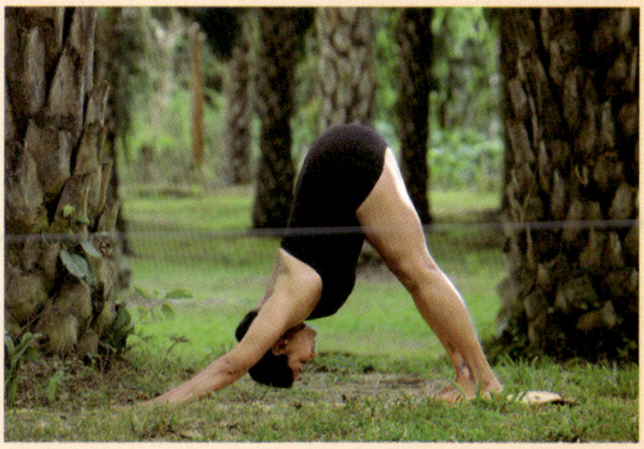

14.

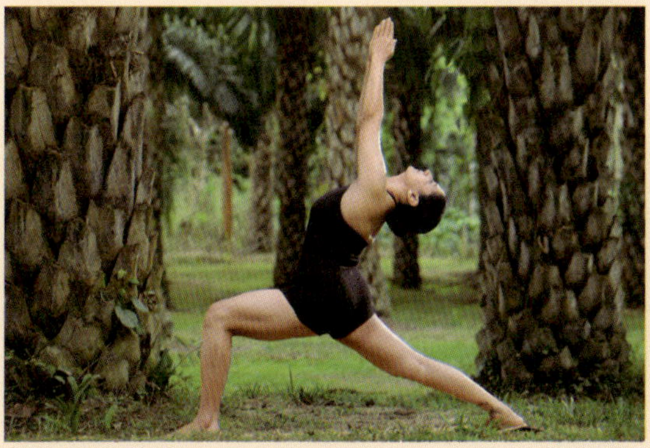

15.

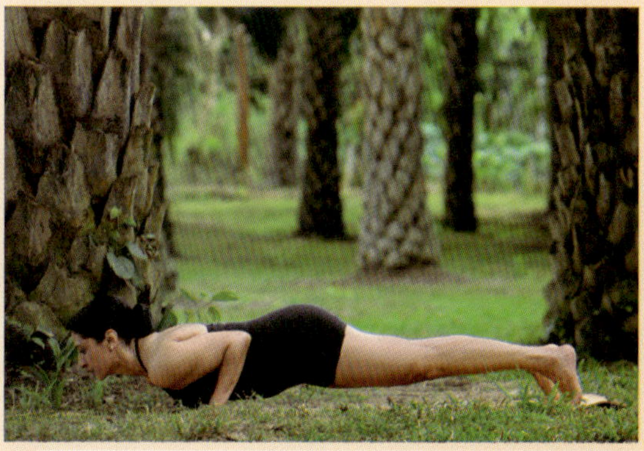

16.

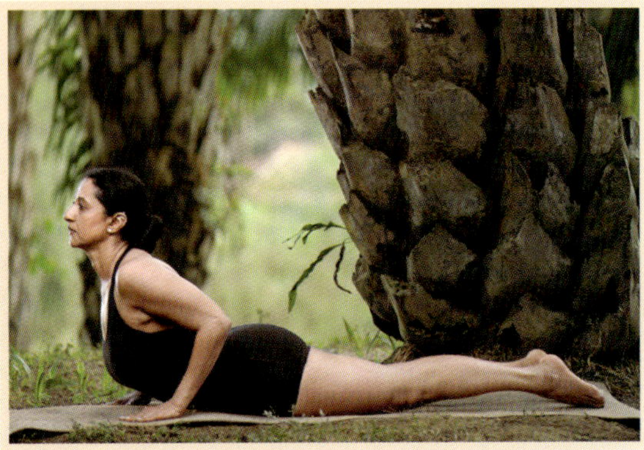
17.

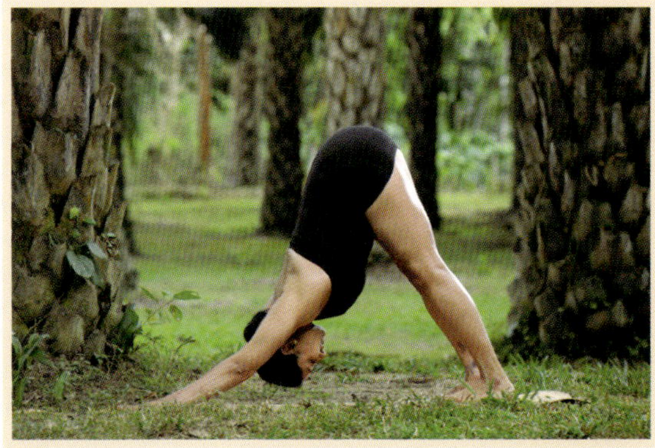
18.

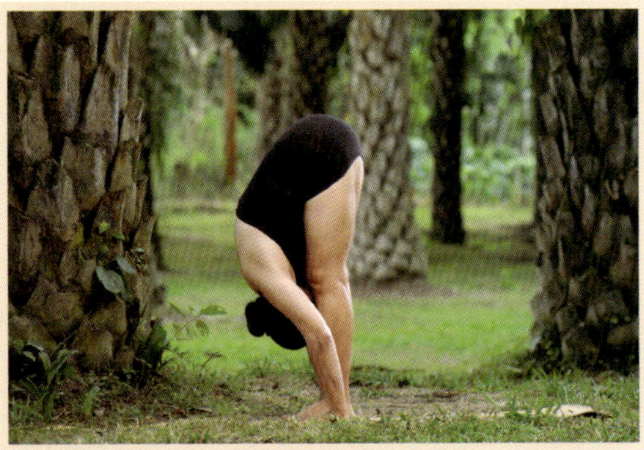
19.

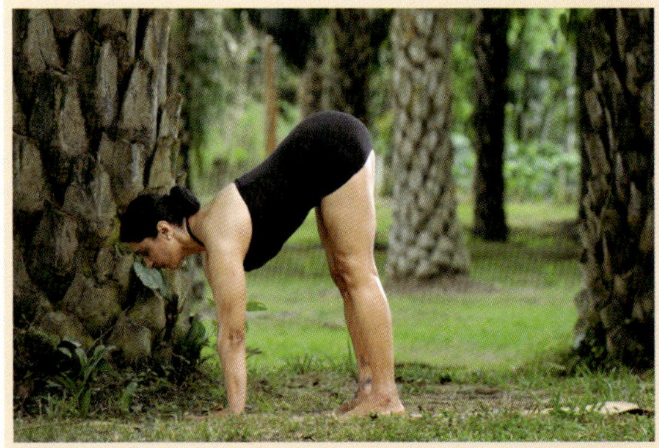
20.

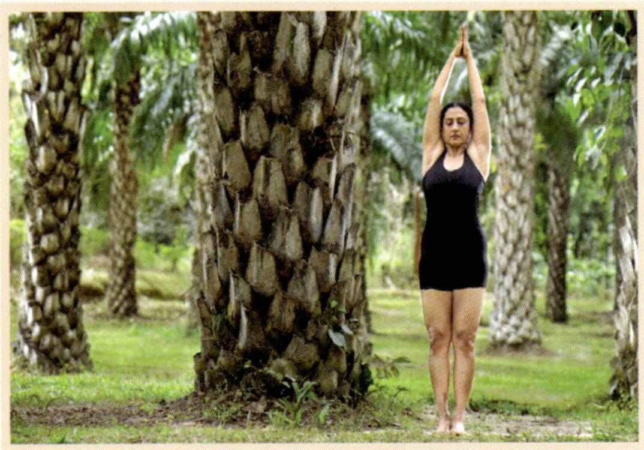
21.

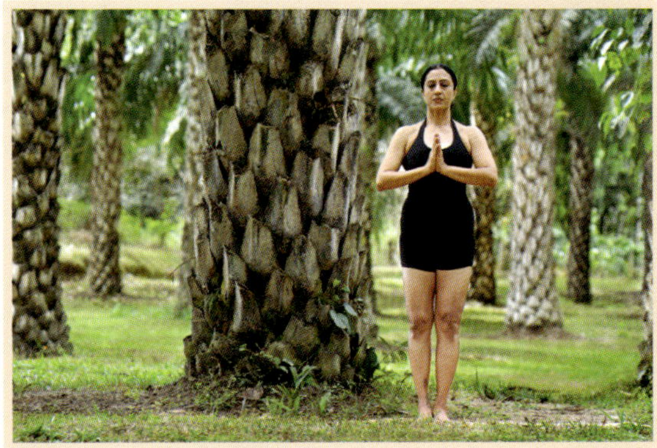
22.

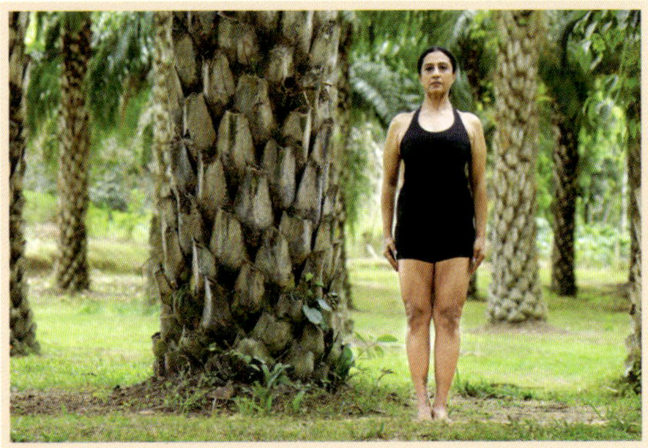
23.

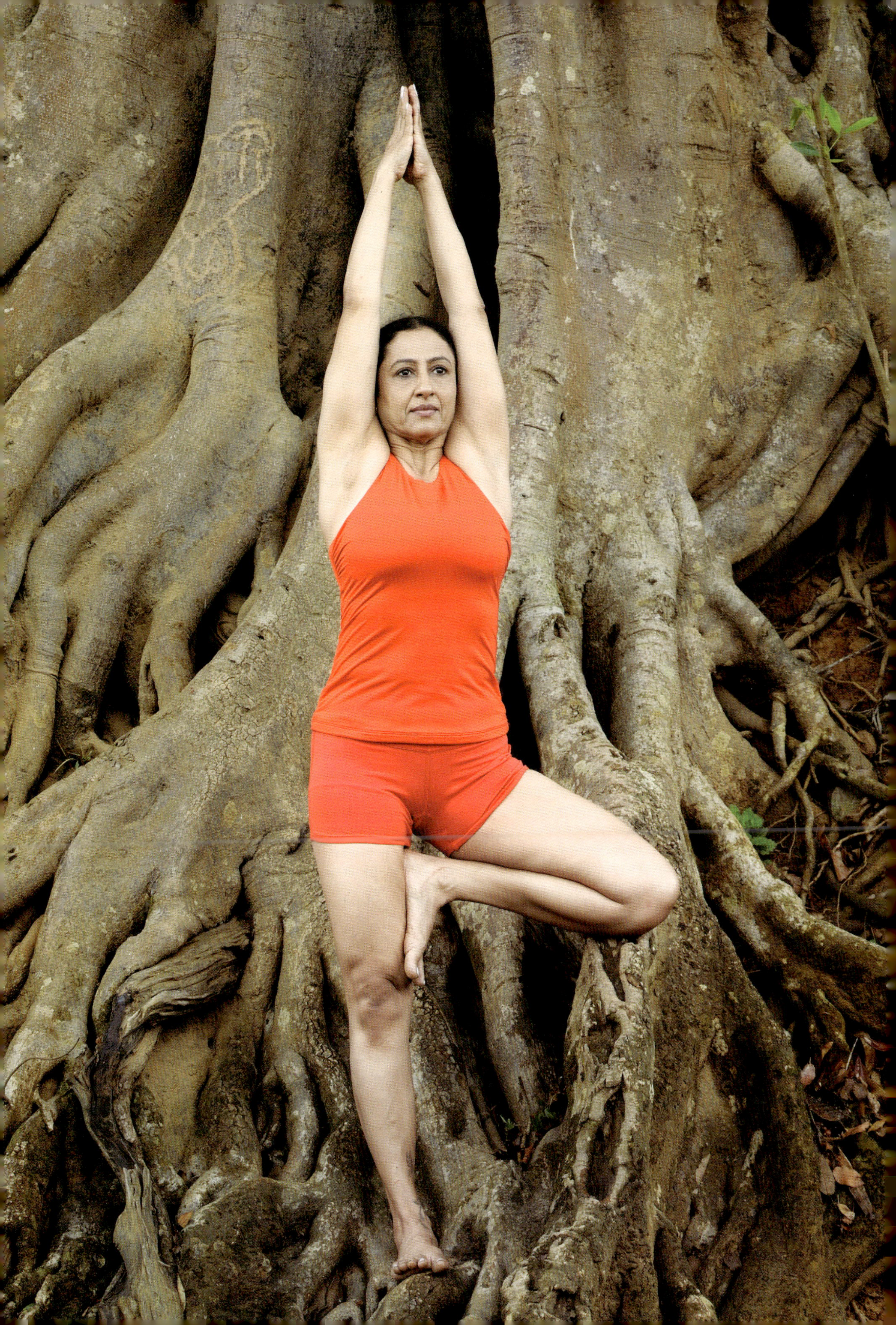

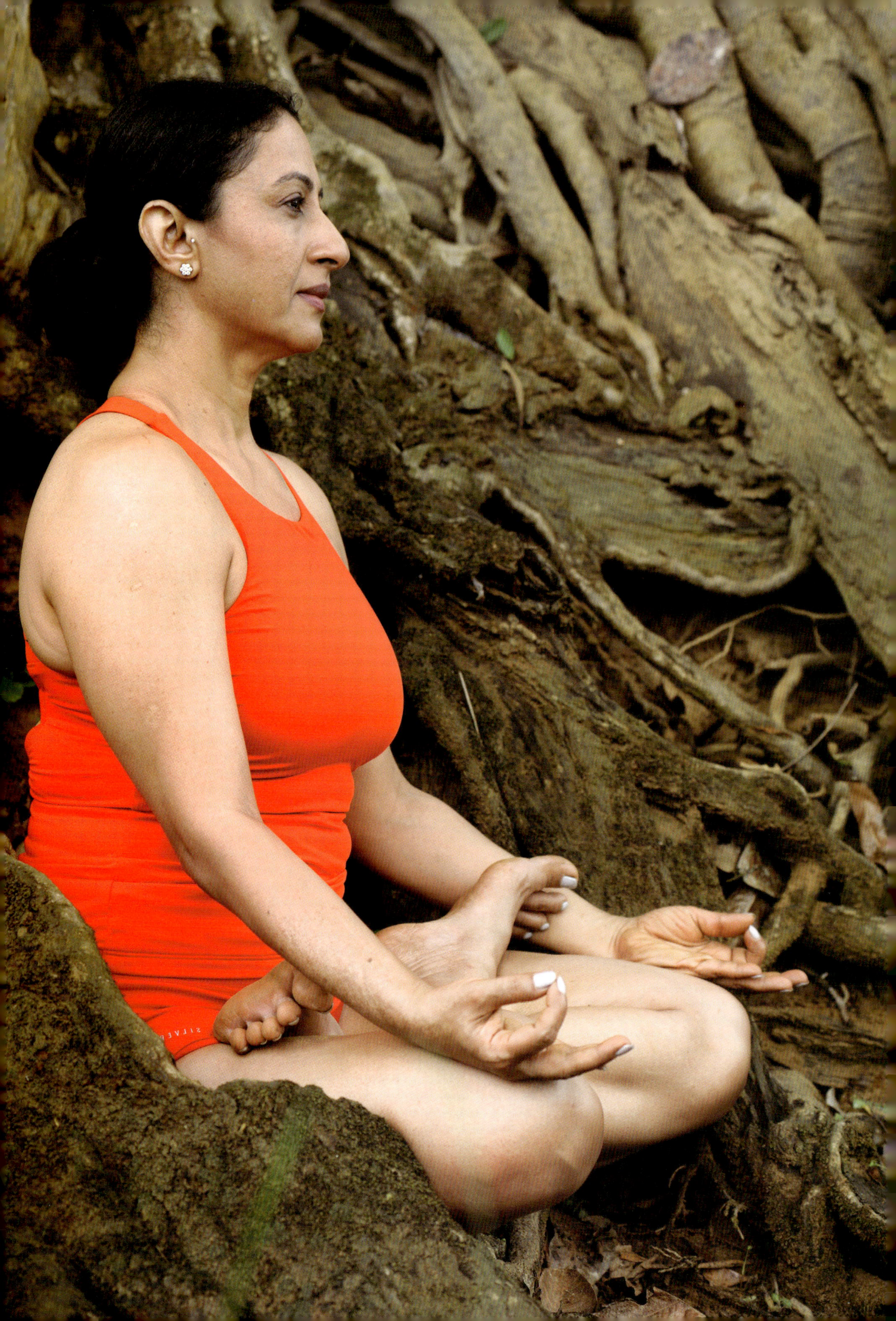

CHAPTER 2

KOSHAS: INNER MAPPING

The ancients described the body as comprising five layers of existence, or *kosha*, each contributing to an individual's unique personality.

In Ayurveda and yoga therapy, the kosha model serves as a vital diagnostic tool to understand an individual holistically. It helps identify and address disturbances within the body by examining imbalances across these layers. Achieving health and well-being depends on maintaining harmony and balance within each kosha.

> **AUTHOR'S NOTE**
>
> Pancha koshas are explained in great detail in the *Taittiriya Upanishad*, which studies the nature of the self and its relationship with the universe. The Pancha Koshas represent the five layers of human existence—physical, energetic, mental, intellectual and blissful. Each kosha is directly connected, layer by layer, to the external world and inner consciousness. The concepts described in the Upanishads are highly symbolic, deeply philosophical and often subtle, thus requiring a guru's guidance for deeper understanding and meaningful realization.

ANNAMAYA KOSHA

The outermost and the visible layer of existence is *annamaya kosha*. It is the physical body that gets nourished by the food we take. This is the most delicate layer amongst the pancha koshas, as any issue in this layer can manifest as imbalances in the other layers too.

The practice of yoga begins with the annamaya kosha, the food sheath, which represents the physical body. This layer is sustained by the food we eat, and its health is reflected in our physical strength, energy and vitality. The practice of asana plays a key role in strengthening this kosha. However, asana alone isn't enough. A balanced lifestyle, including adequate sleep and a nourishing, well-planned diet, is essential for maintaining the health of this layer.

Since annamaya kosha literally means the food sheath, the quality of food we consume has a direct impact on it. Our physical well-being mirrors the choices we make in our daily lives.

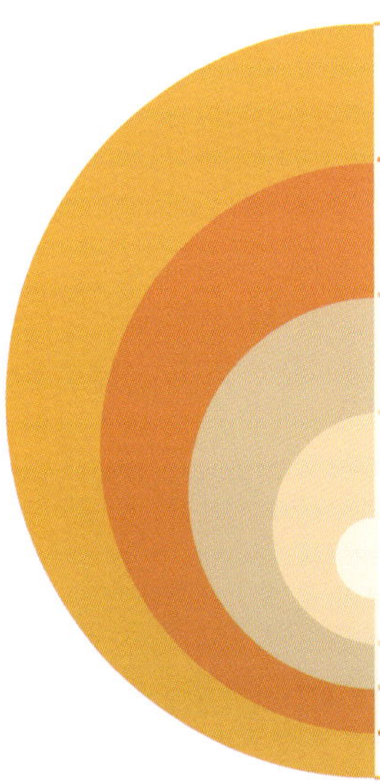

Annamaya Kosha	• Comprises physical or gross body (DNA, cells, tissues, nerves and organs) • Primary function involves ageing and hunger
Pranamaya Kosha	• Comprises vital body (energy field, *nadi*s and chakras) • Primary functions involve illness and fatigue
Manomaya Kosha	• Comprises thoughts, feelings and emotions • Primary functions involve fear and agitation
Vijnanamaya Kosha	• Comprises reaction, intuition and inner consciousness • Primary functions involve confusion and awareness
Anandamaya Kosha	• Marks bliss and liberation

PANCHA KOSHA: THE FIVE LAYERS OF EXISTENCE

The scriptures caution against identifying this kosha as the true self, as it is merely a temporary vehicle that we inhabit. While this physical body is tangible and visible, it is impermanent and constantly changing. Ultimately, the quality of our life experiences is deeply influenced by how we treat this kosha. By nurturing it with mindful living, we lay a strong foundation for deeper exploration of the inner layers of existence.

The annamaya kosha also carries *guna*s (inherent qualities) that an individual is born with. Gunas are divided in three categories: *sattvik, rajasik* and *tamasik*.

GUNAS

Guna can be translated as 'quality', as mentioned in Sankhya philosophy. The three gunas are said to be constantly entangled and interacting with one another, sometimes bringing calmness, at other times energy, and occasionally restlessness. With awareness and conscious regulation, one can positively influence these energies for personal growth.

- Gunas represent the subtlest qualities inherent in all forms of energy.
- Every form of energy contains these three gunas in a unique ratio, defining its nature and function.
- The doshas, which form the body's grosser energies, also contain all three gunas in varying proportions.
- Together, the gunas manifest in all aspects of the world, giving rise to *prakriti*
- The influence of the gunas can be recognized through their impact on our thoughts, emotions and actions.

Sattvik Guna

Sattvik guna represents a state of harmony, clarity and balance within the body, mind and intellect, leading to inner peace and joy. It is considered the purest of the three gunas, fostering spiritual growth and well-being. Sattvik qualities are happiness, peace, wellness, freedom, love, compassion, comfort, empathy, friendliness, focus, hard work, trust, gratitude and selflessness.

Anyone can aim to live a sattvik life by altering a few habits that have the potential to change the nature of the person. To do so, it is important to keep the other two gunas under control.

Lifestyle Changes

- Eating seasonal, regional, fresh and organic food is the first step towards adopting a sattvik lifestyle. Vegetarian food is largely sattvik. Ingredients should be locally sourced and seasonally appropriate to maintain harmony with nature and support overall well-being.
- There should be a fixed timetable for everyday activities, such as sleeping, eating, meditating and exercising.
- Being mindful of your surroundings and making conscious efforts to maintain a clean, harmonious environment support a sattvik mind. A clutter-free space fosters calmness and peace, while disorganized surroundings can disrupt mental clarity and inner balance.
- Studying and reading ancient texts will offer a depth of knowledge that will help maintain mental clarity and calmness.
- Understanding the auspiciousness of the present moment and being mindful about it is very helpful.
- Practising yoga asanas and pranayama helps create the calmness that is vital to lead a sattvik lifestyle.
- A simple relaxing walk in the midst of nature can also prove to be very helpful in bringing out the inherent sattvik nature of the mind.

Asana Practice

Yoga practices, such as asanas and pranayama, have the power to balance energy patterns, which is essential for cultivating sattvik guna.

(Please note: Uncomfortable asanas can be skipped as it will not affect the sequence pattern)

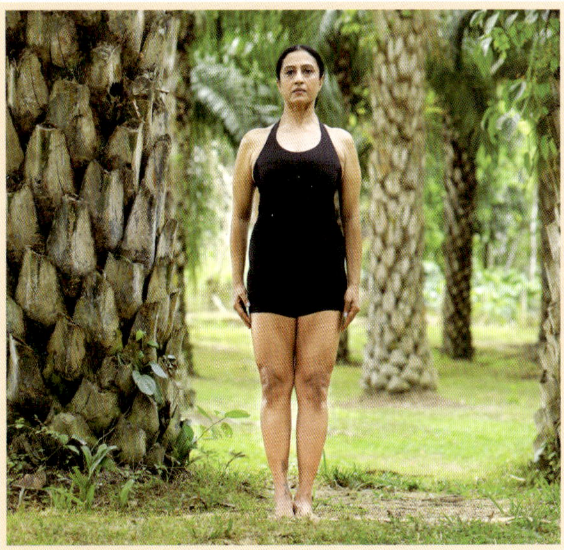

TADASANA

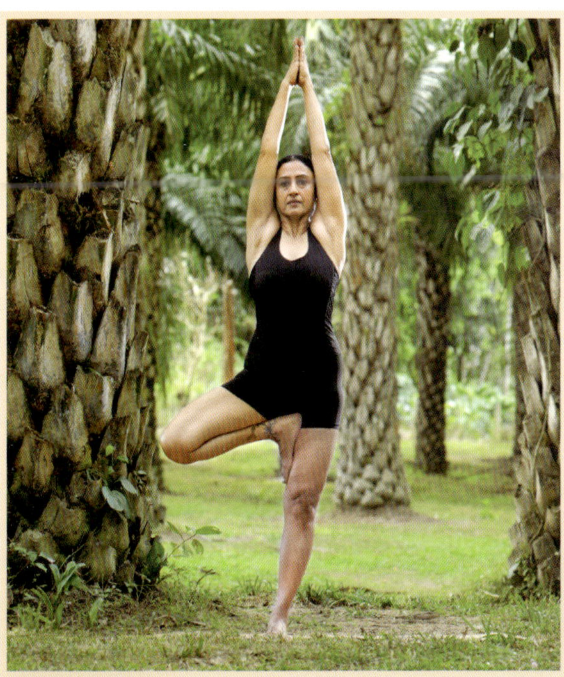

VRIKSHASANA

SURYA NAMASKARA A (FOR REFERENCE, SEE PP. 4–5)

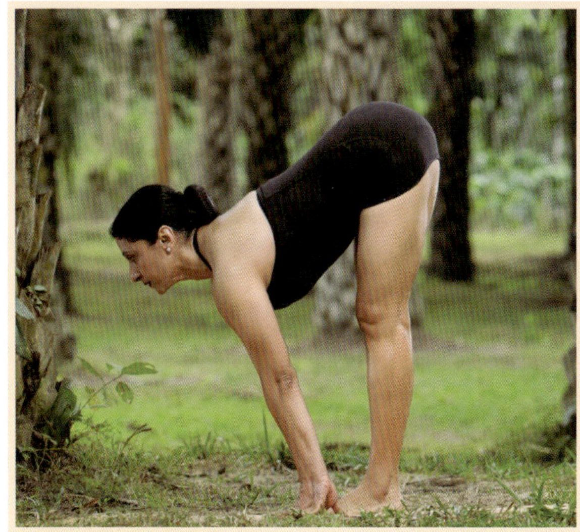

HASTA PADASANA

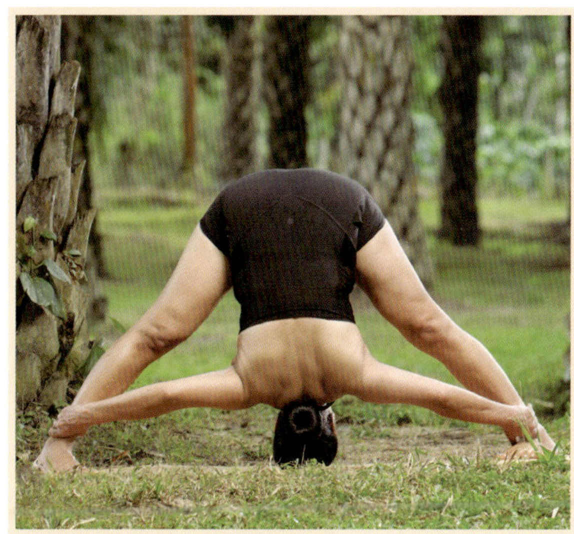

PRASARITA PADOTTANASANA

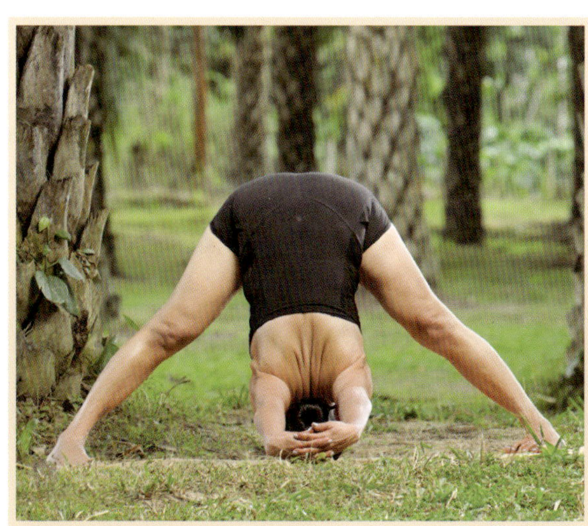

PRASARITA PADOTTANASANA

Standing Asanas

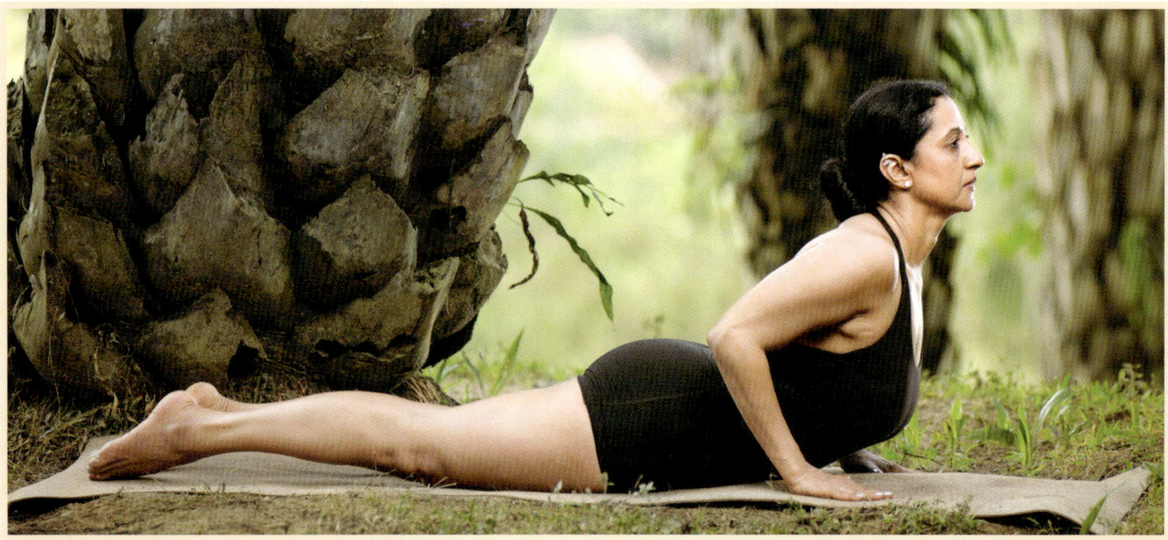

BHUJANGASANA

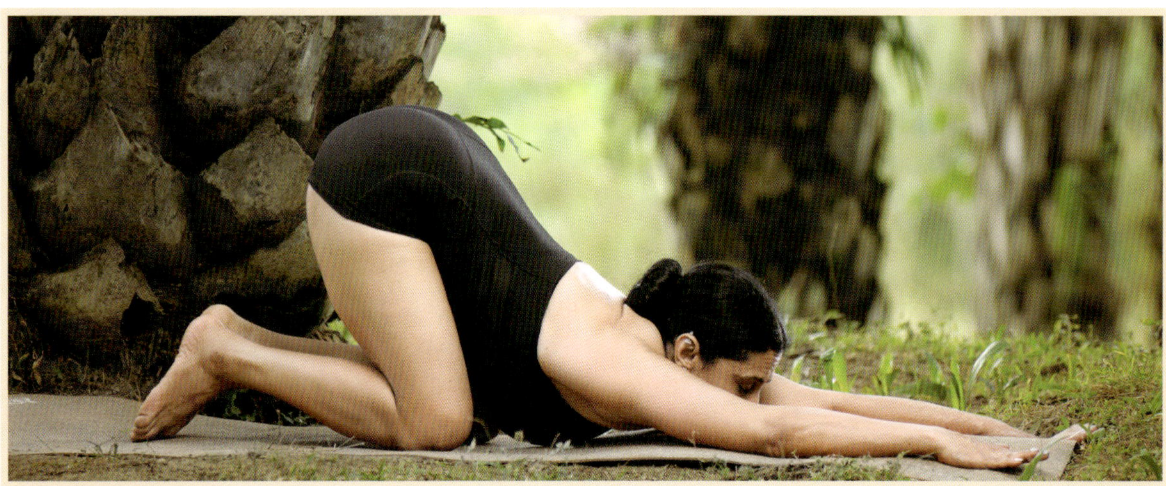

SHESHANKASANA

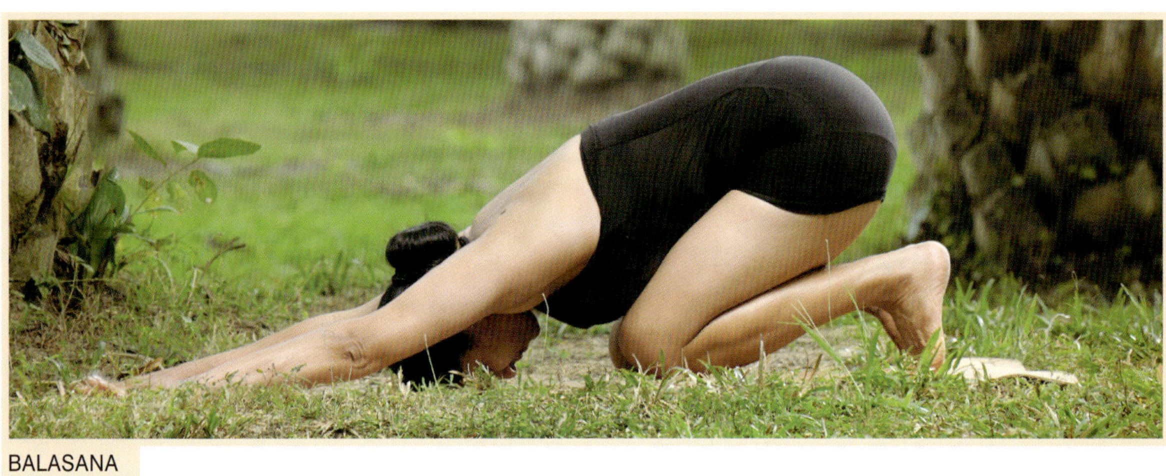

BALASANA

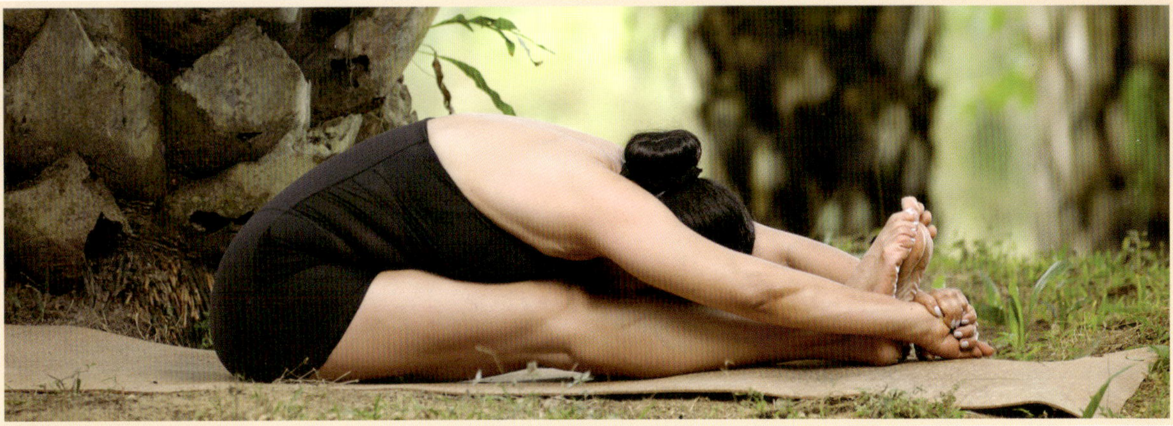

PASCHIMOTTANASANA

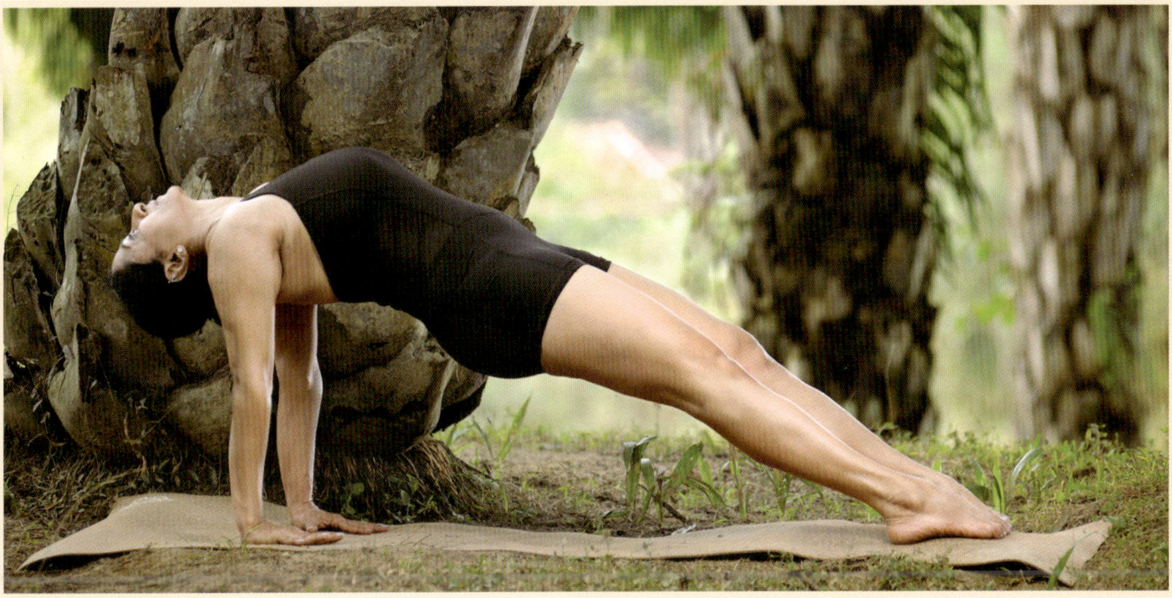

PURVOTTANASANA

Floor Asanas

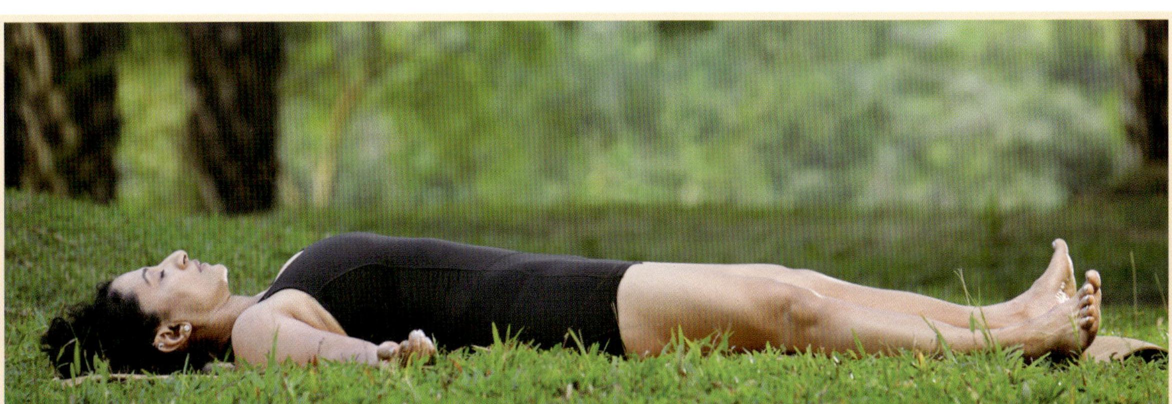

SHAVASANA FOR 10 MINUTES

Cooling Down Asanas

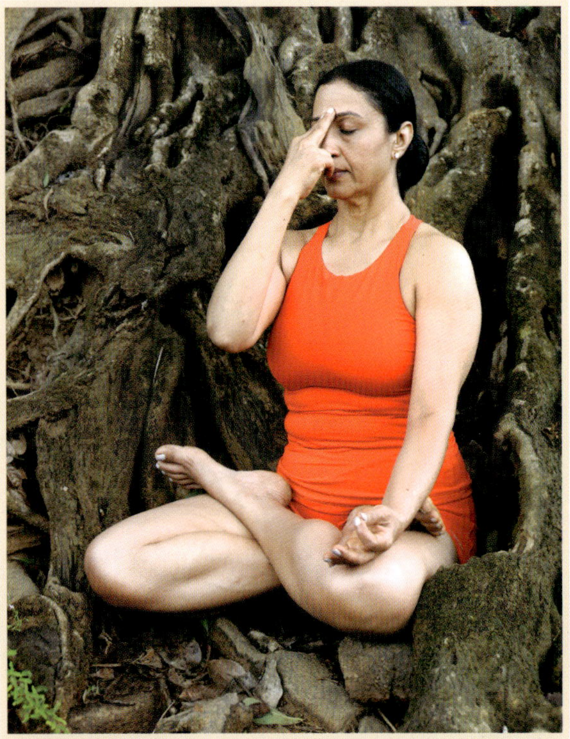

ANULOM VILOM

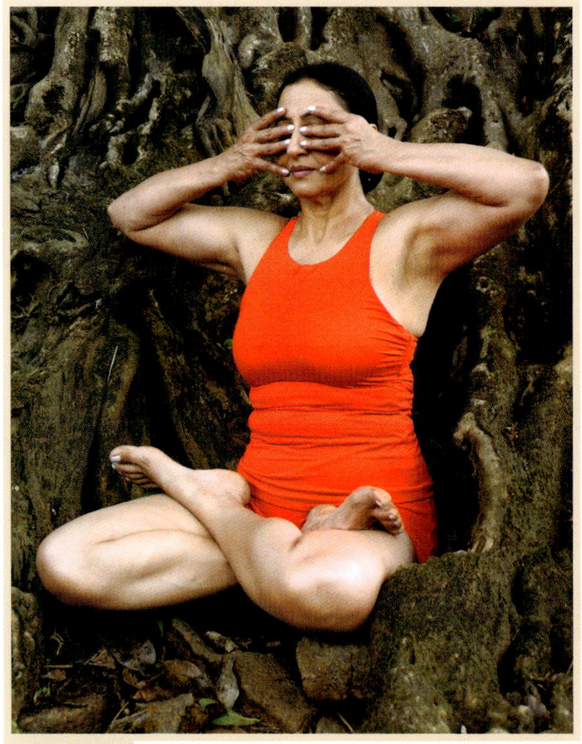

BHRAMARI

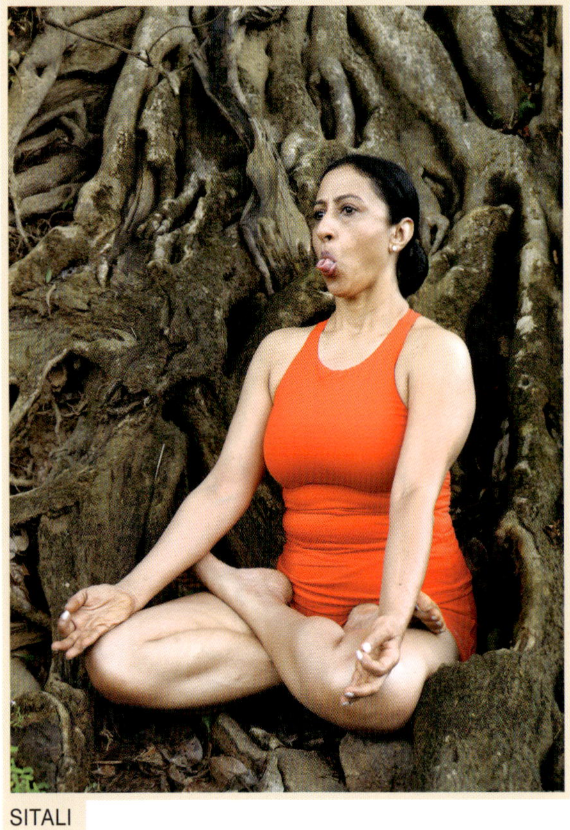

SITALI

Pranayama

Rajasik Guna

This guna is the driving energy of the body. It puts all energy into motion. Keeping this energy under control and balance is important. Gunas can both be negative and positive, depending on how they are managed. Rajasik guna has an active quality, which can be a driving force to pursue life with passion. The negative side can be excess desire which may subsequently lead to greed and uncontrolled restlessness. People with rajasik quality have a deep attachment to their desires. In extreme cases, they could end up being self-centred and egoistic. Noticeable negative characteristics of rajasik guna are anxiety, fear, irritation, worry, stress, over-confidence and chaos.

Rajasik guna can be adjusted by making some lifestyle changes. It is not entirely negative.

However, the extremities of this guna need to be controlled, else they can be harmful to the body and mind.

Lifestyle Changes

- Making dietary adjustments is important to manage this guna. Rajasik foods generally include heavily fried, salty dishes with stimulants and preservatives. These need to be avoided as they can lead to uncontrollable rajasik traits.
- Bringing about self-awareness, self-analysis or introspection can help calm down the rajasik nature of the mind and body.
- Certain professions, such as those in sports or artistic and creative fields, may require individuals to maintain a predominantly rajasik nature at all times.
- Over-exercising and overworking do not work out well for people with dominant rajasik guna.
- Having a home-cooked meal can help decrease indigestion and any tension in the body.
- Meditation will help sort out and compartmentalize the brain and reduce the clutter of thoughts.
- Cooling asanas can help increase focus in daily routine activities.

Asana Practice

Overworking the body with a strenous routine will not help balance rajasik energy. Practising pranayama before the asana routine helps pacify the rajasik guna, promoting a calmer and more focused practice.

(Please note: Uncomfortable asanas can be skipped as it will not affect the sequence pattern)

ANULOM VILOM (FOR 5 MINUTES) (FOR REFERENCE, SEE PREVIOUS PAGE)

SITALI (3 TIMES) (FOR REFERENCE, SEE PREVIOUS PAGE)

BHRAMARI (5 TIMES) (FOR REFERENCE, SEE PREVIOUS PAGE)

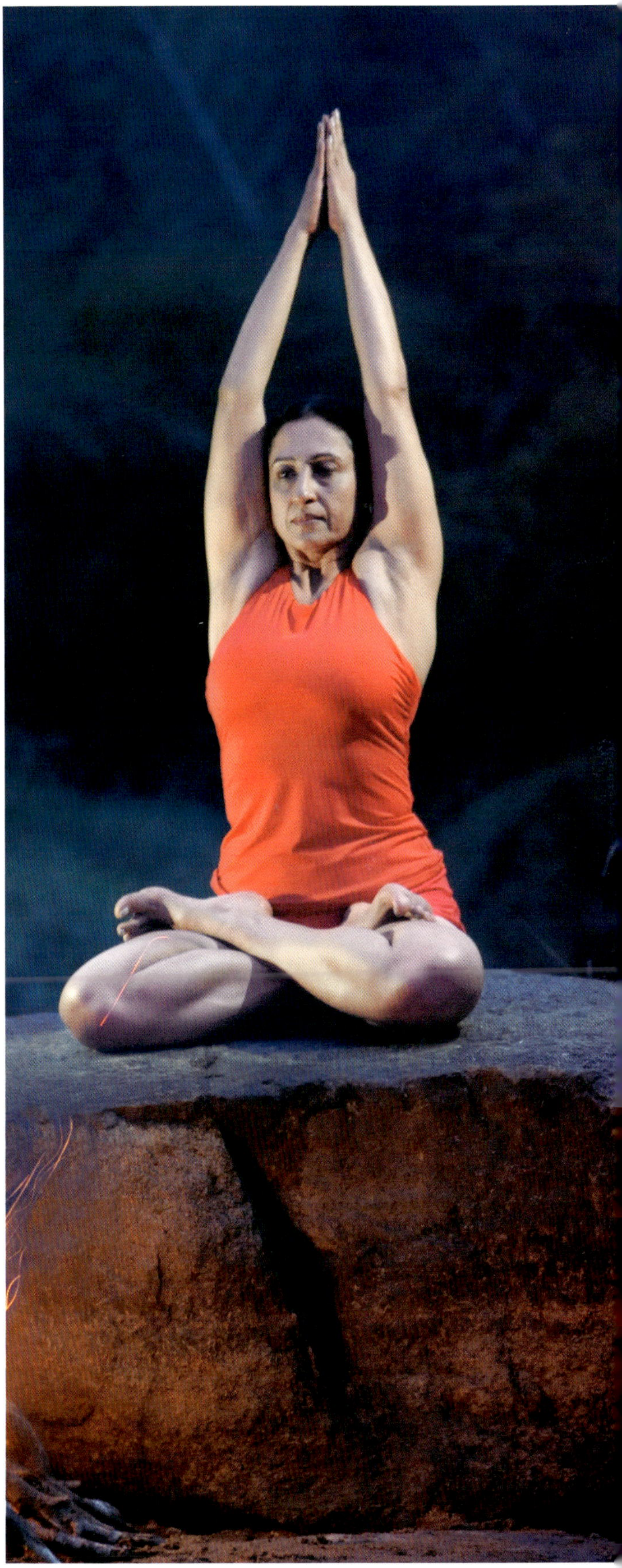

Pranayama

SURYA NAMASKARA A (5 TIMES) (FOR REFERENCE, SEE PP. 4–5)

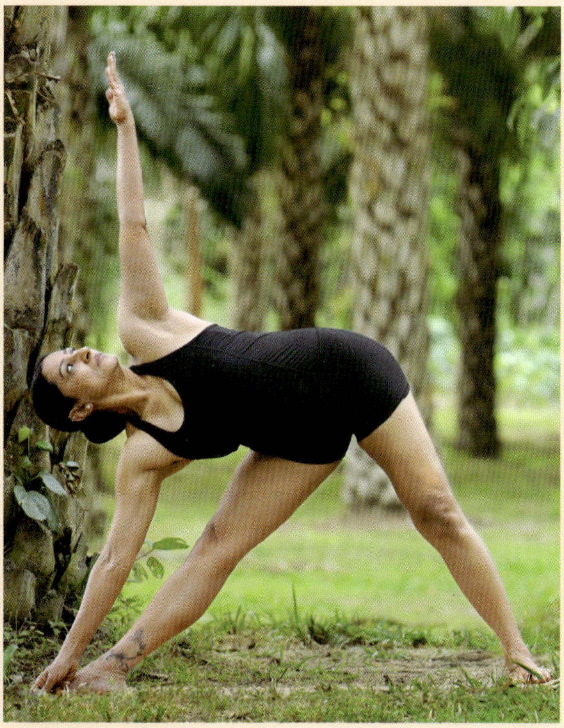

TRIKONASANA 1

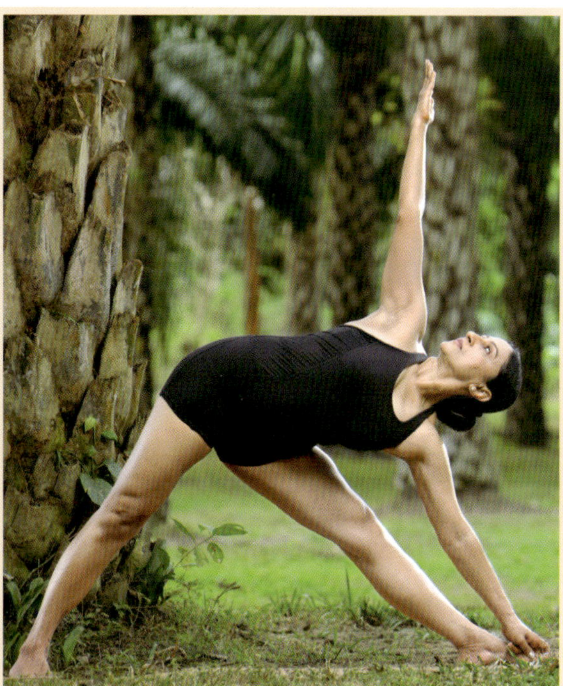

TRIKONASANA 2

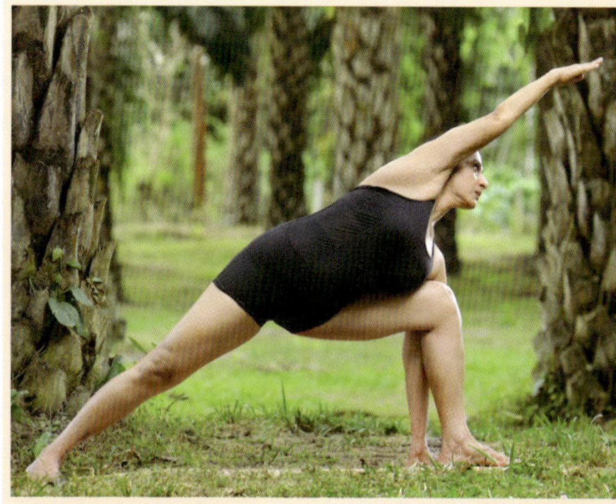

PARSHVAKONASANA

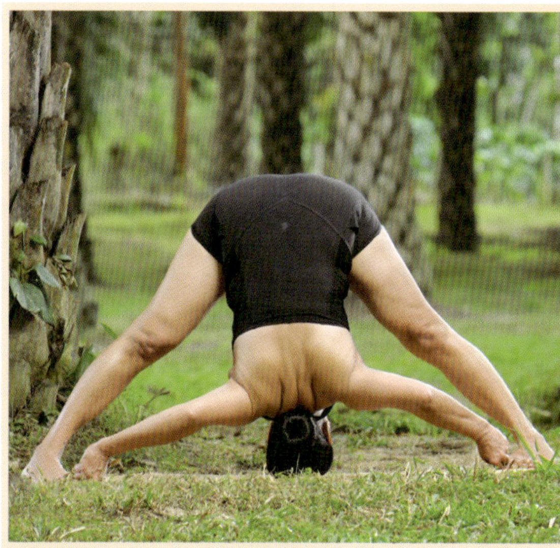

PRASARITA PADOTTANASANA

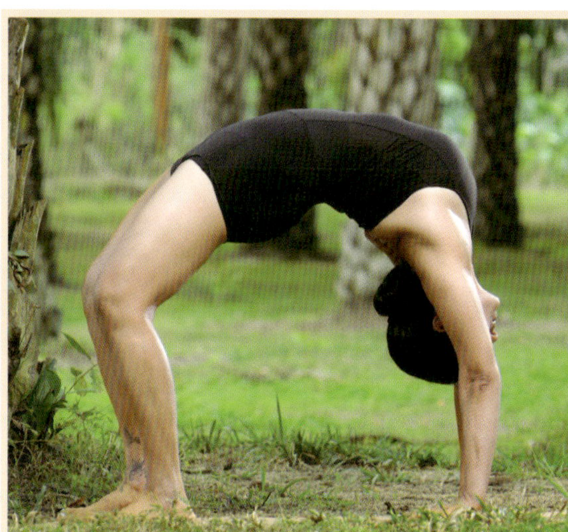

CHAKRASANA (OPTIONAL)

Standing Asanas

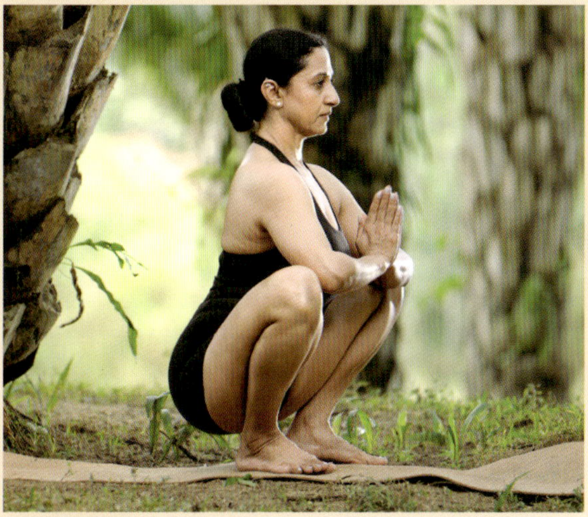

MALASANA

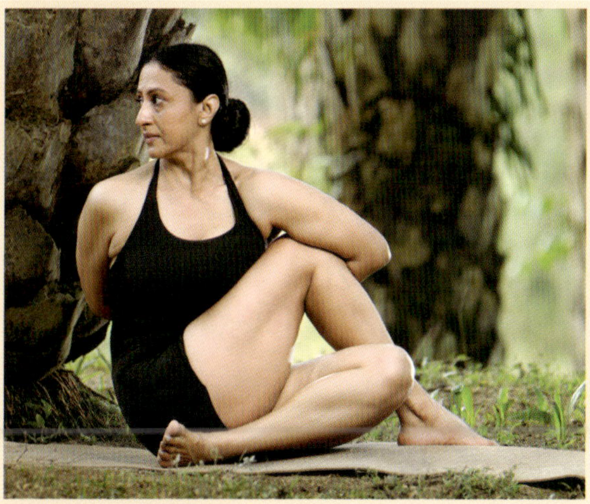

MATSYENDRASANA

Floor Asanas

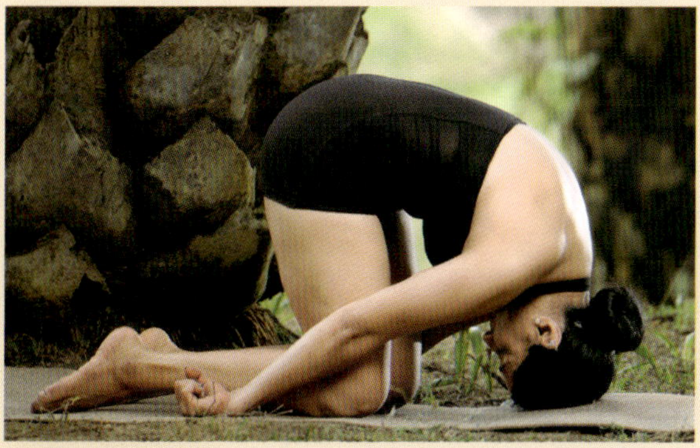

MARJARASANA

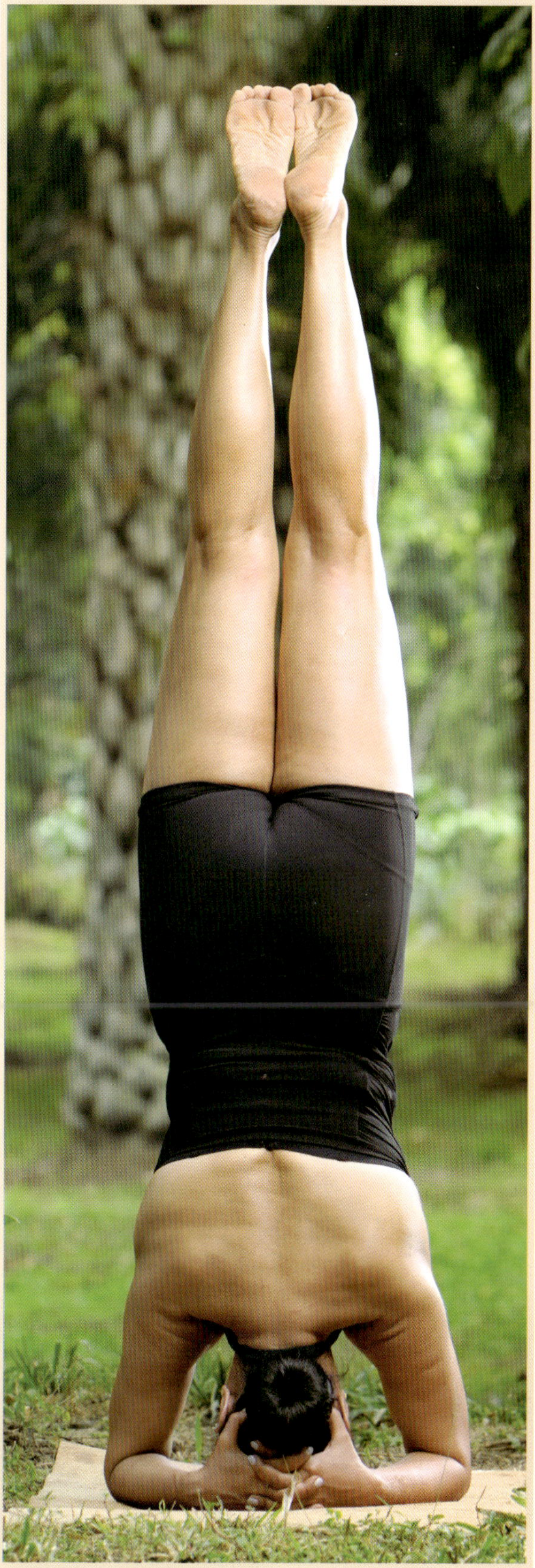

SHIRASANA (OPTIONAL)

Inverted Asana

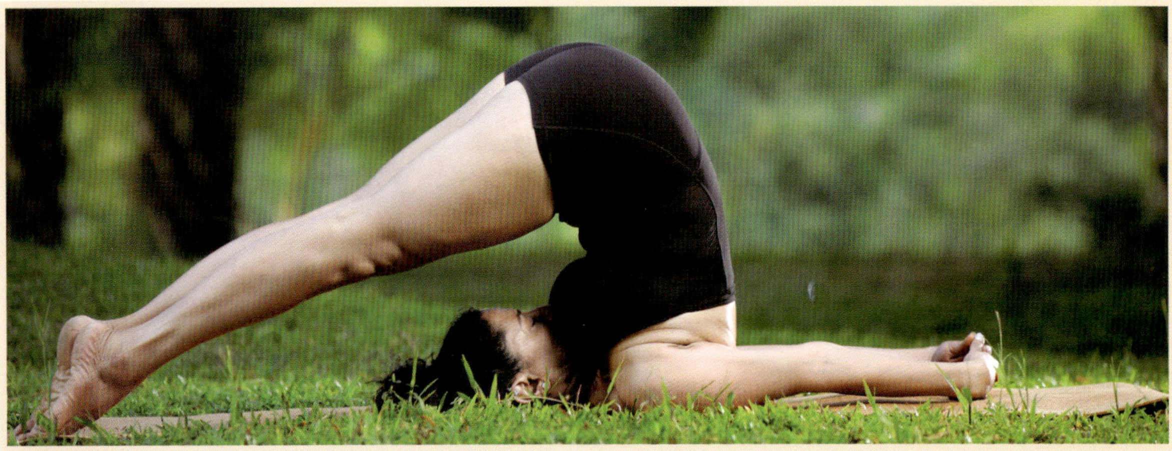

HALASANA

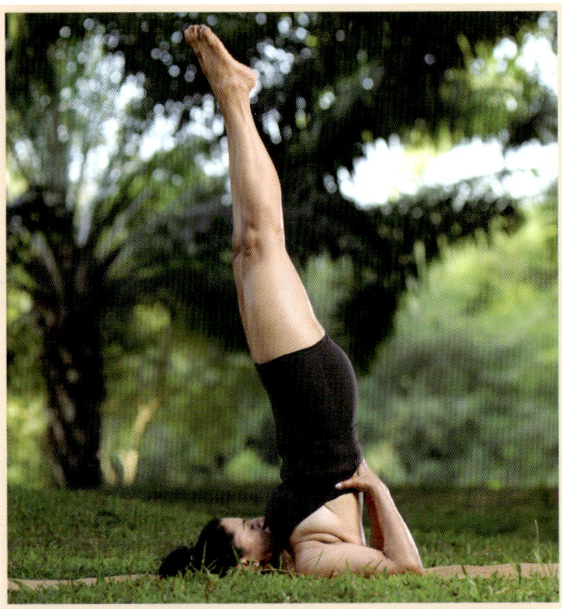

SARVANGASANA 1

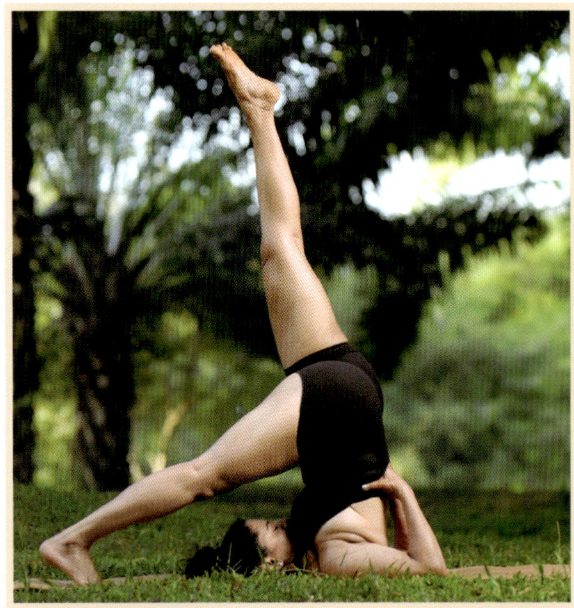

SARVANGASANA 2

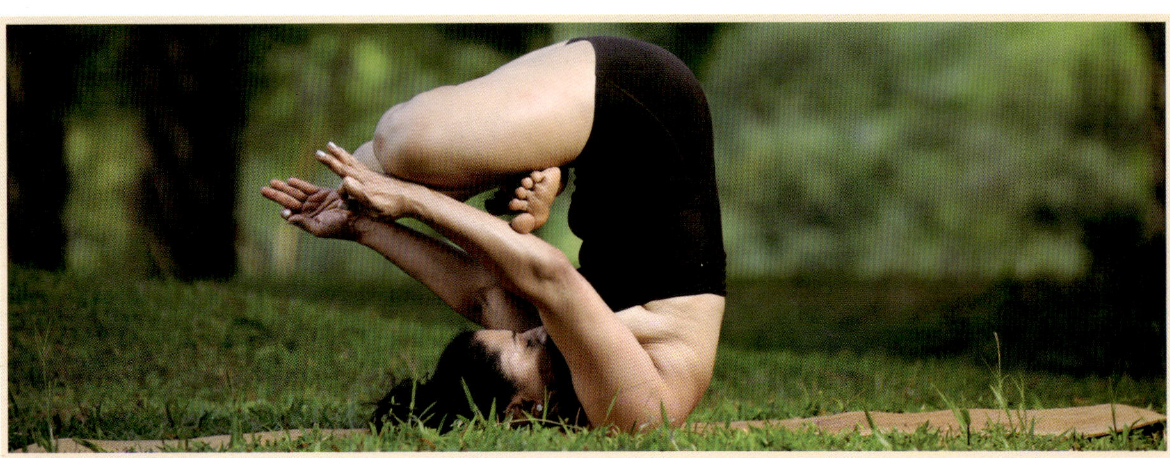

SARVANGASANA 3

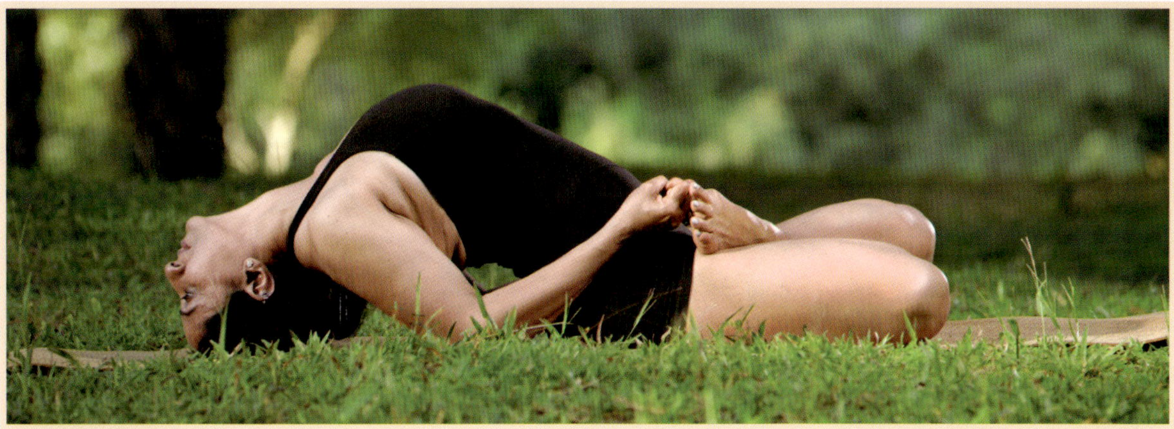

MATSYASANA 1

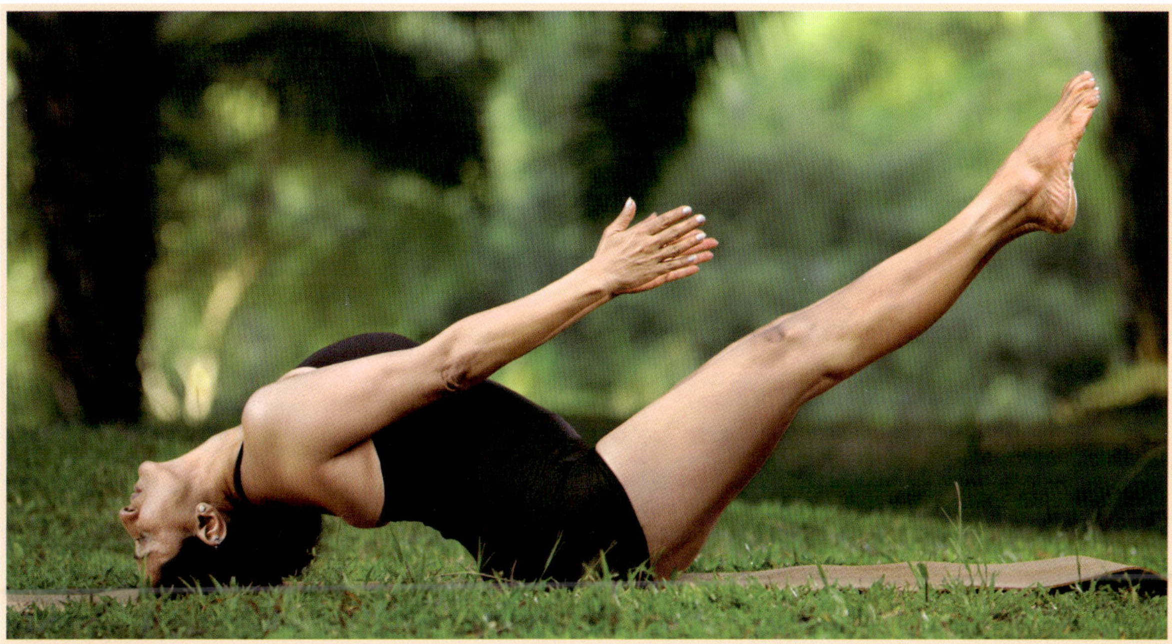

MATSYASANA 2

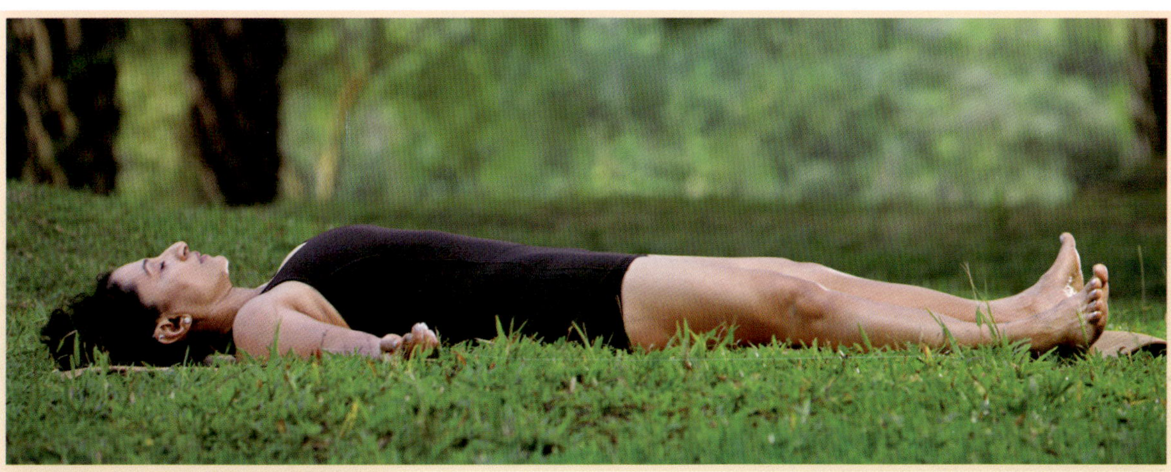

SHAVASANA (10 MINUTES MINIMUM)

Cooling Down Asanas

Tamasik Guna

Tamas means 'darkness' or 'ignorance'. Noticeable tamasik qualities include sluggishness, laziness, anger, attachment, fear of change, depression, self-doubt, guilt, boredom, irritation, addiction and grief.

Tamasik energy in the body is predominantly found in the muscles, bones and flesh. In the mind, it manifests as lethargy and depression.

It is believed that when tamasik guna takes dominance, it is difficult to grow spiritually and reach higher levels of consciousness. To balance this guna, practising yoga in a *vinyasa* pattern (coordinated flow of breathing while moving from one asana to another) with energizing asanas is recommended. Standing asanas are especially beneficial. Pranayama can also help clear the stagnant tamasik prana. Tamasik people find it difficult to sit into dhyana (meditation), therefore it is suggested that they do mindful movement, like walking, climbing and swimming.

Lifestyle Changes

- Consuming fresh and energizing foods helps reduce tamas. Mildly spiced foods, such as those containing ginger, turmeric and cumin, are recommended in moderation for individuals with tamasik tendencies, as they stimulate digestion and boost energy without causing restlessness.
- Nature walks and outdoor activities are important.
- Exercises play an important role in changing the pattern of tamasik energy in the body.
- Sleep and meal timings have to be strictly monitored. Excessive sleeping increases tamas guna.
- Commitment to a goal can drive tamasik people to action.
- Being surrounded by supportive friends and engaging in group activities can help reduce tamas.
- Along with a committed asana practice, getting into a habit of walking everyday has a very positive effect on the tamasik nature of an individual.
- Group meditations and sound meditation are more effective for tamasik individuals than meditating alone.
- Engaging in a variety of interesting activities and continuously learning new things can help transform tamasik tendencies into a more positive and dynamic state.

Asana Practice

A strong and focused Hatha Yoga practice is ideally suited to balance tamas. A consistent practice focusing on movements and deep breathing will help shift the energy pattern. Slightly longer practice of asanas and pranayama will promote greater activity and alertness, hence proving to be beneficial for people with dominanat tamasik traits.

(Please Note: Uncomfortable asanas can be skipped as it will not affect the sequence pattern)

SURYA NAMASKARA A (3 ROUNDS) (FOR REFERENCE, SEE PP. 4–5)

SURYA NAMASKARA B (3 ROUNDS) (FOR REFERENCE, SEE PP. 6–8)

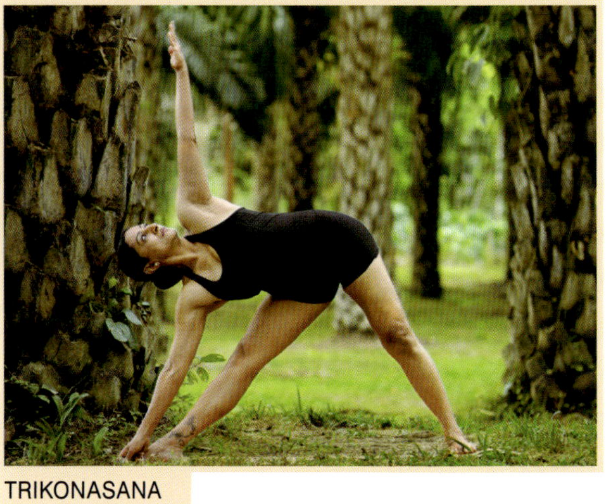

TRIKONASANA

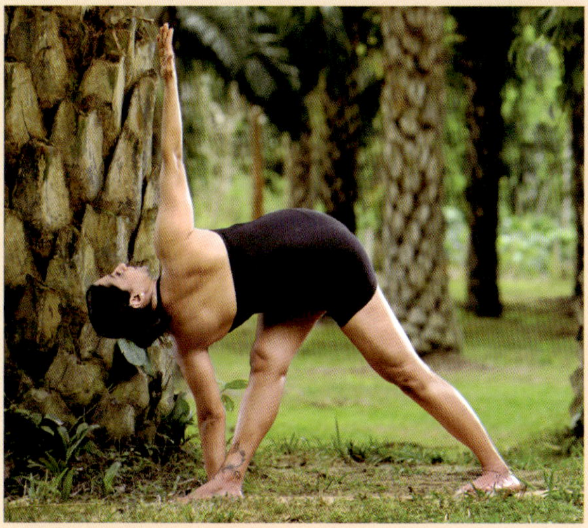
PARIVRITTI TRIKONASANA

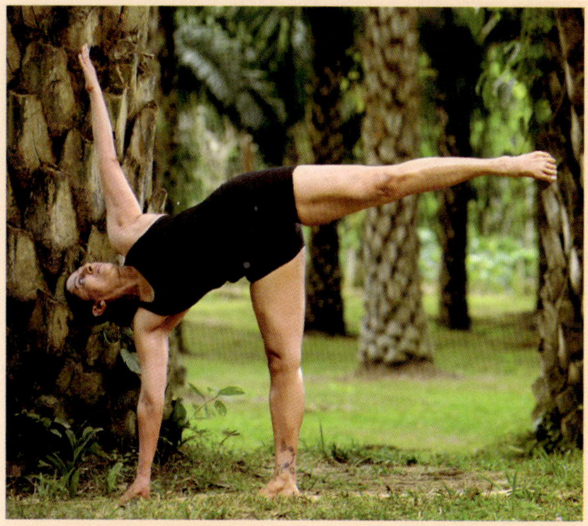
ARDHA CHANDRASANA

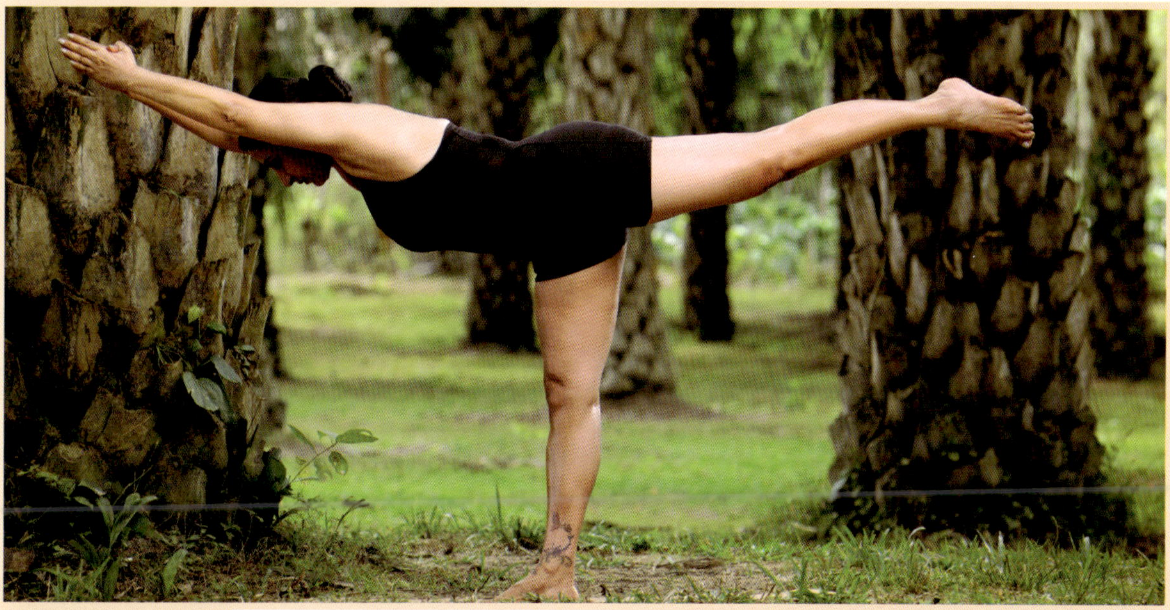
VEERABHADRASANA

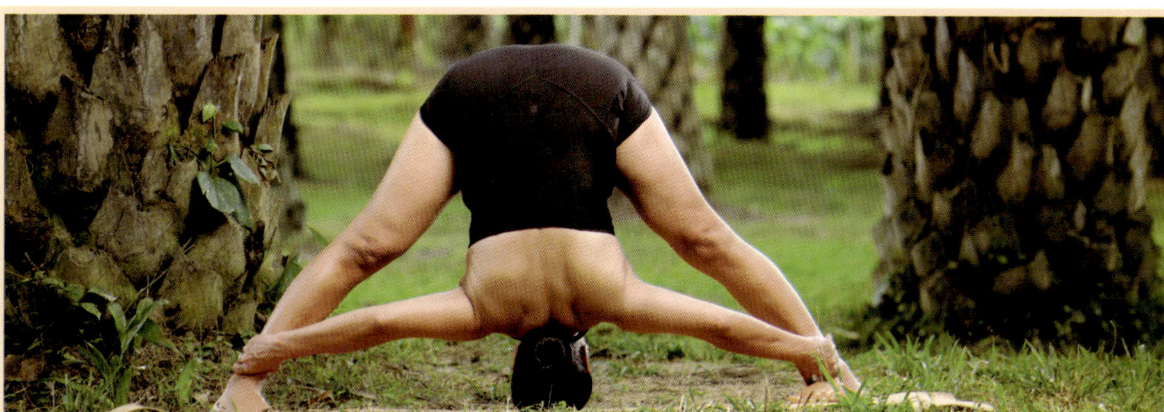
PRASARITA PADOTTANASANA

Standing Asana

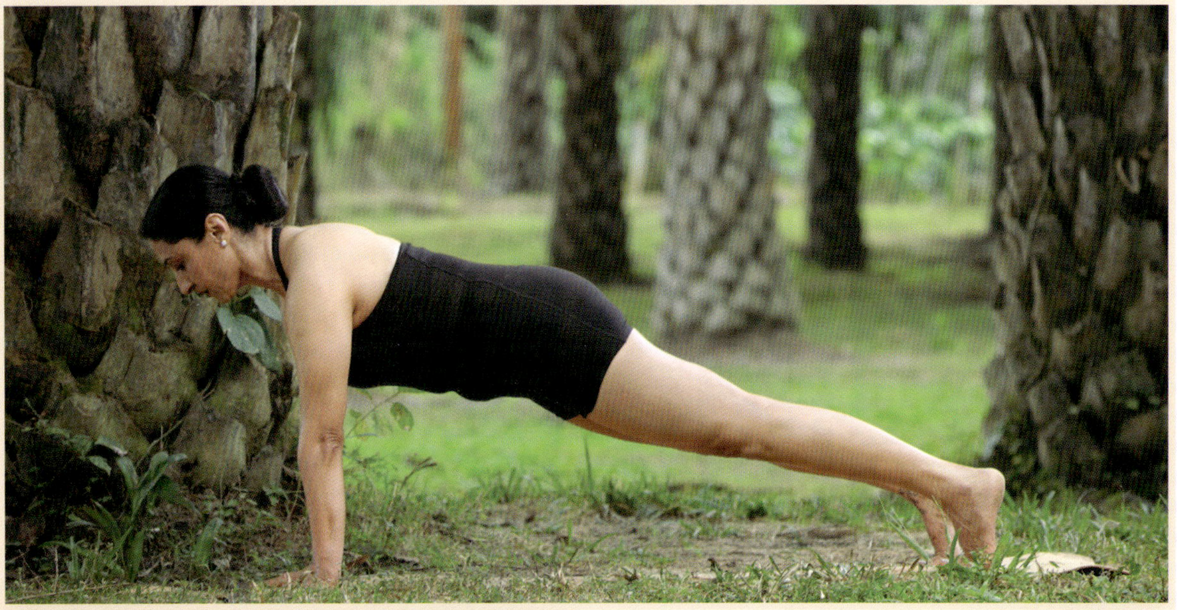

CHATURANGADANDASANA (HOLD FOR 30 SECONDS)

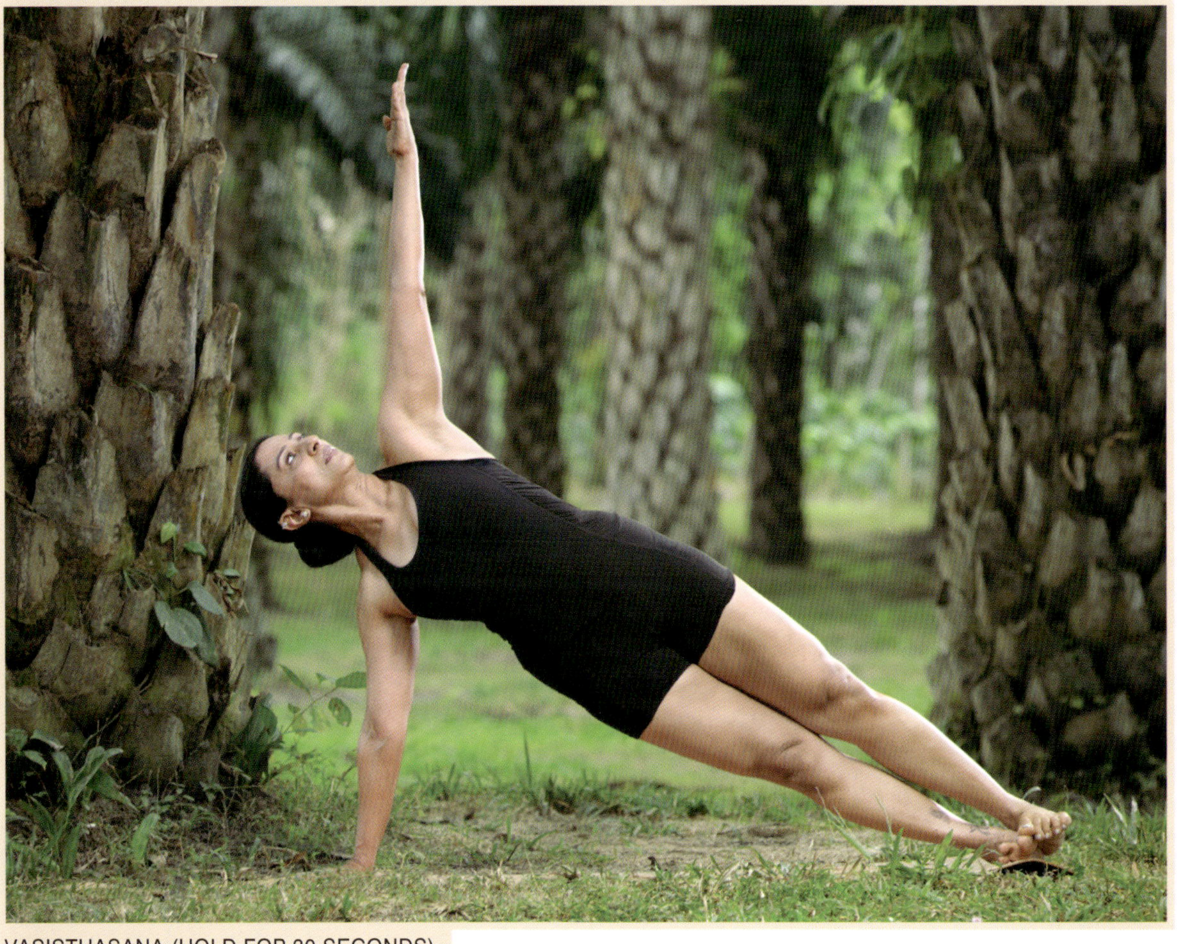

VASISTHASANA (HOLD FOR 30 SECONDS)

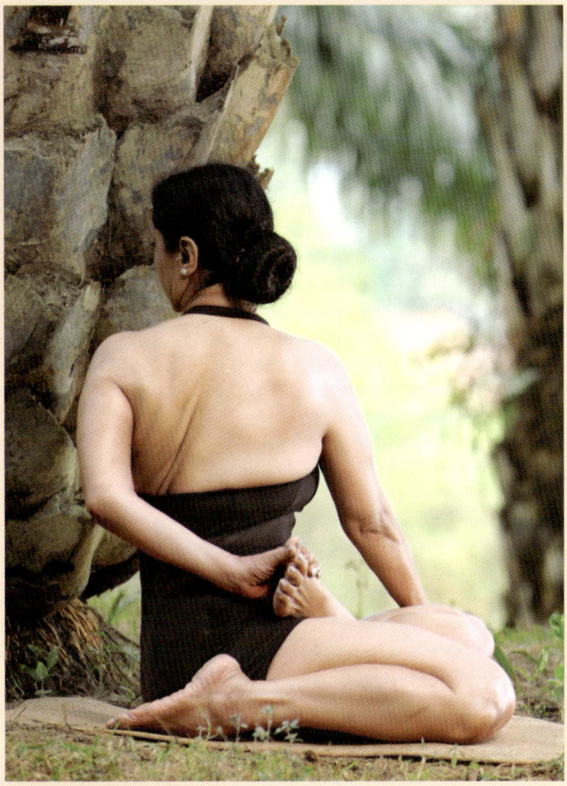

BHARADWAJASANA

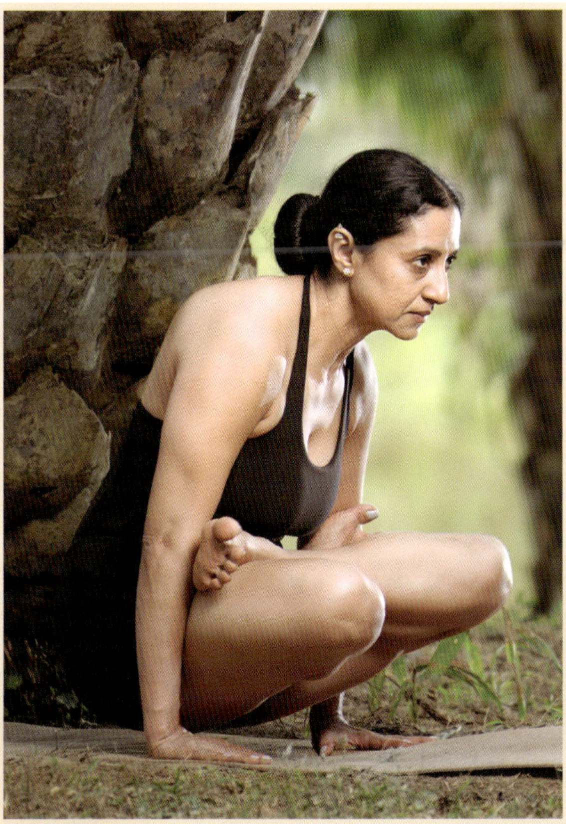

THOLASANA

Floor Asanas

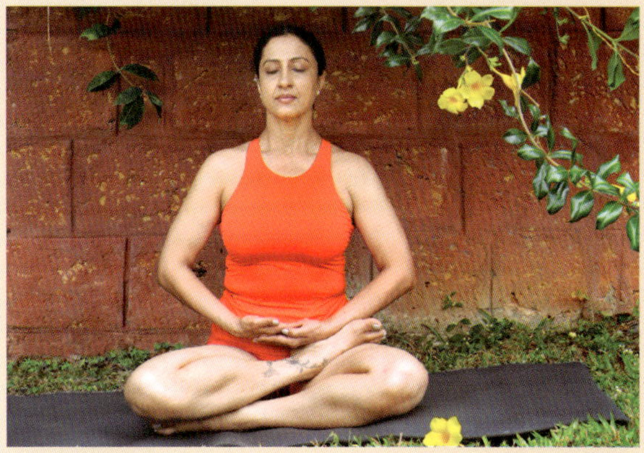

KAPALBHATI

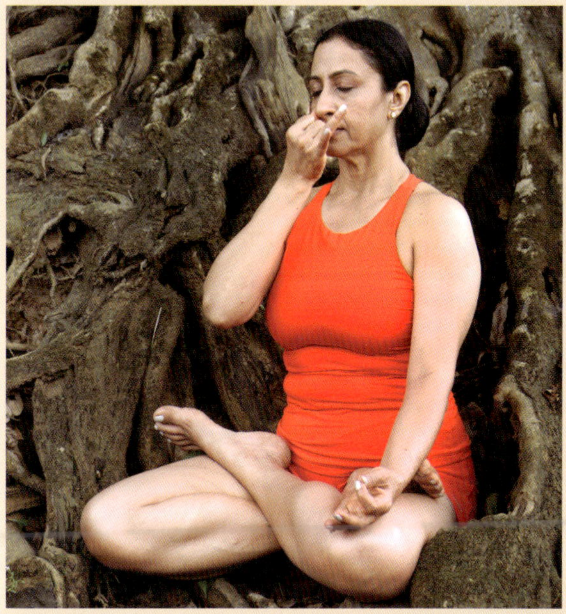

ANULOM VILOM (WITH ANTAR KUMBHAKA)

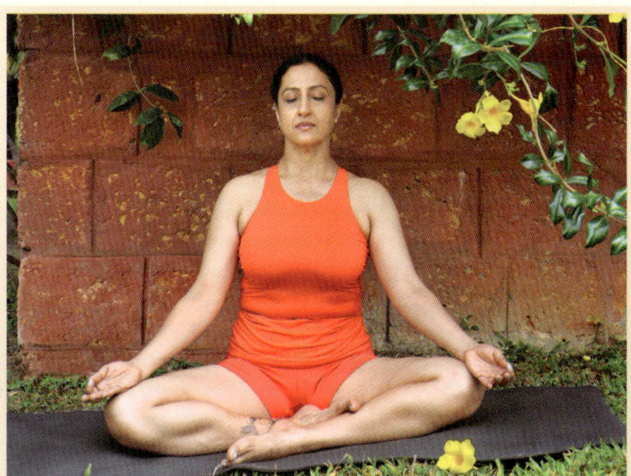

UJJAYI

Pranayama

HALASANA (FOR REFERENCE, SEE P. 20)

SARVANGASANA (FOR REFERENCE, SEE P. 20)

MATSYASANA (FOR REFERENCE, SEE P. 21)

SHAVASANA (FOR REFERENCE, SEE P. 21)

Cooling Down Asanas

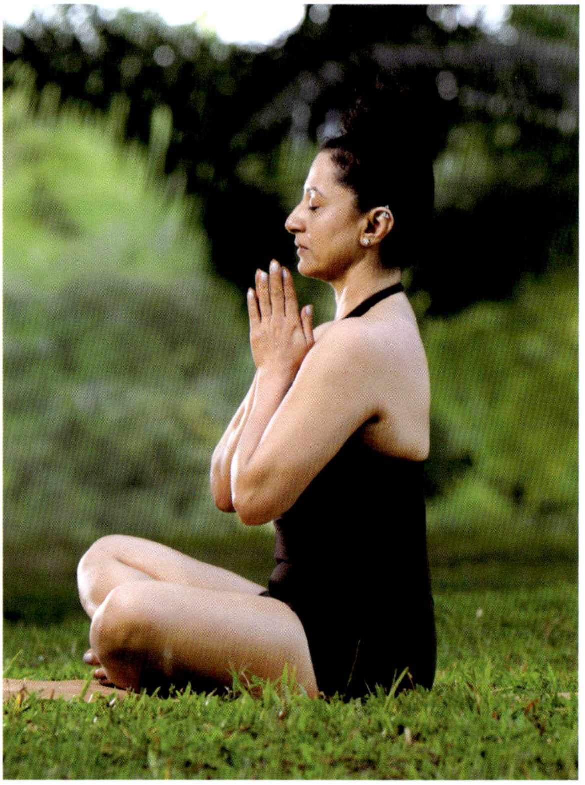

PRANAMAYA KOSHA

This is the second layer of existence, where the air is in circulation. Directly connected with annamaya kosha, this sheath is responsible for the working of the physical body. *Pranamaya* kosha is composed of prana, or life force. Practising different asanas, with focus on breathing, will keep this kosha vital and powerful.

VAYU FUNCTIONING IN THE BODY			
VAYU	**LOCATION**	**MOVEMENT**	**FUNCTIONS**
Prana	Chest and head	Inward	Inhalation
Apana	Lower centre	Downward	Elimination
Samana	Navel	Unites upward vayu with downward vayu	Digestion, assimilation, absorption of thoughts, etc.
Udana	Throat	Upward	Growth, speech and expression
Vyana	Heart and lungs	Circular	Cardiac activity, circulation and nervous system

MANOMAYA KOSHA

This is the third layer of existence, where an individual's personality takes shape. *Manomaya* kosha holds subtle memories, which may manifest through genetic influences or karmic impressions. It is within this layer that thought patterns, understanding and behaviours develop and evolve.

Maintaining mindfulness and alertness is crucial for the optimal functioning of this kosha.

A balanced routine that includes disciplined living, along with the practice of yoga asanas and pranayama, helps keep this layer responsive.

This kosha also forms mental maps, embedding experiences, decisions and behavioural patterns. These imprints, in turn, shape a person's health, conduct and spiritual growth, influencing the overall journey of self-realization.

This kosha has four sections

- Manas
- Buddhi
- Chitta
- Ahamkara

MANAS

A major part of the manomaya kosha, manas is the everyday mind. It is the coordinator of the senses and the mental screen on which thoughts and images arise. There are many layers to it. The workings of manas, or the mind, are not confined to the mind alone; their effects extend and influence the entire body. During meditation, manas becomes still, with its energies concentrated rather than dispersed. Sensory distractions fade, wandering thoughts subside, and attention sharpens with focus.

BUDDHI

Buddhi is the intellect. It assigns meaning, value and reflection to the experience the mind captures. Buddhi is awakened as the mind provides it information and doesn't do anything beyond giving a perspective. Manas sends the first wave of thought, and buddhi carries it further to reflect a meaning to it. Bhuddhi gives the power to discriminate and decide what is good and what is not. It is the force behind the wisdom and our reactions depend on its reflection. It influences the way we understand and interpret our experiences, take decisions, and act.

CHITTA

Chitta is the unconscious storehouse of past thoughts and experiences, the pool of all memories. It accumulates impressions and blends them with the newly formed metal imagery to add richness to experience. These stored impressions are propelled back and forth in our minds in the form of habitual behaviours, desires, intensions, etc. This activity becomes especially noticeable during meditation, when thoughts may arise as fantasies, disturbing memories, simple desires, or intense emotional urges.

However, meditation can shift these impressions, holding the power to transform and reshape their patterns, leading to deeper clarity and inner change.

AHAMKARA

Ahamkara is the activity of attributing objective existence to self or ego. *Aham* means 'I' and *kara* means 'doing' or 'making'. It is the 'sense of identity'. Once ahamkara takes on an identity, the rest of the divisions starts to functions in that context. Buddhi or intellect is the most to get influenced by ahamkara. Ancient and sacred texts prescribe many ways to overcome the influence of ahamkara. One of the most efficient ways is to surrender to the faith of divine energy which is referred to as *Ishwara pranidhana*. Following the principles of ashtanga from the *Yoga Sutra*s is a very powerful way to overcome ahamkara.

DISCLAIMER

The sections discussed in this chapter are profound and vast. They are based on the information collected from various texts that explain the essence and function of each of these mind fields. Most of the interpretations you have read so far are from my personal understanding. The above points have been expressed following the explanations offered by my Guruji and my own research. I continue to explore into this aspect of knowledge and further understand these valuable concepts.

VIJNANAMAYA KOSHA

This fourth layer is connected to wisdom and deeper states of consciousness. This kosha deals with inner well-being and growth. With a balanced *vijnanamaya kosha*, an individual will get knowledgeable and wise. Understanding the ashtanga principles and living a disciplined life will enhance the growth of this kosha.

This is the place of discernment and a space for enquiry. This kosha receives its information from the *indriyas*, meaning 'organs of perception' or the sense organs. The indiriyas collect information and help acquire knowledge and perspective about a certain object. Whatever information we receive from the indriyas are taken into the manas, and is then judged and processed by buddhi, which results in knowledge.

THREE DIVISIONS OF INDRIYAS

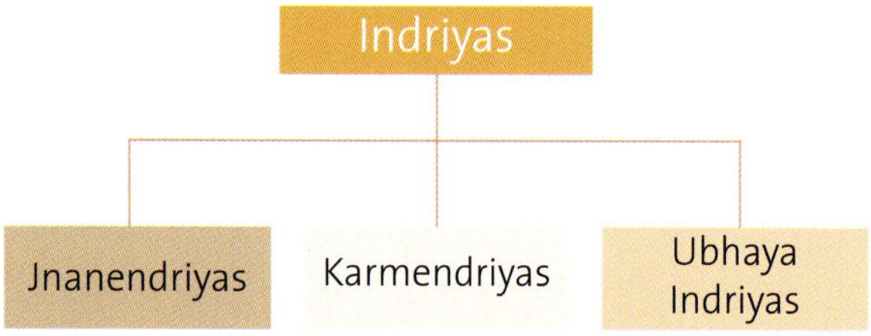

JNANEDRIYAS

Jnanedriyas are five in number and governed by the five elements of pancha bhootas.

JNANEDRIYAS AND THEIR FUNCTIONS		
ORGAN	**FUNCTION**	**ELEMENT**
Chakshu	*Drishti*	Agni
Karna	*Shabda*	Akasha
Nasika	*Gandha*	Prithvi
Jihva	*Rasa*	Jal
Twak	*Sparsha*	Vayu

These organs facilitate communication, directly interacting with the manas and buddhi. Subsequently, chitta processes this information, while ahamkara shapes the response based on identity and ego.

KARMENDRIYAS

These are organs of action.

- *Hasta* (palm/hands): Their function is to receive (*grahana*) and to give (*dana*)
- *Paada* (foot): The function is movement (*gamana*)
- *Guda/Paayu* (anus): The function is defecation (*mala visarga*)
- *Linga Upasta* (penis): The function is sex (*ramana*) and urination (*mootra visarjana*)
- *Vak* (tongue): The function is speech (*vachana*)

UBHAYA INDRIYA

Ubhaya indriya encompasses both sensory perception and motor functions, serving as the vital link between the creation of a thought and the entire experience of that creation. It is not a physical organ but the manas itself, orchestrating how we perceive, process, and respond to the world.

AUTHOR'S NOTE

- The Ashtanga Yoga system outlined in the *Yoga Sutras* highlights the last four limbs as essential practices for mastering the indriyas.
- Pratyahara is withdrawal of senses, like a turtle pulling its limbs into its shell. By actively turning our awareness and attention away from the indriyas, we conserve prana and cultivate a focused mind. Ideally, pratyahara is practised during meditation or Hatha Yoga practices.
- *Svaadhyaya* (self-enquiry) is a yogic practice which is a part of pratyahara, recommended to create a distinction between self-conscious awareness and body sensations. This in turn helps disentangle the soul's misidentifications with the sense organs.
- *Vairagya* (non-attachment) is the conscious control of our attraction to the external world of sense objects. This detachment allows to choose what is good for our mind to be drawn towards, with the ideal goal of experiencing both sweet and bitter fruits. Vairagya in simple terms is 'letting go'.

Mastering control of the indriyas is both challenging and rewarding experience. Minimizing and reducing the powerful influence senses have on the mind will cultivate inner peace, mental focus, clarity of mind, and happiness.

ANANADAMAYA KOSHA

This is the fifth sheath which is often referred to as the atma of a being. This is the innermost kosha, where our supreme self resides. This kosha transcends all others, surpassing the physical body and the thinking mind. Learned yogis explain that this kosha can be experienced in states of meditation. Many interpret *ananda* as 'equanimity' and some explain it as a blissful state. It is peace, joy and love beyond perception, independence beyond any reason or stimulus.

When the *anandamaya kosha* is experienced with practice, it is a state of complete bliss. This experience remains stable and does not change. When one can deal with all kinds of circumstances life has to offer and yet maintain peace and harmony within, that is ananda or supreme bliss.

AUTHOR'S NOTE

Texts explain that the transition from the vijnanamaya to anandamaya kosha is an important stage in the heightening of super consciousness, and this is the actual essence of the practice of yoga. Sage Patanjali in the *Yoga Sutras* has devoted an entire section to this event where the consciousness becomes capable of perceiving the four dimensions of time: past, present, future and eternity. Sage Patanjali explains how to go about this transition in the chapter 'Vibhuti Pada' in the *Yoga Sutras*. He refers to it as the important accomplishment of yoga.

The scriptures have prescribed three important practices that are helpful to train anandamaya kosha. They are:

- *Seva*: This opens our heart, revealing our innate unity with other beings.
- *Bhakti*: This opens and cleanses the karmic block to a large extent.
- *Samadhi*: This is intensely focused meditation which opens our heart to our own divine being.

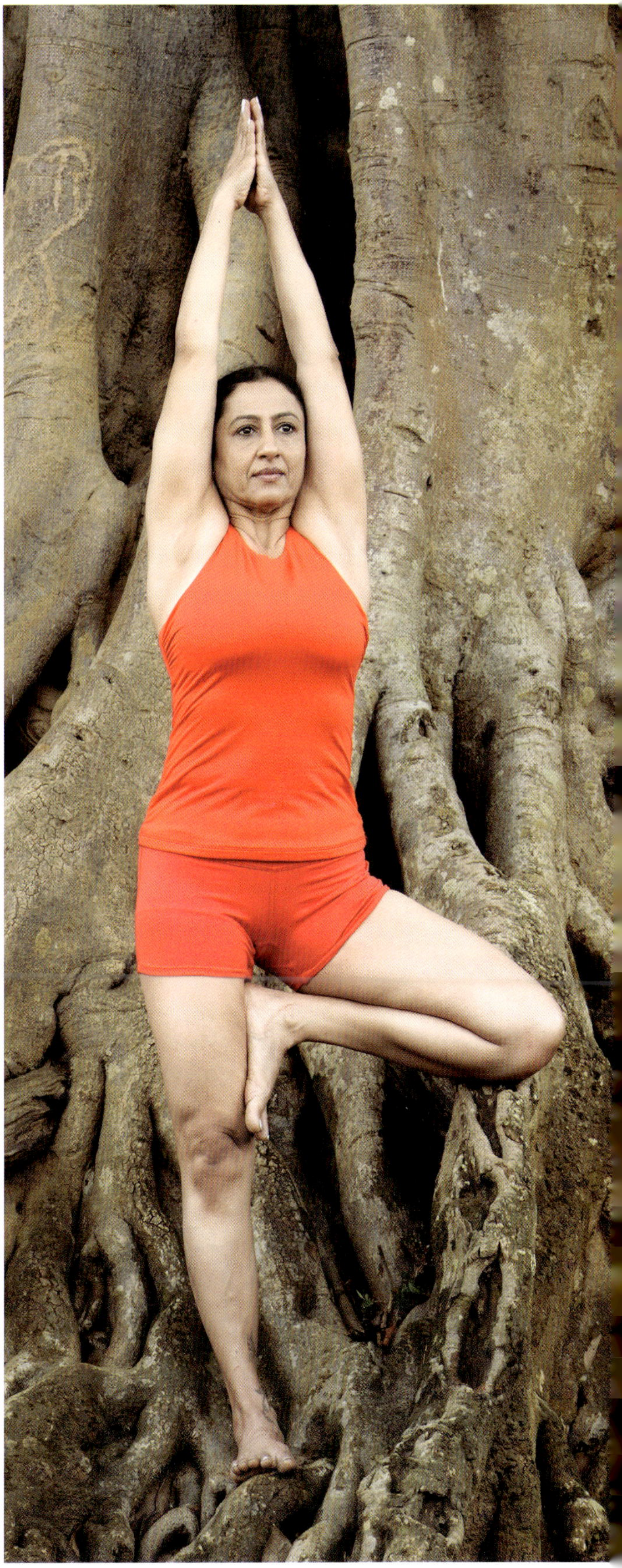

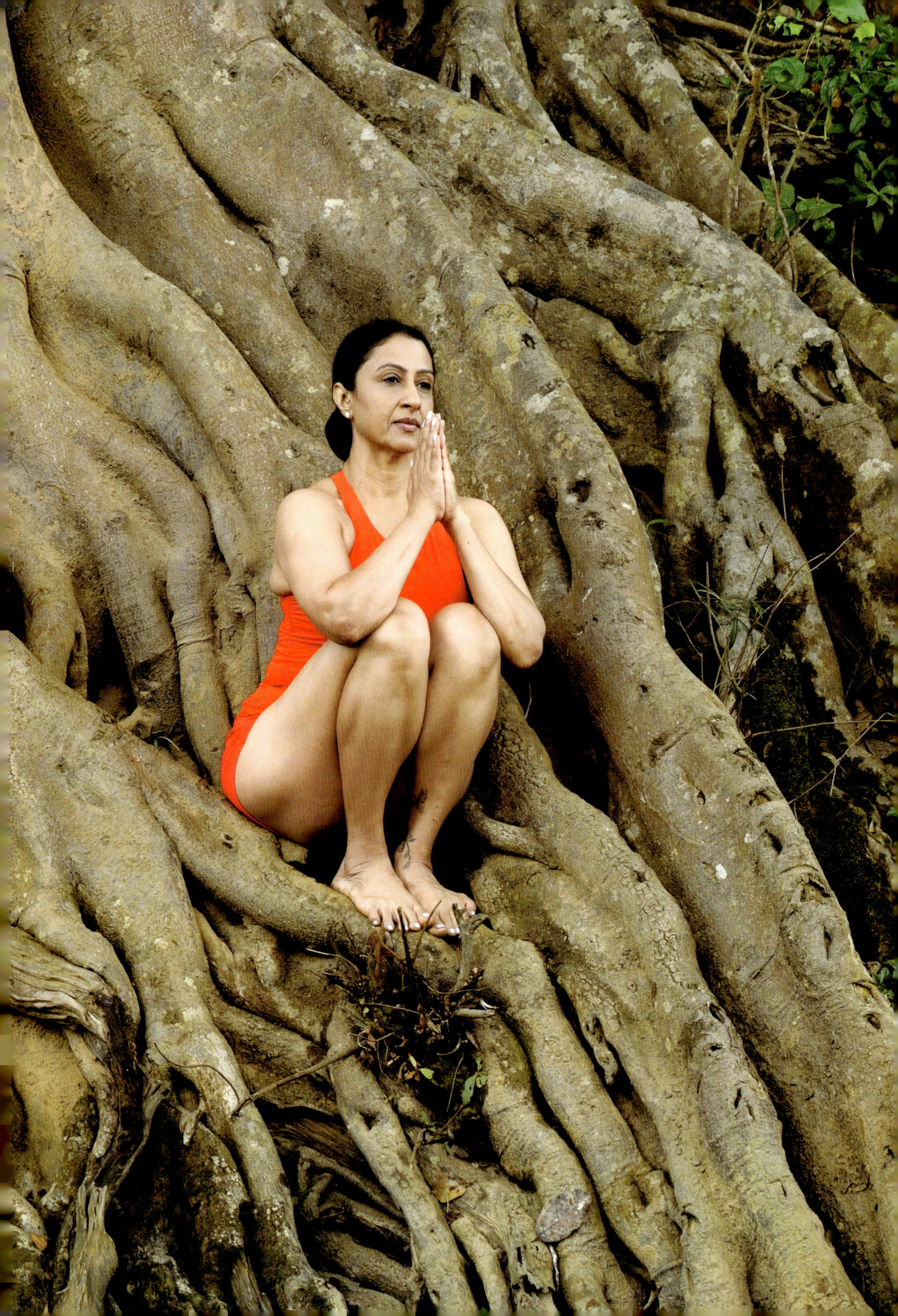

CHAPTER 3
CHAKRAS: ENERGY CENTRES

The energy centres of the body are centres of information, which have their own frequency and expression. They do not have a form or a structure. They can be only felt. They have their own functions with associated organs, glands, chemicals and hormones. These clusters of information form the personality of an individual. These energy centres can be activated in various ways in the form of consciousness.

The activations of the centres need not be in the order of its arrangement in the body, but it can be in the order of the individual's requirement or purpose. These centres are called chakras. The energy that flows through these chakras is called *kundalini*. The movement of this energy is always present in the body and that's what makes the body function. However, there are specific yogic techniques that can be practised to activate specific energy residing in these chakras. The primary goal of activating the chakras is to facilitate spiritual growth and to understand one's true nature and connection to the universe. With this connection, there is increased awareness, greater emotional stability and resilience.

KUNDALINI

Kundalini is a widely discussed subject amongst yoga practitioners. It is also sometimes referred to as 'yoga of awareness'. The study of kundalini comes from the texts on *Tantra Yoga*. This is a powerful energy that carries unmanifested potential within us—beyond the limits of our mind. *Kunda* means a 'pit', and the coiled-up energy (*ilini*) within this pit is known as kundalini. This is often depicted as a serpent wrapped three-and-a-half times. There are various methods prescribed to wake up the kundalini energies. It can be awakened by the physical and spiritual practices of yoga, such as chanting of mantras, practising specific asanas, specific pranayama and mudra. When awakened, the kundalini energy rises through vortices of energy called the chakras, which leads to spiritual awakening that gets manifested as liberation.

It is believed and experienced by practitioners that awakened kundalini allows one to live a life with more awareness. It helps develop unique qualities that offer:

- *Jnan*: Limitless knowledge and insight that help in solving challenges of life with ease and calmness,
- *Ichchha*: Strong will and determination, a quality that helps one see things through until the end,
- *Chitta*: Greater awareness with insight into the happenings in life, and
- *Kriya*: Doing the right thing at the right time.

Kundalini practice has the potential to expand an individual's capacity and opens doors to more possibilities with greater potential. However, the main purpose of practising Kundalini Yoga is to promote spiritual enlightenment. Scientific research has found that this practice has great therapeutic benefits. It helps decrease stress, anxiety, depression; improves cognitive functions, self-confidence, self-esteem and feelings of self-worth.

BASIC METHODS TO AWAKEN KUNDALINI

- Bhakti: To bring in a sense of self-surrender, humility and gratitude to all energies in the universe and the Creator
- Dhyana: To cultivate clarity in the mind and awareness through self-assessment and observation

- Hatha Yoga: To build a strong and healthy body
- Pranayama: To cultivate awareness and control of the prana

Awakening kundalini is an integral part of yoga practice. However, to do so, a separate set of practices are followed, all of which are more austere than general yoga practice. This has to be done with the guidance of a qualified guru.

AUTHOR'S NOTE

In modern times, Kundalini Yoga is often misunderstood as an experience-driven practice, overlooking its true potential. Scriptures highlight that kundalini awakening is meant to expand consciousness and wisdom, not merely to provide fleeting experiences. Its real purpose lies in achieving profound spiritual growth and higher states of awareness.

ASANA PRACTICE

Asana sequence performed to clear the path of Kundalini:

Standing Asanas

SURYA NAMASKARA A (FOR REFERENCE, SEE PP. 4–5)

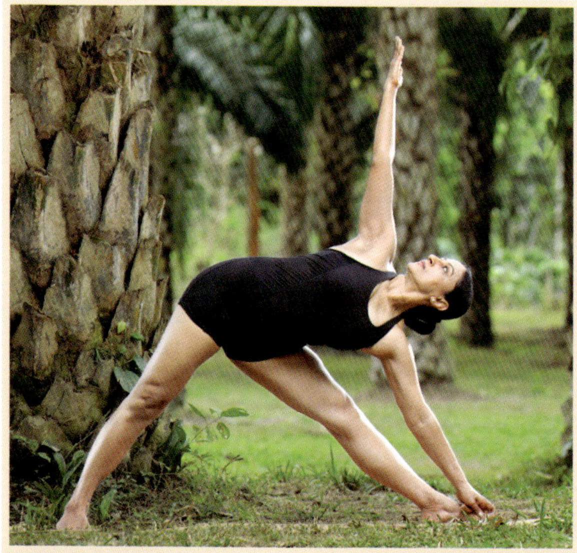

TRIKONASANA

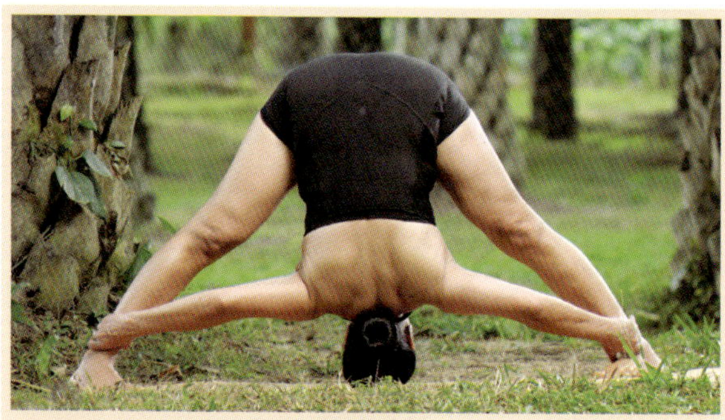

PRASARITA PADOTTANASANA

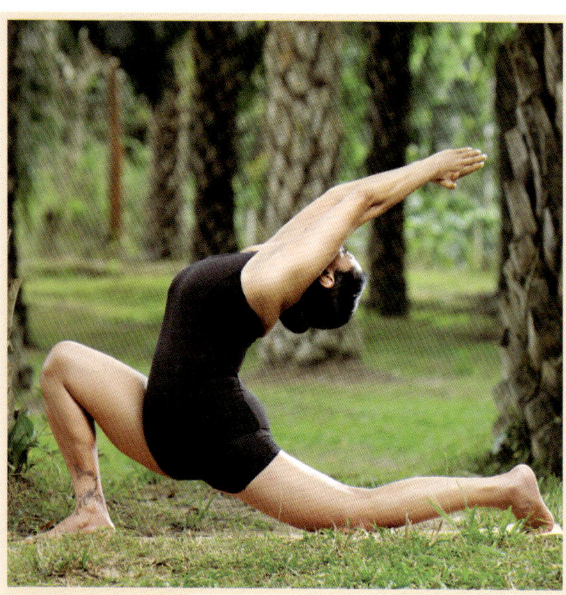

ASHWACHALANA

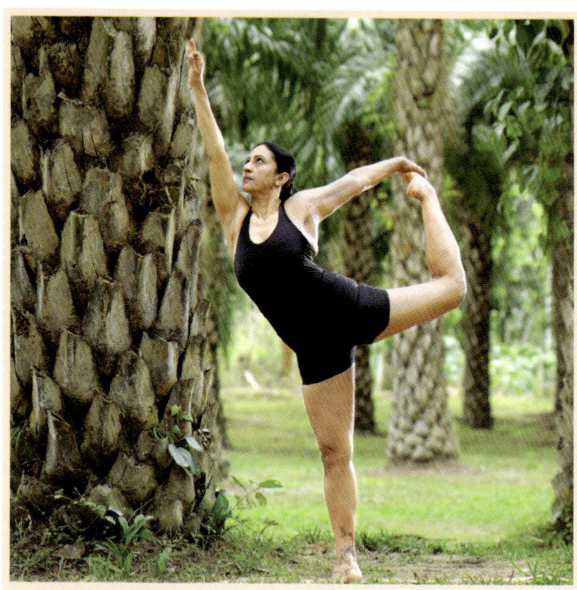

NATARAJASANA

Sitting Asanas

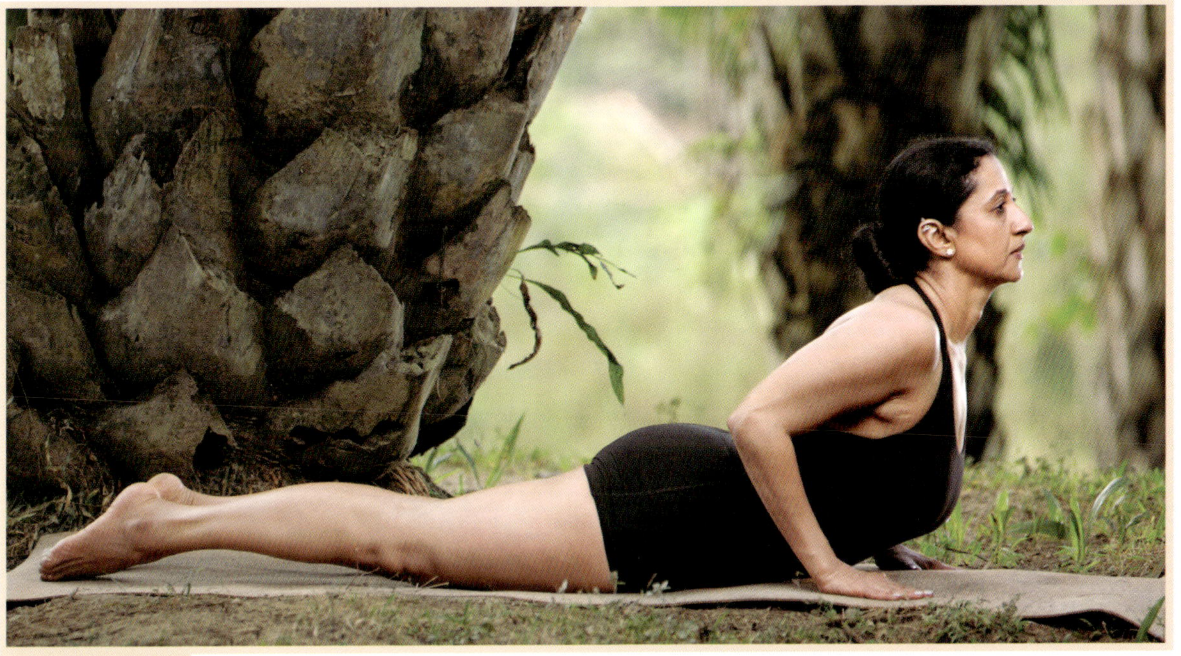

BHUJANGASANA

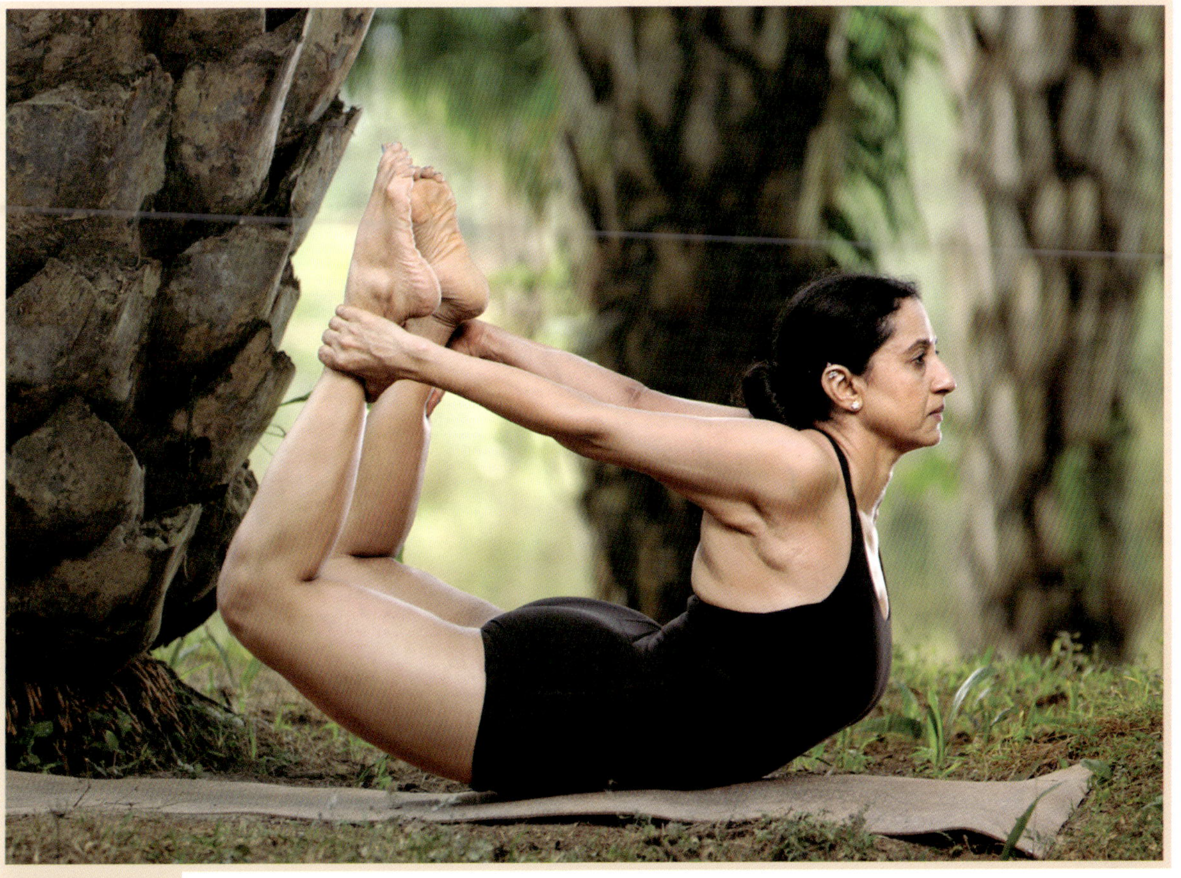

DHANURASANA

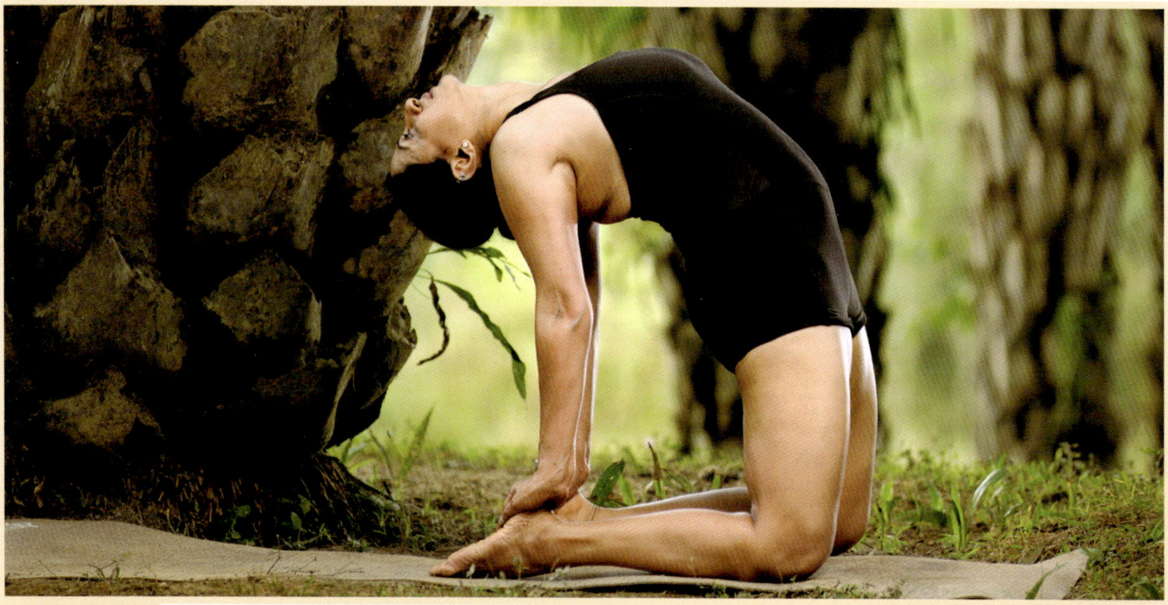

USHTRASANA

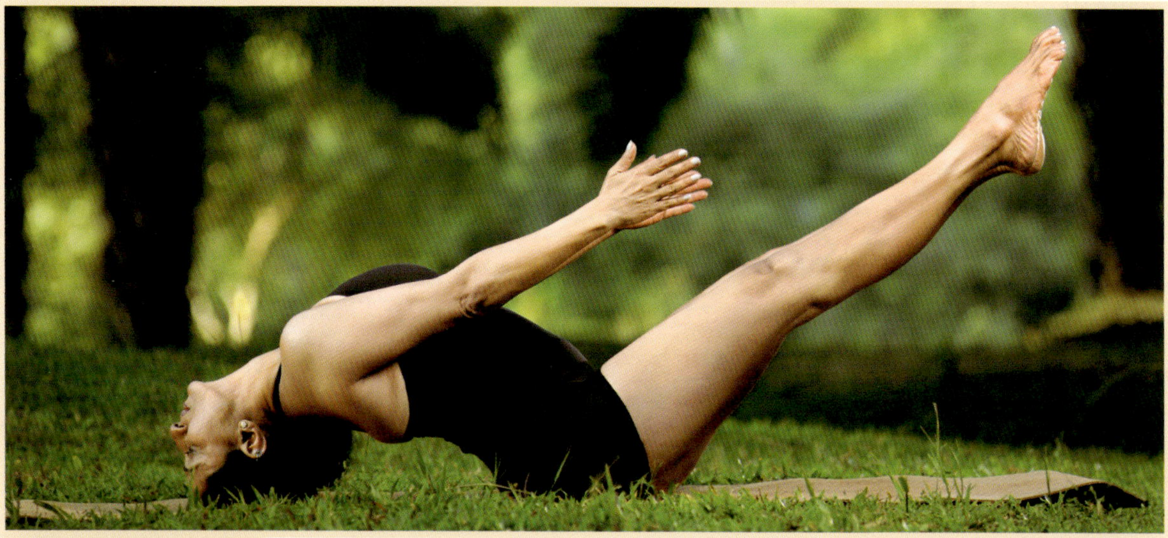

SAMPURNA NAVASANA

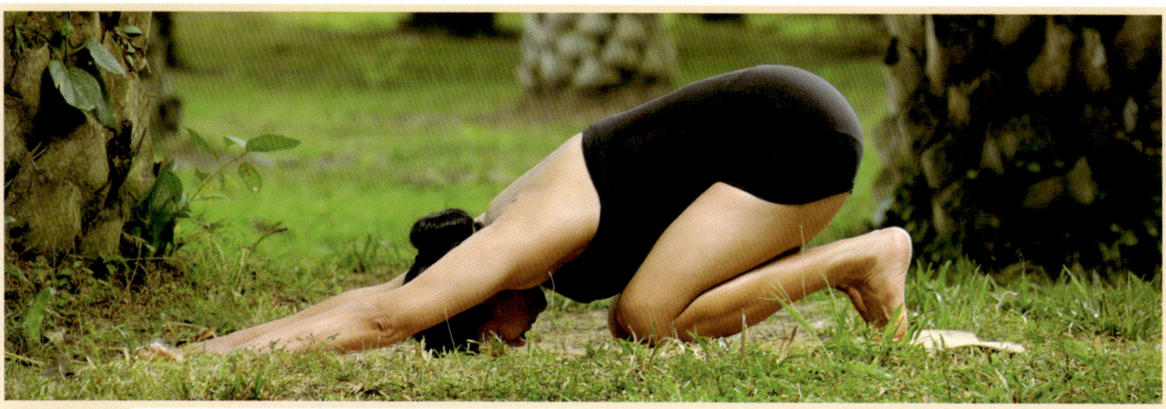

BALASANA

Cooling Down Asanas

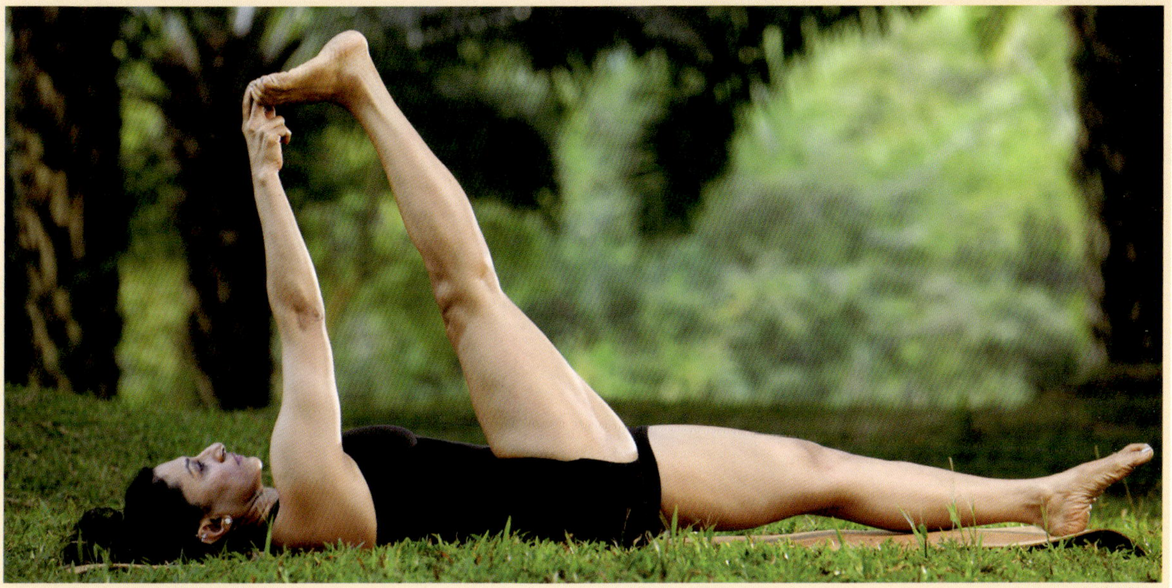

SUPTA HASTAPADANGUSHTHASANA 1

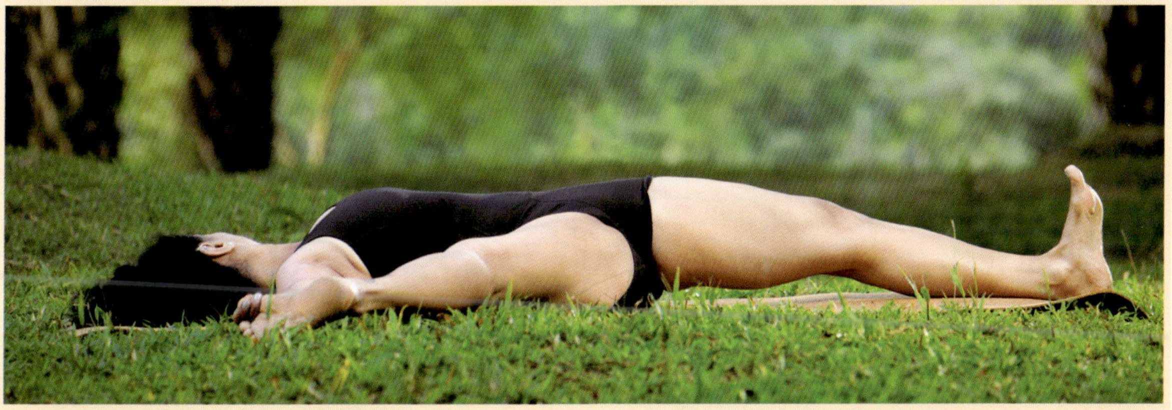

SUPTA HASTAPADANGUSHTHASANA 2

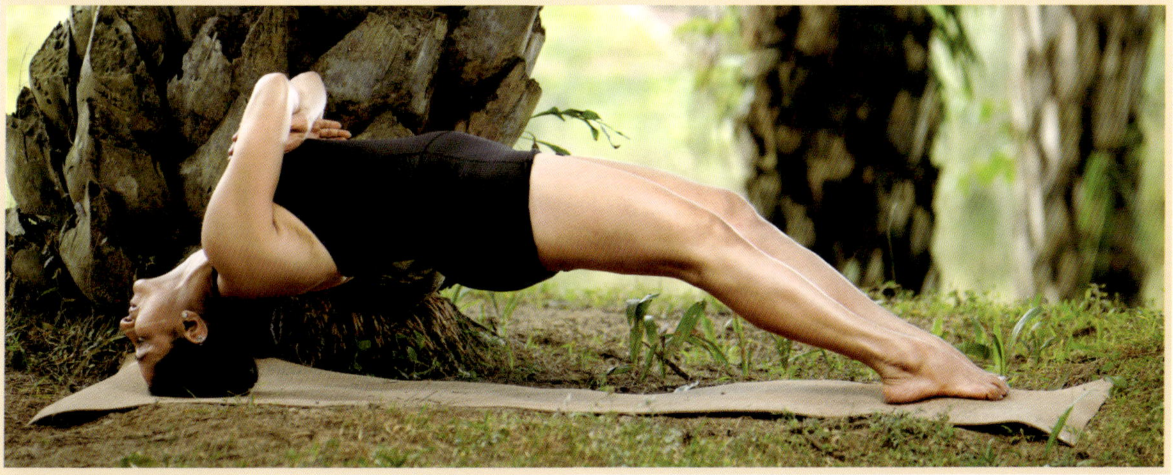

SETHUBANDHASANA

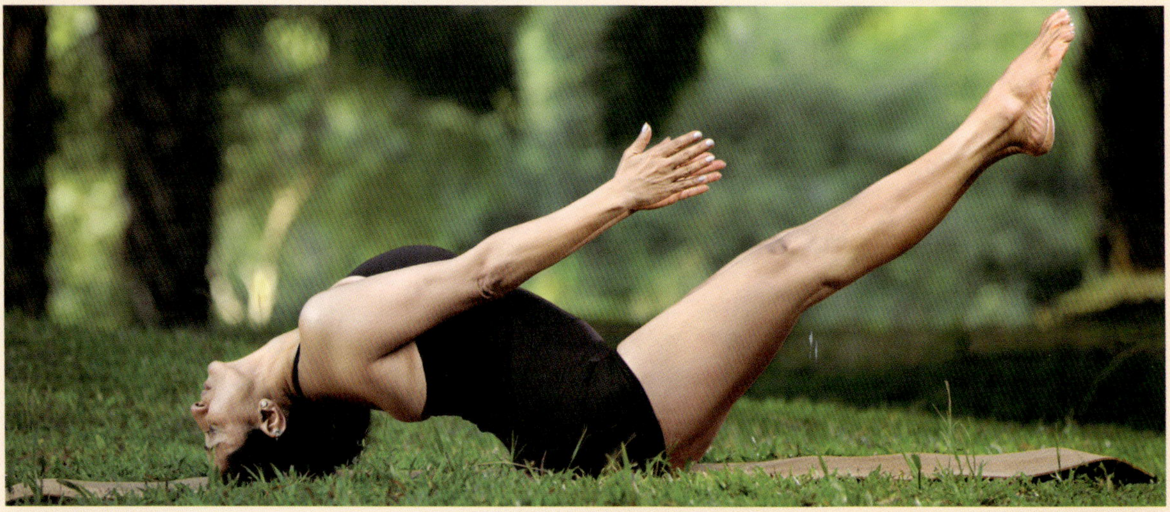

MATSYASANA

Pranayama

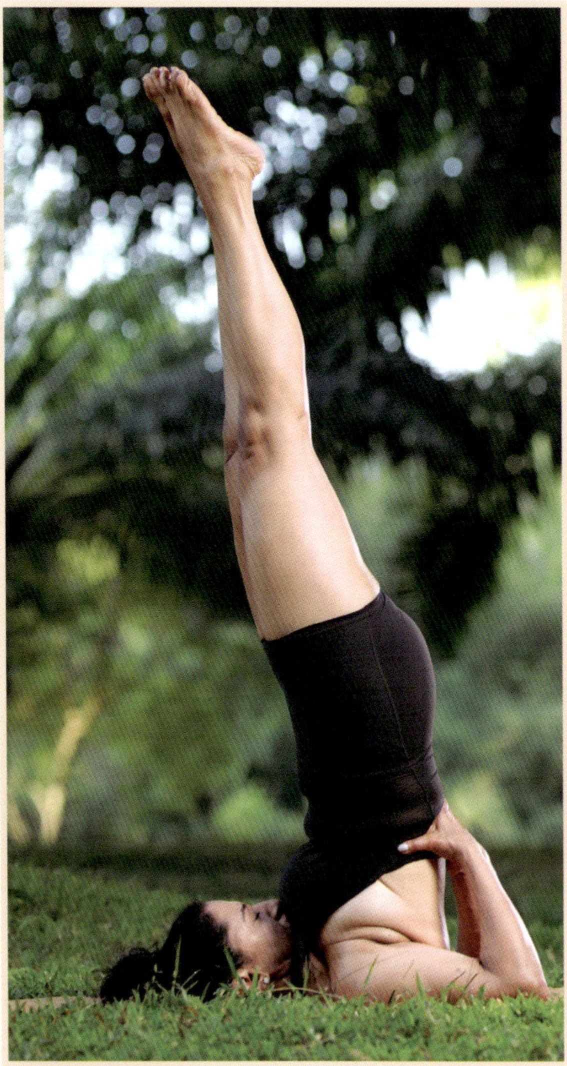

SARVANGASANA

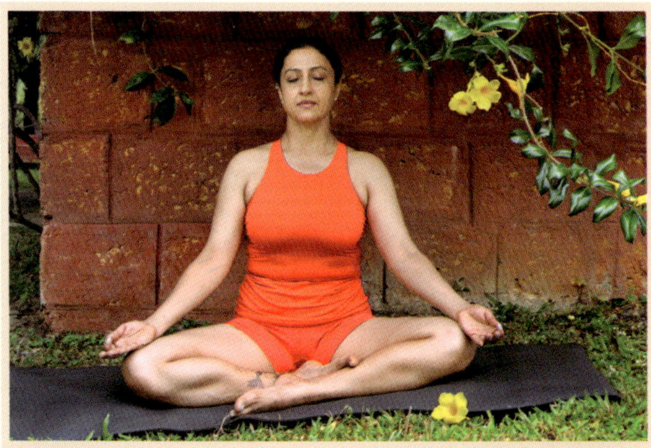

UJJAYI

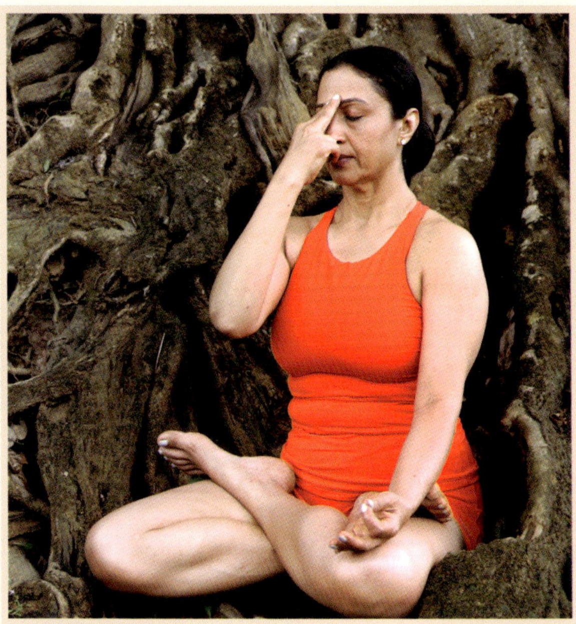

ANULOM VILOM

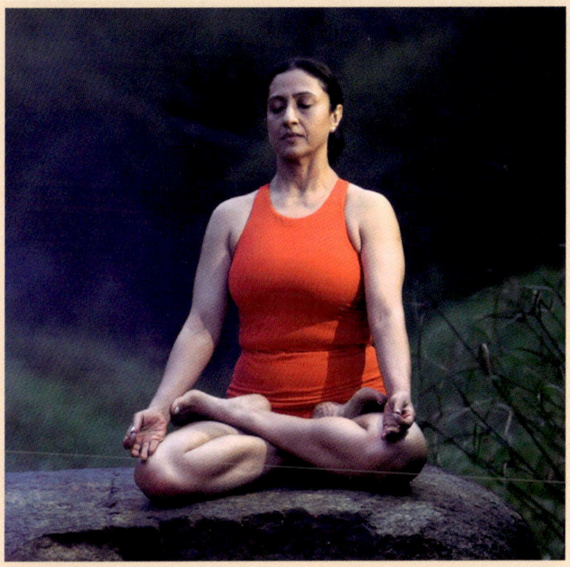

BHASTRIK

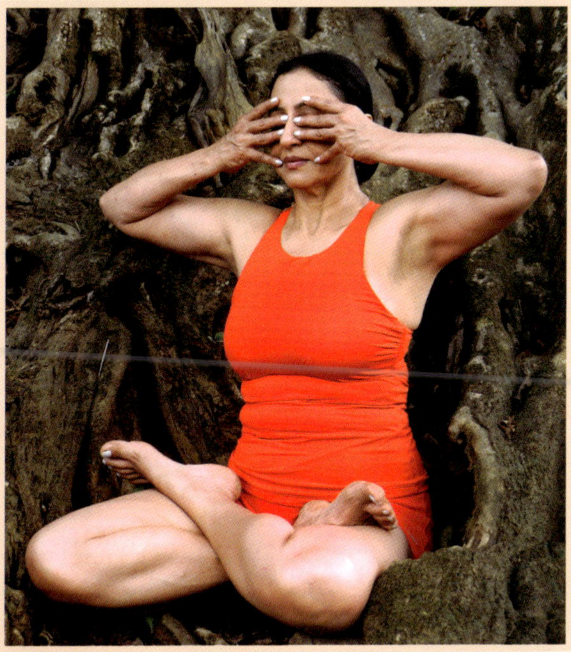

BHRAMARI

CHAKRAS AND NADIS

Many ancient texts suggest that the rishis, in their deepest states of meditation, perceived the presence of spinning wheels of energy and meticulously documented the various stages of this profound experience. These documented scriptures provide great guidance to a practitioner to understand and record the stages of their progress of the awakening energy centres. The knowledge of the chakras in the scriptures provides visualizing techniques to focus on the different levels of energy, all of which exists within the body from the lower to the higher realms. It can be said that only a serious practitioner of yoga will be able to experience the energy emanating from the chakras.

There are seven recognized chakras, located along the spinal cord. These energy centres are activated by the flow of prana in the energy channels called nadis. The main three nadis are along the length of the spine called *ida*, *pingala* and *sushumna*. These nadis cross along the spine where the central nadi, or the sushumna, is located, and at every intersection of the nadis a chakra is formed. The movement of the chakras is influenced not only by the flow of prana during breathing but also by the prana derived from food, the environment, and thoughts, all of which direct energy from the nadis into the chakras. However, chakras are powerful energy points that have direct or indirect influences on the koshas.

AUTHOR'S NOTE

The scriptures also warn about the high potential of these energy channels. They are to be chanelled for attaining spiritual wisdom only by using proper knowledge. If these practices are not done with careful monitoring, it can create imbalance and psychological problems.

According to some ancient manuals, there are about 72,000 nadis (some even refer to about 350,000). Of the three main nadis, sushumna has three more layers: the first being *vajra nadi*, the second, *chitrini nadi*, and the third, *bhrahma nadi*. Brahma nadi is the subtlest and contains the main chakras of life. The sushumna nadi, representing the central channel of consciousness, is activated when both nostrils flow freely and unobstructed.

Our right nostril (called pingala) is governed by the sun, providing heat to the body, and the left nostril (called ida) is governed by the moon. The central nadi, sushumna, becomes active when the ida and pingala are balanced. There are yogic techniques that can bring in the balance and clear the sushumna nadi channel to facilitate the flow of kundalini energy.

NADI

Nadi Vijnan (the science of nadis) explores how these energy channels function. By applying the techniques outlined in Nadi Vijnan, one can facilitate the free flow of prana throughout the body.

Nadi is said to originate at the base of the spine and connect to the *nabhi*. To ensure overall well-being, nadis must be kept clear of obstructions. Blocked nadis can lead to imbalance, discomfort or illness. Since nadis are highly sensitive, they can become blocked due to various factors, such as unhealthy habits, stress, trauma and toxin accumulation.

The scriptures prescribe various methods to cleanse the nadis and unblock energy pathways, ensuring a smooth flow of prana. These include:

1. Asana: Enhances circulation
2. Pranayama: Clears the three major energy pathways
3. Shatkriya: Includes six purification exercises
   - *Jal Neti*: Nasal cleansing using salted water
   - *Trataka*: Gazing steadily without blinking until the eyes tear up
   - *Nauli*: Abdominal churning to strengthen and cleanse the digestive organs
   - *Kapalbhati*: Forceful exhalation using abdominal contraction
   - *Dauti*: Swallowing a long, thin strip of wet muslin cloth and then pulling it back out to cleanse the stomach and esophagus
   - *Basti:* Yogic enema
4. Mudras: Energy seals that balance the elements of the body
5. Mantras: Reciting sacred phrases
6. Kumbhaka: Breath retention techniques that enhance pranic control
7. Bandhas: Energy locks that regulate and redirect prana within the body

Though these cleansing techniques have limited healing powers, their ability to promote good health can never be underestimated.

IDA AND PINGALA NADI

Before delving into the central nadi, let us first understand about ida and pingala.

Ida is the subtle energy channel that flows along the left side of the body, connected to the left nostril. It corresponds to the right hemisphere of the brain and is associated with emotional well-being, intuition and calmness. Often described as the embodiment of lunar energy, ida represents the feminine aspect within the energetic body. When breathing predominantly through the left nostril, ida becomes activated, promoting relaxation and introspection. This energy channel begins at the Muladhara Chakra and ascends along the left side of the spine, eventually terminating at the right hemisphere of the brain.

Pingala is the energy channel that flows along the right side of the body, connected to the right nostril. It is linked to the left hemisphere of the brain and governs solar energy, vitality, and masculine qualities such as action, logic and focus.

Breathing primarily through the right nostril activates pingala, stimulating alertness and energizing the system. Like ida, pingala also begins at the Muladhara, but it ascends along the right side of the spine, terminating at the left hemisphere of the brain.

SUSHUMNA NADI AND KUNDALINI

The stored energy of kundalini resides in the sushumna nadi. There are techniques of pranayama that are specifically aimed at awakening the dormant energy residing in the sushumna nadi. Kumbhaka, which means retention of breath, is one of the main techniques. This is practised by blocking the left and the right nostril channels, thus allowing the prana to flow through this middle channel, or the sushumna nadi. With dedicated practice of kumbhaka, a practictioner will be able to wake the kundalini from the base of the Muladhara Chakra. This tremendous energy can be then guided upwards along the sushumna nadi, piercing in through the six chakras, making way to the seventh and the final chakra, the *Sahasrara*.

Muladhara Chakra (Root Chakra)

- **Location:** The base of the spine
- **Origin:** Muladhara originates at the sthula sharira
- **Pancha Bhoota:** Prithvi, the realm of innate matter, such as plants, animals and humans
- **Strength:** Muladhara Chakra can be experienced as a feeling of stability, security, endurance and stamina
- **Tanmatra:** Gandha
- **Vayu:** Apana
- **Jnanendriya:** Nose
- **Karmendriya:** Feet
- **Colour:** Red
- **Cosmic Realm:** None

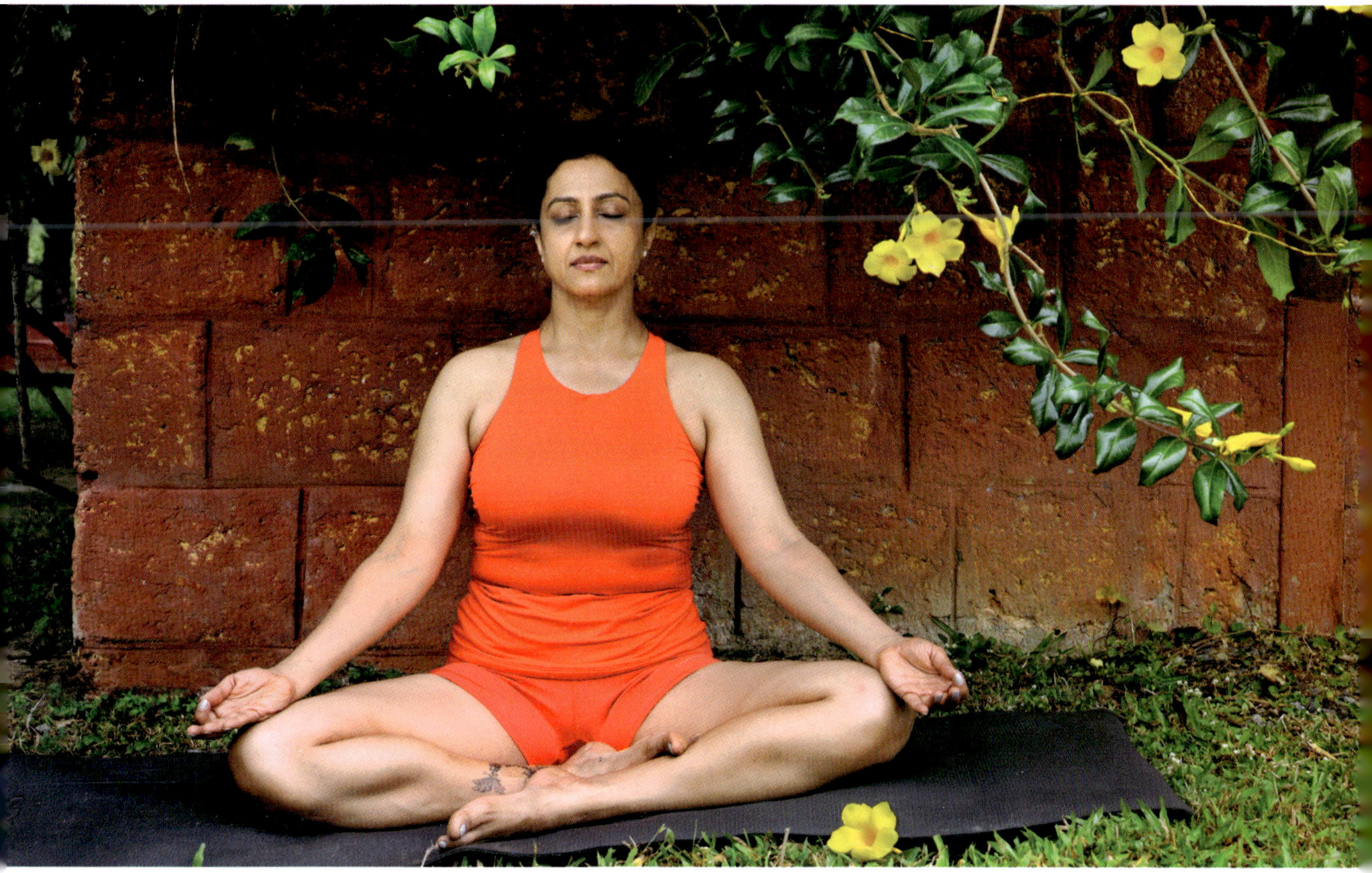

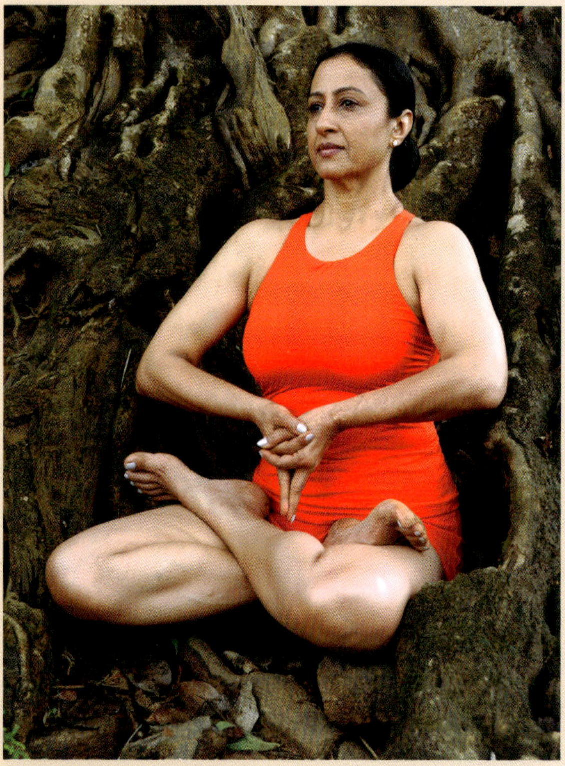

MULADHARA CHAKRA

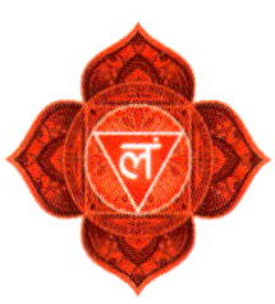

Muladhara is the 'root' or the support chakra. It is the first of all chakras to take form within the subtle body at the base of the spine, and thus it is the base of our existence and survival.

Kundalini and Muladhara Chakra

In deep state of meditation, the kundalini energy appears in the form of a red dot. When awakened, it is seen as a reddish aura, with the energy travelling upwards through sushumna nadi.

In order for the kundalini to rise, one has to overcome the knots which bind the ida, pingala and sushumna. To be able to achieve this, all attention must be focused on inner awakening of the consciousness by shutting down all external experiences and stimulation.

A guru's guidance plays an important role for mastering these advanced techniques. This forms a basic and brief introduction to the very austere practice of Tantra Yoga.

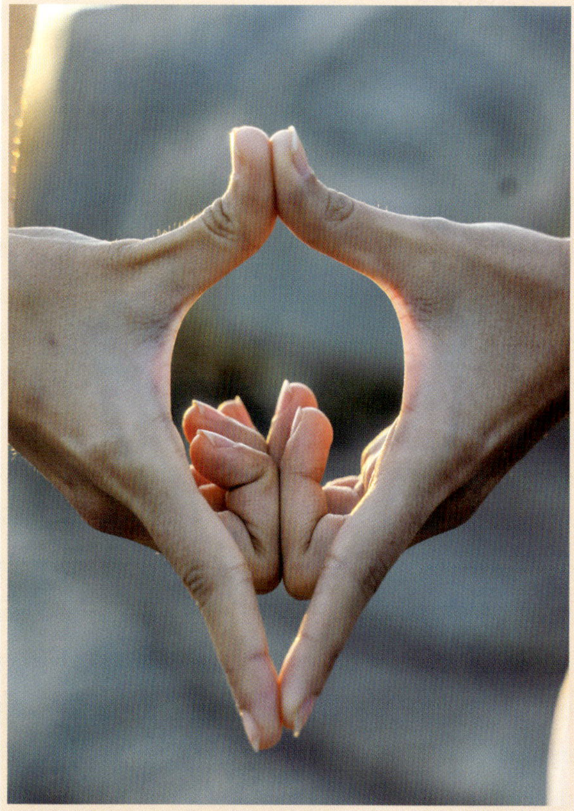

YONI MUDRA (ALSO USED FOR AWAKENING MULADHARA)

TANMATRA

The tanmatras are the subtle elements that form the basis of our physical existence. Each of the pancha bhootas are linked to specific tanmatras, which together govern the functions of the sense organs. These links are as follows:

- Akasha: Linked to shabda and the sense of hearing
- Vayu: Linked to shabda and sparsha, governing hearing and touch
- Agni: Linked to shabda, sparsha and *rupa*, governing hearing, touch and vision
- Jal: Linked to shabda, sparsha, rupa and rasa, governing hearing, touch, vision and taste.
- Prithvi: Linked to shabda, sparsha, rupa, rasa and gandha, governing all five senses

Svadhisthana Chakra (Sacral Chakra)

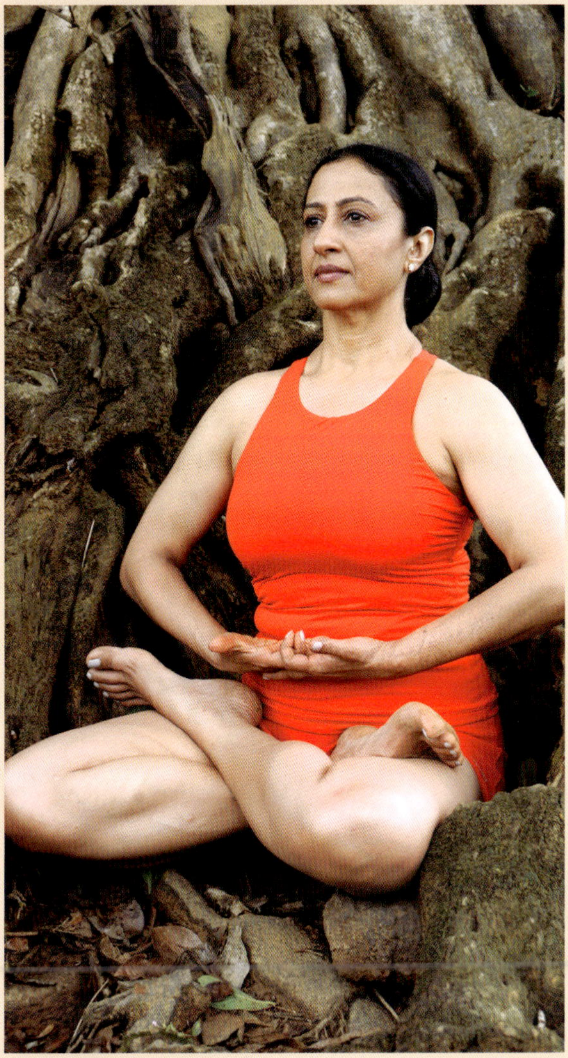

SVADHISTHANA CHAKRA

- **Location:** Two inches below the navel; around the area of sacral nerve plexus
- **Origin:** Svadhisthana Chakra originates in the sthula sharira
- **Pancha Bhoota:** Jal
- **Strength:** Svadhisthana Chakra manifests as longevity, good digestion and balanced sexuality
- **Tanmatra:** Rasa
- **Vayu:** *Vyana*, responsible for circulations of blood and nutrients
- **Jnanendriya:** Tongue
- **Karmendriya:** Genitals
- **Colour:** Orange
- **Cosmic Realm:** *Bhuvarloka*, the space between Earth and Sun

Svadhisthana Chakra is the centre of self-expression. The Sanskrit word *sva* means 'one's own', reflecting the chakra's connection to individuality and personal desires. Svadhisthana Chakra functions in the lower abdomen and is closely linked to the sacral nerve plexus, testis, ovaries and the urogenital system. Governing the element of water, it influences the bladder, symbolizing the chakra's role in the cleansing and purification of the body, mind and spirit. The colour of this chakra is described as orange.

Kundalini and Svadhisthana Chakra

The Svadhisthana Chakra is often seen as a vessel that holds and filters our desires, guiding us in choosing the kind of life we wish to cultivate. It is within this energy centre that decisions related to passion, pleasure and personal growth take shape. Discipline and goal setting feeds the rhythms of this chakra. Our patterns of sleep, food and sex, all contribute to the integrity of this chakra.

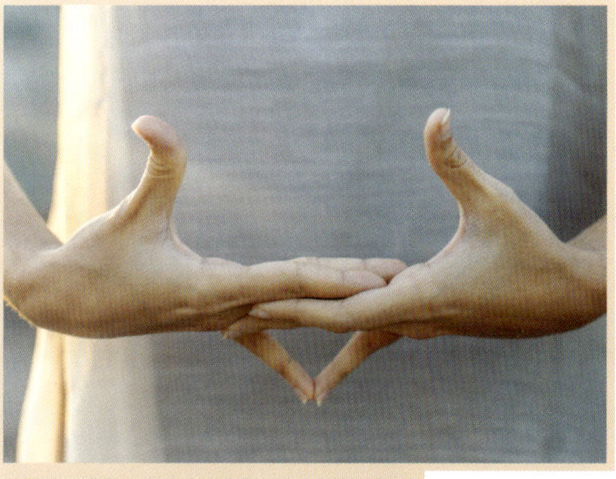

SVADHISTHANA MUDRA (VARIATION)

Manipura Chakra (Navel Chakra)

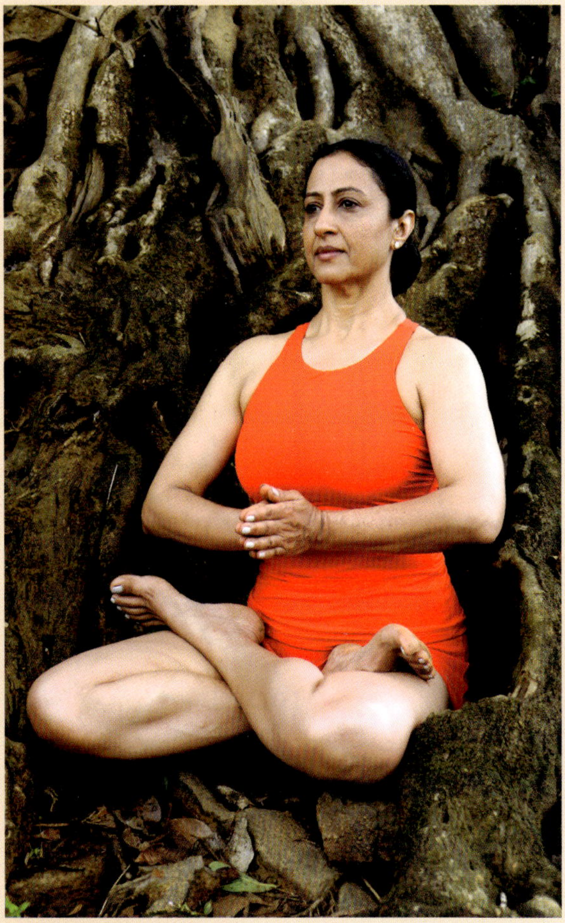

MANIPURA CHAKRA

- **Location:** At the level of solar plexus
- **Origin:** This chakra originates in sthula sharira
- **Panch Bhoota:** Agni
- **Strength:** This chakra manifests as emotional stability, good appetite and a general feeling of well-being
- **Tanmatra:** Rupa
- **Vayu:** *Samana*, responsible for digestion
- **Jnanendriya:** Eye
- **Karmendriya:** Bowel
- **Colour:** Green
- **Cosmic Realm:** *Svargaloka* (heaven or the space between Sun and the Pole Star)

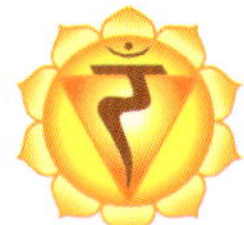

Manipura Chakra has the power to hold or contain all the five elements. *Manipura* literally means the 'place of precious gems'. This chakra holds the database or an inbuilt map of the universe of creation that is you. It forms the network of our existence, where the physical aspects of the body manifest and reflect the transformative and consuming qualities of fire. Its functions cover the nervous system, immune system and digestive system, as well as the nerve plexus and the pancreas. It handles the regulatory functions of the body that helps maintain stability and balance in life.

In the sthula sharira, the energy presents itself in the nervous system, establishes links in the sensory messages, takes charge of the immune system and absorbs nutrition that is supporting our entire system. Manipura Chakra organizes and catalogues our experience. The fire element in this chakra 'burns' both food and experience, providing the driving force for digestion and cognition.

Kundalini and Manipura Chakra

The awakening of kundalini at this chakra grants mastery over the element of fire, empowering transformation, willpower and inner strength. The physical aspects of the body in which this chakra manifests reflect the consuming qualities of fire.

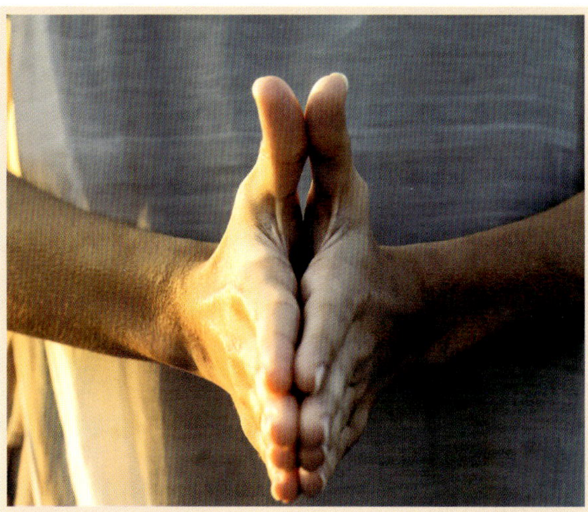

MANIPURA MUDRA

Anahata Chakra (Heart Chakra)

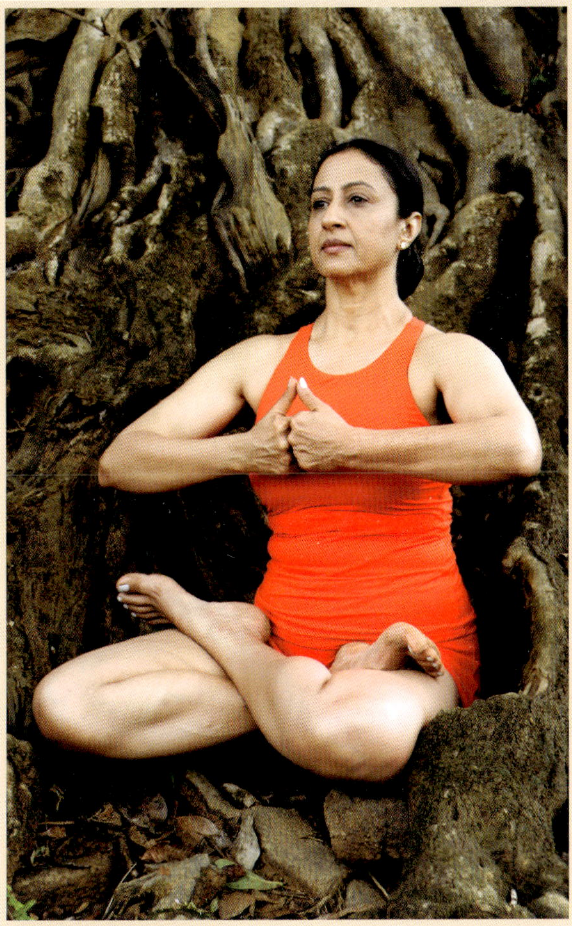

ANAHATA CHAKRA

- **Location:** At the level of cardiac plexus
- **Origin:** This chakra originates in the sthula sharira
- **Pancha Bhoota:** Vayu, the external air
- **Strength:** This chakra manifests as kindness, love and compassion
- **Tanmatra:** Sparsha
- **Vayu:** Prana, responsible for respiration
- **Jnanendriya:** Skin
- **Karmendriaya:** Hands
- **Colour:** Green
- **Cosmic Realm**: *Maharloka*, or the abode of the great sages

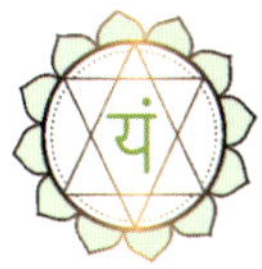

Anahata Chakra literally means 'the sound that comes without striking of two things'. It is often referred to as the sound of life. This chakra originates from the sukshma sharira.

Anahata Chakra manifests in the sthula sharira through the rhythms of the heart and lungs, the activity of the cardiac plexus, and the vibrations from the glands. It represents our expression of the heart, where the senses expand into spiritual love. Through deep identification with all forms of life, this chakra connects us to the greater family of the universe. It holds the power to expand consciousness, opening the mind to appreciation, compassion and love for all life.

Kundalini and Anahata Chakra

Granthis (explored in detail in another chapter) are energetic knots or bundles of energy that embody the challenges of incarnation. These three locks are located at the Muladhara, Anahata and Ajna chakras. They represent the unopened doors within the body, restricting access to higher planes of consciousness—places within the subtle body where the grip of *maya* (illusion) is strong.

Anahata Chakra holds bundles of granthis. Kundalini arrives at Anahata Chakra as it swathes through each of these locks, liberating their power and dissolving the illusions that each one holds.

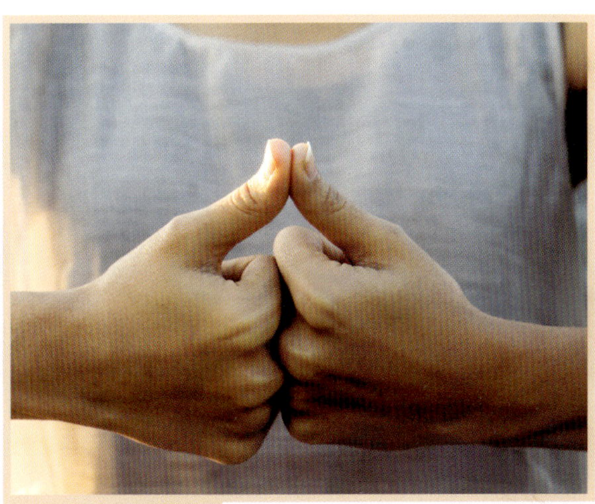

ANAHATA MUDRA

Vishuddha Chakra (Throat Chakra)

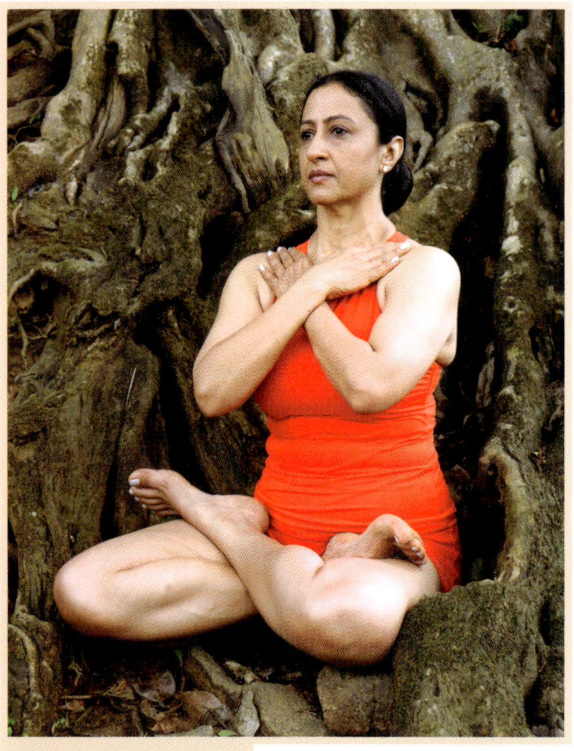

VISHUDDHA CHAKRA 1

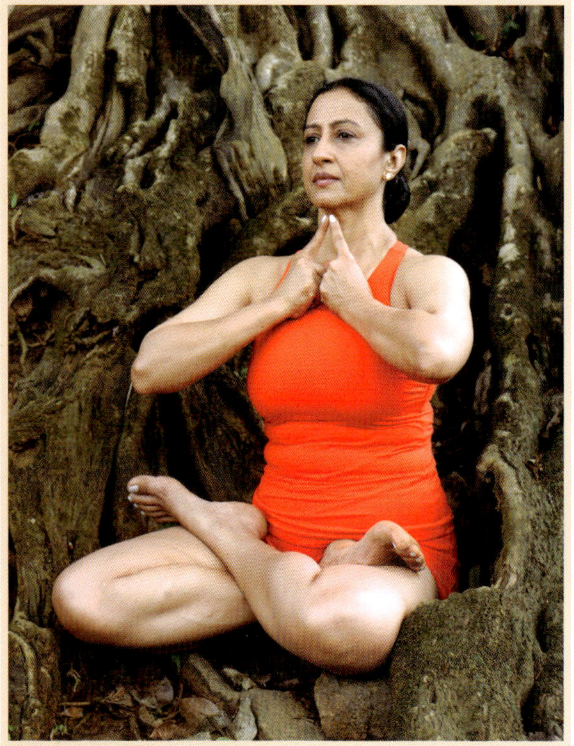

VISHUDDHA CHAKRA 2

- **Location:** At pharyngeal plexus
- **Origin:** The root of the Vishuddha Chakra originates from the sthula sharira
- **Pancha Bhoota:** Akasha
- **Strength:** This chakra manifests as good speech, communication and purity
- **Tanmatra:** Shabda
- **Vayu:** Udana
- **Jnanendriya:** Ears
- **Karmendriya:** Mouth
- **Colour:** Sky blue
- **Cosmic Realm:** *Janaloka*, or the world where humans live

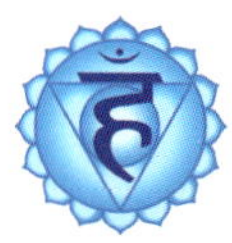

Vishuddha means 'pure'. Vishuddha Chakra represents our ability to express the true sounds of our hearts through speech. This chakra holds all the elements that shape our lives. Acting as a key pathway in the subtle body, it channels the seed syllables of all preceding chakras, guiding the yogi towards pure consciousness. Its energy clears space by aligning the nadi currents in the throat and neck, ensuring a smooth transition to the higher chakras.

Kundalini and Vishuddha Chakra

One of the important texts of yoga, *Hatha Yoga Pradipika*, speaks of the four stages of awakening. This begins with the dissolution of the first bundle of energy which is in the Muladhara Chakra. The next stage is dissolution of the second bundle of energy in the Anahata Chakra as the kundalini passes through and towards the Vishuddha Chakra.

Ajna Chakra (Third Eye Chakra)

- **Location:** At the point where the eyebrows meet
- **Origin:** The root of Ajna Chakra is in the pituitary gland
- **Pancha Bhoota:** Akasha

- **Strength:** This chakra manifests as good perception
- **Colour:** Indigo
- **Cosmic Realm:** *Tapaloka*, or the mansion of the blessed

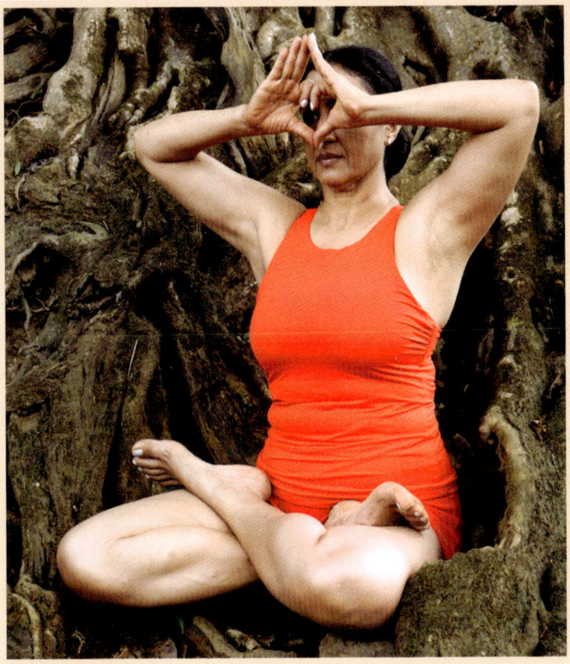

AJNA CHAKRA

Ajna Chakra is beyond the five elements, hence the rest of the factors mentioned for the earlier chakras are not applicable for this.

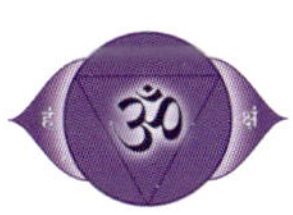

Ajna Chakra transcends the elemental realms governed by the five lower chakras, delving deeper into the perception of consciousness. It houses the final energetic block that the ascending kundalini must overcome on its path to higher awareness.

Known as the 'third eye', the Ajna Chakra opens the gateway to deeper reality, where perception extends beyond the physical. It governs the sensory faculties and cognitive processes, enabling intuition, insight and clarity of thought.

Closely linked to the mind, the Ajna Chakra empowers the ability to form abstractions, conceptualize higher truths, and comprehend that which lies beyond everyday experience.

Kundalini and Ajna Chakra

When Ajna Chakra is activated by the rise of kundalini, the practitioner will be able to see beyond the gross physical realm. The sixth chakra governs the two sheaths: manomaya kosha (mind) and vijnanamaya kosha (intelligence).

Ajna Chakra allows us to find the path to the true self and see beyond the illusions of duality present in our normal lives. It is this path that opens us to the possibility of becoming dispeller of darkness. The seed syllable AUM, resonates with the cosmic sound, connecting us to the combination of A (sun), U (moon) and M (fire).

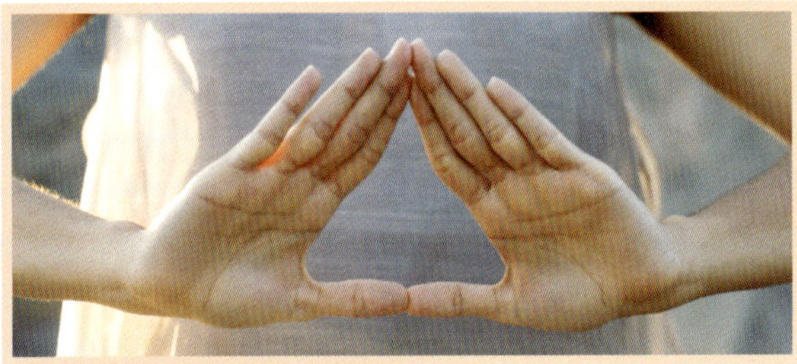

AJNA MUDRA (VARIATION)

Sahasrara Chakra (Crown Chakra)

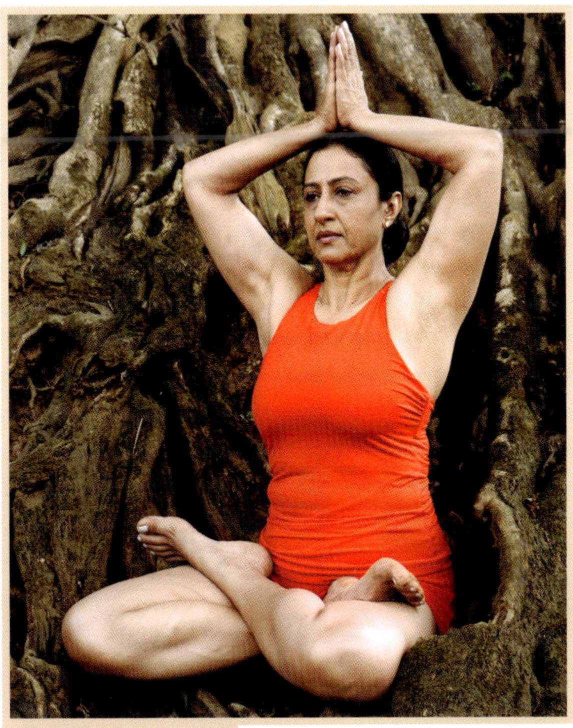

SAHASRARA CHAKRA

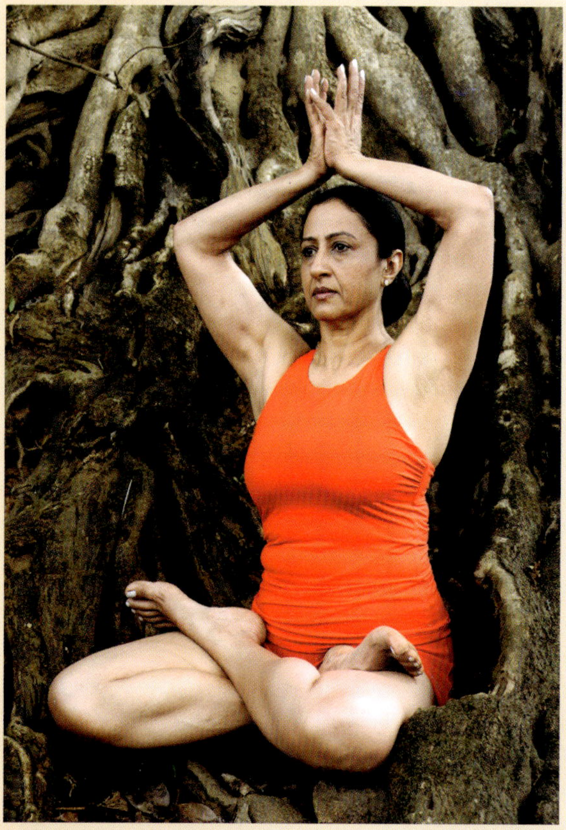

SAHASRARA CHAKRA 1

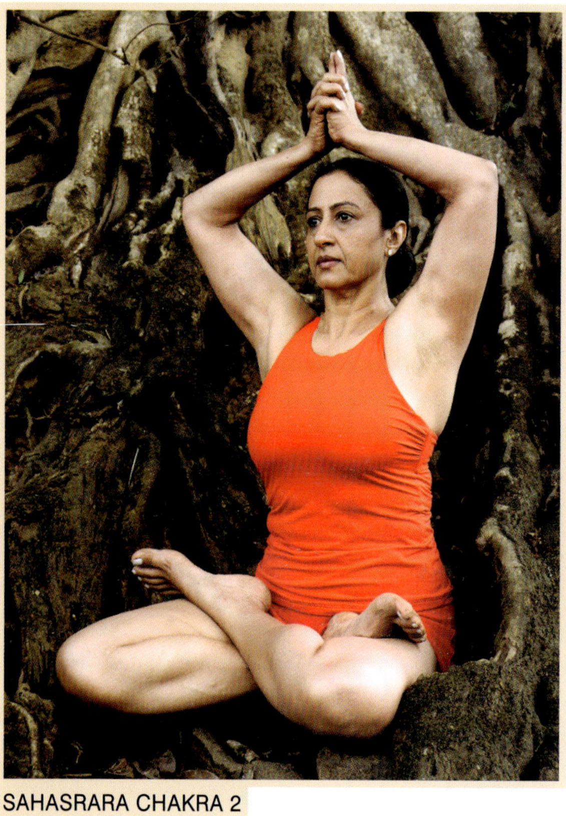

SAHASRARA CHAKRA 2

- **Location:** At the crown of the head
- **Origin:** Pineal Gland
- **Pancha Bhoota:** Akasha
- **Strength:** This chakra manifests as highest state of spirituality.
- **Cosmic Realm:** Satyaloka, or the realm of ultimate truth and pure consciousness.

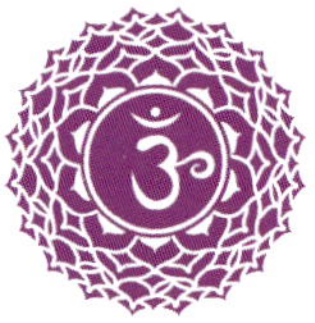

The seventh chakra, known as the thousand-petalled lotus, is the gateway to cosmic freedom. It is located above the crown of the head. For the first time since kundalini has risen and activated each chakra, the lotus of the seventh chakra turns downward. Here, the yogi transcends the cycle of evolution.

The Sahasrara Chakra is not included in the classical listing of the body's six chakras, as it exists beyond the physical form and takes no part in either the gross or subtle body. It corresponds to the fifth and highest sheath of human existence—the anandamaya kosha, which represents the

MAHABINDHU

Within the Sahasrara Chakra is the full moon resplendent as in the clear sky. Inside it, constantly shinning like lightning, is the triangle and further inside shines the great void, well concealed and attainable only by the great effort—the subtle *bindu*, the chief root of liberation. It pulses like a cosmic heartbeat, echoing the stillness that underlies all movement, the silence between every breath. *Mahabindu* is the centre of the Sahasrara Chakra.

Bindu is a timeless yogic symbol of unity, present throughout each chakra. The essence of yoga is often described as a journey—from the seed (potential) to the point (bindu), and ultimately to Mahabindu, the absolute void, where all duality dissolves into pure consciousness.

deepest layer of consciousness. This sheath carries the imprints of past experiences and attachments across lifetimes, dissolving as the yogi attains self-realization.

The root of the Sahasrara Chakra is the pineal gland. The *loka* associated with Sahasrara Chakra is *Satyaloka*. Bathed in radiant stillness, it is also linked to the *Brahma Randhra*, the sacred point where Shiva (masculine energy) and Shakti (feminine energy) unite. This subtle portal is revered by yogis, mystics and sages alike.

This divine meeting signifies the dissolution of duality, leading to transcendence and self-realization. Here, silence becomes sound, and the seeker becomes the seen.

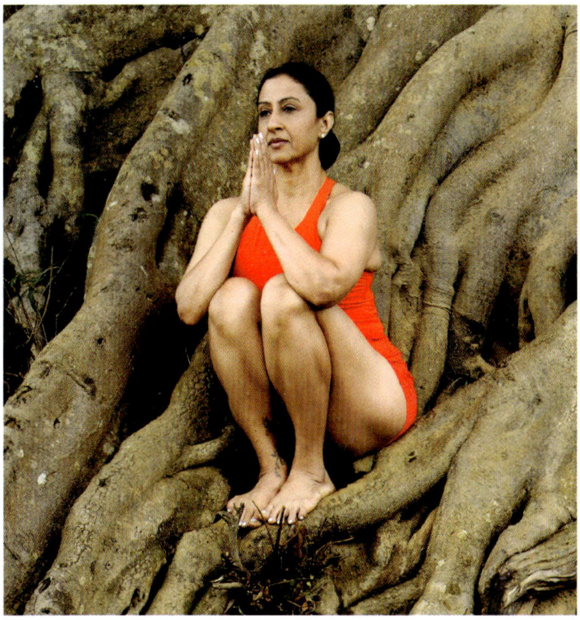

CHAKRA INFORMATION AT A GLANCE

	MULADHARA	SVADHISTHANA	MANIPURA	ANAHATA	VISHUDDHA	AJNA	SAHASRARA
Origin	Sthula Sharira	Sthula Sharira	Sthula Sharira	Sthula Sharira	Sthula Sharira	Sthula Sharira	Pineal Gland
Location	Connected to spinal nerves and the glands	Around the area of sacral nerve plexus, ovaries/ testis and kidneys	Below the midriff	Cardiac nerve plexus, respiratory and cardiac systems and thymus gland	Pharyngeal nerve plexus, vocal cords, trachea and oesophagus, thyroid and parathyroid glands	Forehead	At the crown of the head
Cosmic Realm	-	Bhuvarloka	Svargaloka	Maharloka	Janaloka	Tapaloka	Satyaloka
Pancha Bhoota	Prithvi	Jal	Agni	Vayu	Akasha	Akasha	Akasha
Tanmatra	Gandha	Rasa	Rupa	Sparsha	Shabda	-	-
Vayu	Apana	Vyana	Samana	Prana	Udana	-	-
Jnanendriya	Nose	Tongue	Eye	Skin	Ears	-	-
Karmendriya	Feet	Genitals	Bowel	Hand	Mouth	-	-
Colour	Red	Orange	Yellow	Green	Sky blue	Indigo	-

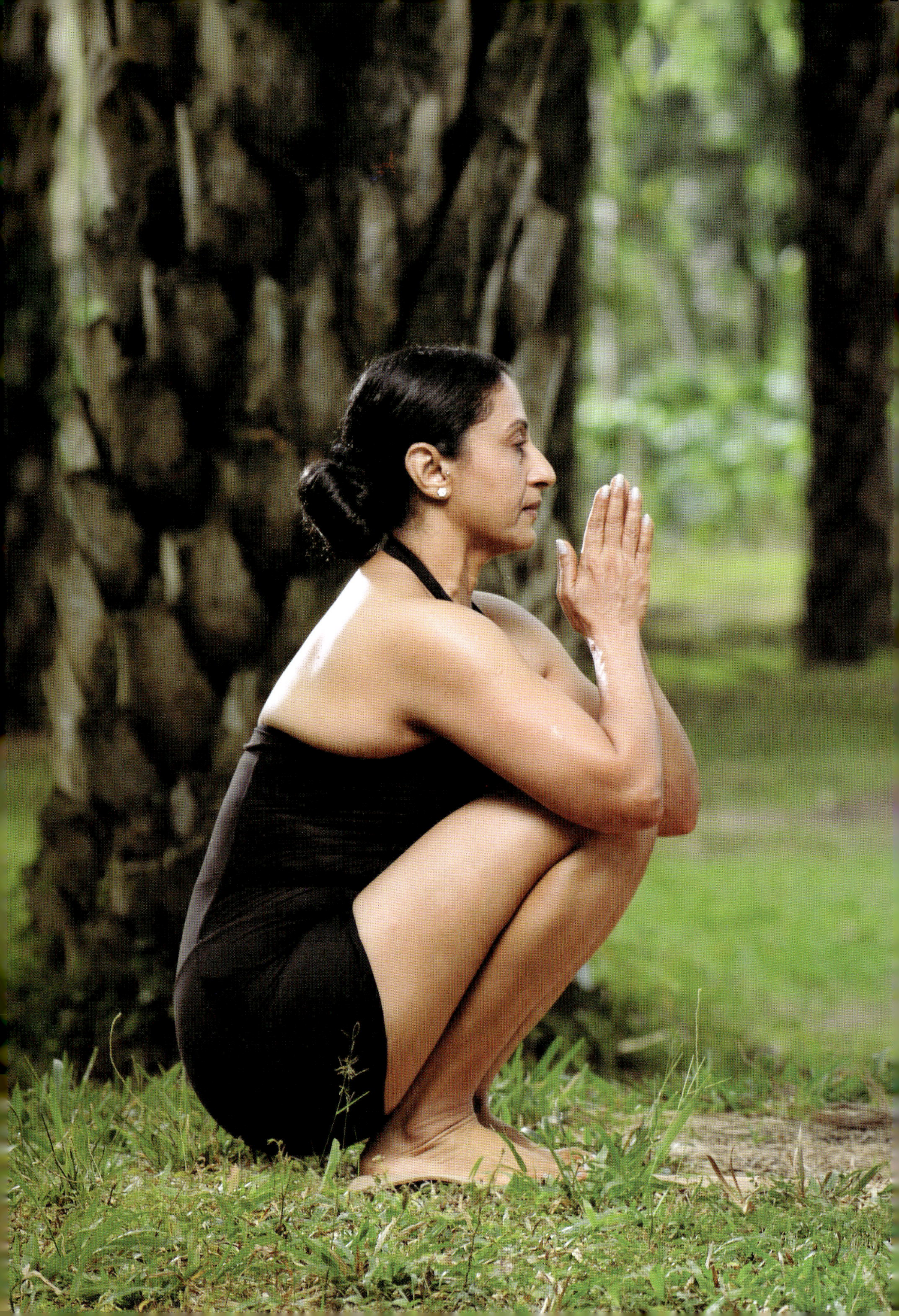

CHAPTER 4
PRAKRITI AND PURUSHA

Prakriti is the fundamental root of all beings and the manifested universe. Prakriti is the primordial feminine energy, the dynamic force of nature that drives creation, sustenance and transformation. It is not merely an abstract concept but a living, ever-evolving principle that animates all existence. It is the nature of the body that is determined by birth. Prakriti is the source of the five elements, which combine in different ratios to form a unique personality. This uniqueness is called guna.

Purusha is the Universal Consciousness that pervades the universe. This is the conscious energy that governs life and reality. Purusha exists beyond the realms of time and space and is present everywhere in everything. It is all-pervasive, eternal and cannot be destroyed. It is also considered as the masculine energy that encompasses the cosmos. It remains unchanged and unaffected by the transformations of the physical world, acting as the silent witness to all action and movement. While prakriti (nature) is dynamic and creative, purusha stands as the stable, conscious observer, the source of awareness that enables perception and existence. Together, purusha and prakriti explain the dual principles of existence. Purusha and prakriti are the essence of creation. In purusha's presence, prakriti manifests the physical universe. Neither exists in isolation.

AUTHOR'S NOTE

The concepts explained in this chapter are complex and based on a vast study of the ancient texts.

Understanding these concepts is vital for studying philosophy and essence of yoga. A guru's guidance can play an important role in this task.

PRAKRITI AND VIKRUTI

The prakriti of a person is predetermined from birth. Factors such as time of conception, environment, surroundings, mental state, food and habits of the mother influence the formation of the prakriti of a person.

Vikruti can be translated as 'after the creation'. In Ayurevda, prakriti is the unique predetermined ratio of *vata*, *pitta* and *kapha*. When this ratio changes due to lifestyle, diet or environment, the body goes through an imbalance, causing discomfort or disease. This state is vikruti, which is basically an imbalanced prakriti.

AUTHOR'S NOTE

Vikruti is not a static state; it changes from day to day, season to season and even in different stages of life. The first step in Ayurvedic treatment is to assess vikruti, which means identifying imbalances in the body. This is done by observing how you breathe, digest food, eliminate waste, sleep, and also by analysing your daily habits and work life. All these factors help understand what is out of balance and guide the right treatment.

PRAKRITI AND CHAKRAS

Chakras are energy centres in the body that affect our physical, mental and spiritual well-being. Each chakra is linked to prakriti, or our natural state. Kundalini Yoga helps balance prakriti, bringing us in tune with our true self. This true nature is made up of five great elements (jal, agni, vayu, prithvi and akasha), which form the foundation of our body and energy. When energy flows properly to the chakras, it provides them with the necessary information to function well.

All six chakras are associated with the five elements:

- The Root Chakra is connected with the earth element.
- The Sacral Chakra is connected with the water element.
- The Navel Chakra is connected with the fire element.
- The Heart Chakra is connected with the air element.
- The Throat Chakra is connected with the space element
- The Third Eye Chakra strengthens when all elements are in balance.

The five elements can be balanced by practising certain mudras.

PRAKRITI AND MUDRAS

Mudras are an ancient practice that uses hand gestures to balance the body's doshas, nadis and chakras. By harmonizing the body's elemental forces, mudras promote stability of the mind and body, enhancing focus, concentration and overall well-being. This balance is essential for meditation, healing and the regulation of energy. Mudras are arrangement of fingers to form a pressure point.

In Classical Indian dance forms, as described in the *Natyashastra*, mudras are used gracefully for storytelling. The expressive movements of the fingers create auspicious patterns in the air, weaving an aura of beauty and tranquility that captivates the audience, delighting both the mind and the senses.

In Ayurveda and other traditional medicine systems, such as Chinese medicine, fingers hold significant importance as they are linked to the five elements of the body. Each finger corresponds to specific organs and plays a crucial role in maintaining health and well-being by influencing energy flow and balance.

Hands and fingers are rich in sensory receptors and have a direct, intricate connection with the brain through the nervous system. This means the way we hold our fingers and hands can influence our emotional states. Yogis and ancient meditators used mudras for various purposes, from enhancing meditation and mental focus to supporting healing and well-being. Ancient rishis developed this practice based on the belief that the human body is composed of five fundamental elements—earth, water, fire, air and space. Each element is associated with specific mudras, which are used to restore balance and harmony within the body.

SIGNIFICANCE OF PRACTISING MUDRAS

Physical Level

In yoga, *hasta mudras* are often practised alongside pranayama and are typically performed while seated in postures such as Padmasana, Sukhasana, or Vajrasana. Mudras help stimulate different parts of the body involved in breathing, influence energy flow, and even impact one's mood. Specific hands guide energy pathways and reflexes to the brain. By curling, crossing, stretching and touching the fingers and hands, we can enhance the mind–body connection, as each area of the hand corresponds to different aspects of the body and mind.

Spiritual Level

On a spiritual level, practising specific mudras is an outward representation of one's inward intentions. There are many different mudras and it is said that mediating on a specific mudra can help manifest hopes and realize energies. When your hands come into a mudra, it allows a physical connection with an intangible energy.

These subtle hand gestures are more than symbolic; they are ancient codes, unlocking flows of energy within the body. With regular practice, mudras can calm the mind, awaken awareness, and deepen one's meditative state. In that quiet stillness, a sacred dialogue begins—between the self and the universe.

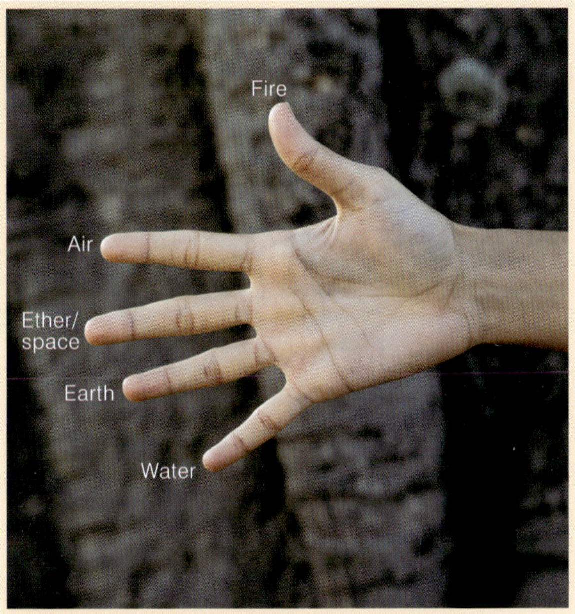

FIVE FINGERS PRESENTING FIVE ELEMENTS

AGNI MUDRA (CONNECTED TO MANIPURA CHAKRA)

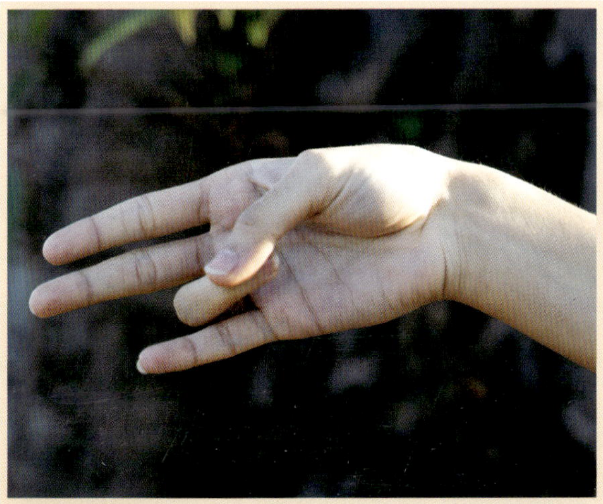

AGNI MUDRA

Agni Mudra is formed when the tip of the ring finger touches the base of the thumb, while the thumb gently presses down on the ring finger. The remaining fingers are kept straight and relaxed.

Benefits

- Helps in weight loss and balancing hormones
- Controls anxiety
- Aids digestion
- Eases vertigo
- Improves clarity of voice
- Gives relief from ear pain

The thumb is associated with the fire element, agni, and the Manipura Chakra located in the solar plexus. Practising this mudra generates a sense of warmth, as fire represents energy, strength, vitality and transformation.

On a psychological level, an excess of the fire element can manifest as restlessness, anger, fear, or anxiety. Physiologically, fire is essential for a strong immune system and a healthy metabolism. When balanced, it helps burn impurities in both the body and mind.

To practise this mudra, find a comfortable place, preferably outdoors, and hold the hand gesture. Breathe in and out evenly, counting to eight for both inhalation and exhalation, for about 5–10 minutes. As you breathe, visualize the warmth of the sun, allowing yourself to relax and absorb its energy.

VAYU MUDRA (CONNECTED TO ANAHATA CHAKRA)

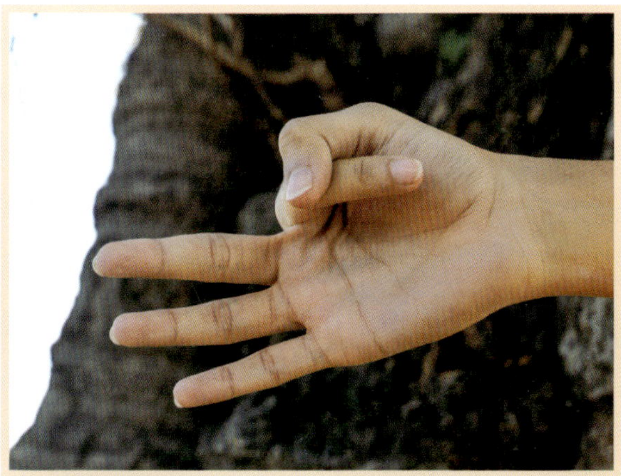

VAYU MUDRA

It is formed by joining the tip of the index finger to the base of the thumb and letting the thumb rest lightly on index finger, with a gentle pressure. Keep all other fingers straight and relaxed.

Hold this mudra for 12 deep breaths in Ujjayi Pranayama. Sit in a quiet place and practise alone. Practising this mudra regularly builds up energy resource in the body.

The air element, associated with the index finger and linked to the Anahata Chakra, represents prana, movement, rhythm and connection.

When in excess, it can lead to psychological imbalances, such as instability, anxiety, weakness, disassociation and disorientation. Physiologically, it may manifest as bloating, indigestion and body aches.

Benefits

- Eases vayu-based diseases, like sciatica, cervical spondylitis, abdominal discomfort and knee pain
- Eliminates air accumulated in body that might be causing discomfort
- Helps control restlessness and indecisiveness
- Improves eyesight
- Boosts the immune system and increases body's resistance against diseases

AKASHA MUDRA (CONNECTED TO THE VISHUDDHA CHAKRA)

The middle finger is linked to the space element and the Vishuddha (Throat) Chakra. Space represents openness, clarity, stillness and self-expression, creating space for other elements to exist.

In excess, it can lead to feelings of emptiness, insecurity and disconnection.

To practise this mudra, warm up the body with an easy stretching and sit in a quiet place and practise lengthy and restful breathing for 5–10 minutes.

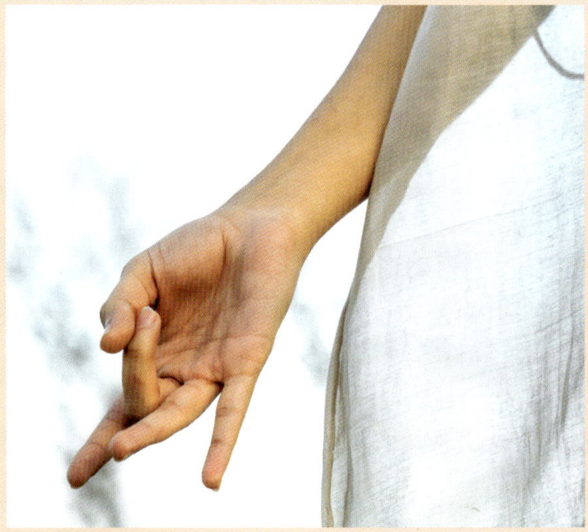

AKASHA MUDRA

Benefits

- Increases calcium content, makes bones stronger
- Boosts intuitive power and analysis
- Cures locked jaw due to yawning
- Good for all heart-related problems
- Controls high blood pressure
- Reduces anger and fear
- Improves alertness and sensory powers

BHOOMI MUDRA (CONNECTED TO THE MULADHARA CHAKRA)

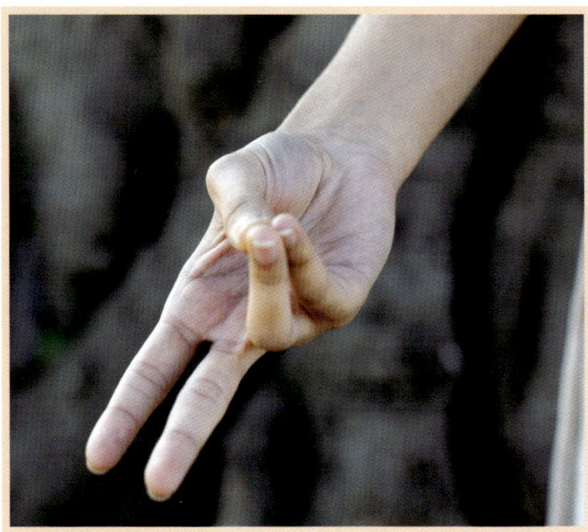

BHOOMI MUDRA

This mudra is held with index and the middle finger opened straight and the rest of the fingers held together.. This mudra is held downwards, ideally touching the floor while staying in a seated position.

The mudra can be practised in standing positions too, and also in other asanas, such as Vajrasana, Veerasana, Padmasana and Sukhasana. Breathe from the nose. Choose a quiet place with traces of strong wind blowing.

The ring finger is associated with the Muladhara Chakra and prithvi, the earth element which represents our connection to the physical body, inner stability and the earth itself.

The earth element is linked to grounding, security, stability and a strong foundation. It helps us feel centred, well rooted, and in tune with our basic needs such as food and shelter.

An excess of the earth element can lead to feelings of heaviness, sluggishness, dullness, or a lack of energy and motivation.

Benefits

- Removes weakness
- Boosts stamina and energy
- Reduces digestion-related issues
- Clears toxins from the body
- Promotes inner happiness, kindness and thoughtfulness
- Regular practice enhances stability, security and inner strength

JAL MUDRA (CONNECTED TO THE SVADHISTHANA CHAKRA)

Also called Buddhi Mudra, it is formed when the tips of the little finger and the thumb are joined, with the thumb applying gentle pressure, and the rest of the fingers are kept straight.

The water element is associated with the little finger and the Svadhisthana Chakra. It embodies flow, softness, fluidity, flexibility, movement and curiosity.

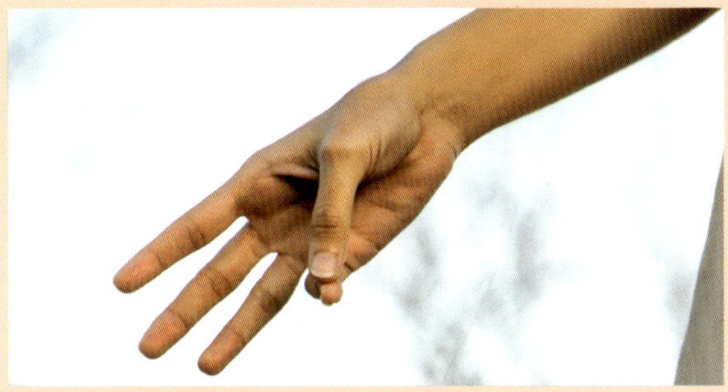

JAL MUDRA

Benefits

- Improves blood circulation
- Helps restore water balance in the body, especially during diarrhoea, dehydration and gastroenteritis
- Purifies blood and skin disorders
- Hydrates dry skin and eyes

HOW TO PRACTISE THE MUDRAS

- Start each mudra session by washing hands and letting them dry thoroughly.
- Clap your hands five times, feeling the impact of the clap against your palms.
- Rub your hands together firmly for 30 seconds while maintaining a relaxed breath.
- Hold the hands in front of the navel chakra, around one inch away from the navel. This will allow the energy to flow into the hands.
- Then place the palm in front of the heart, with both hands slightly cupped and held as if you are holding a football.
- Steady your breath to calm down your mind.
- Select the mudra required.
- Do not exert too much pressure on the hands to feel the energy.
- To reap best benefit of the mudra, hold the specific hand gesture for atleast 15 minutes. These 15 minutes can be stretched along the course of the day—spending five minutes in the morning, five in the afternoon and five in the evening.

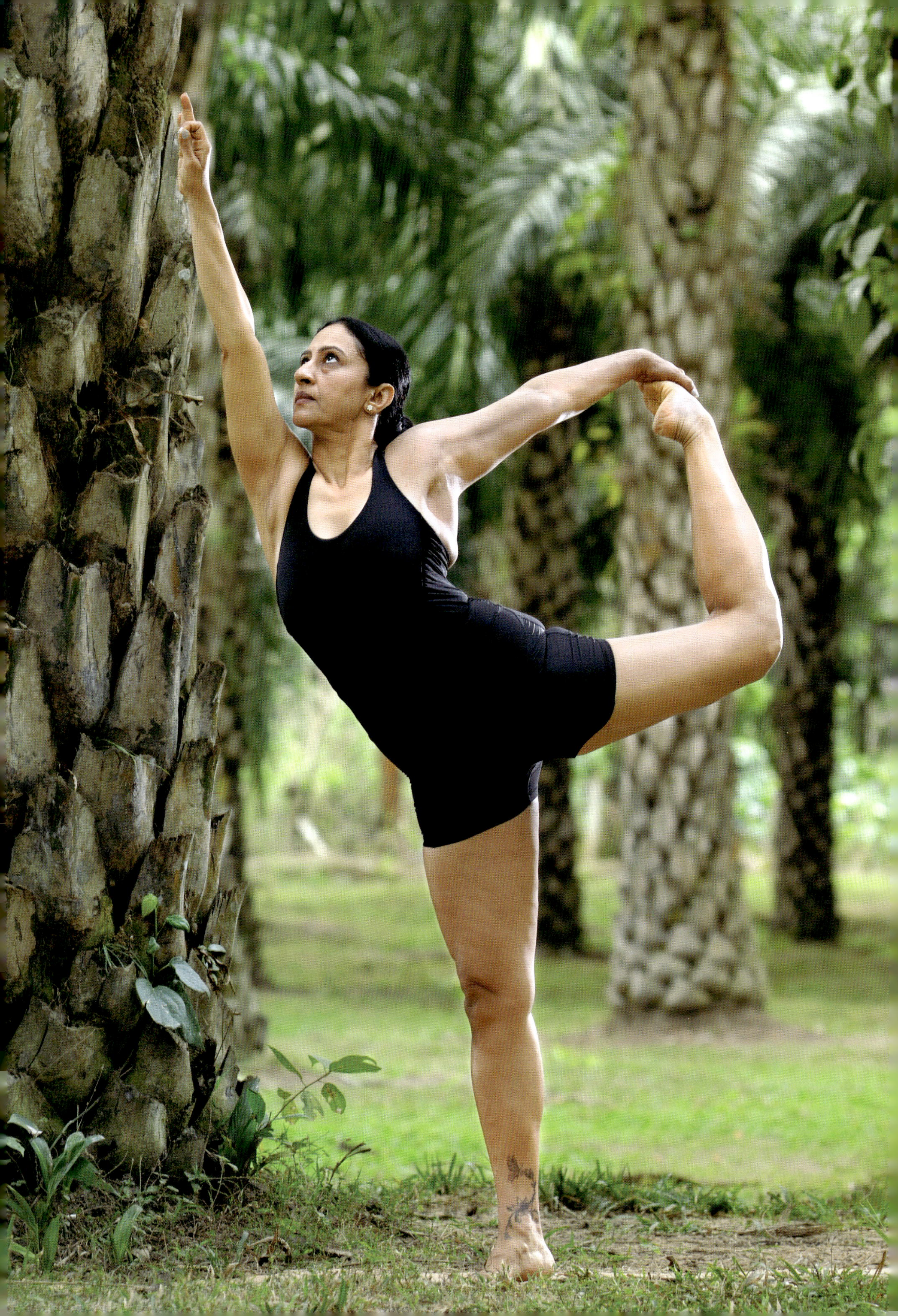

CHAPTER 5

PRAKRITI AND DOSHA

Prakriti is an individual's inherent body constitution, determined at birth, remaining constant throughout life. Vikruti is the current state of balance or imbalance in the body, influenced by factors such as diet, lifestyle, environment and emotions.

Both prakriti and vikruti are governed by doshas—vata, pitta and kapha—each representing different combinations of the five fundamental elements: space, air, fire, water and earth. Doshas define an individual's physiological and psychological tendencies and, like fingerprints, are unique to each person.

Recognizing one's dosha and its current state is the foundation of self-awareness in Ayurveda. Understanding this balance or imbalance helps guide lifestyle choices, diet and wellness practices to support health and healing.

The three doshas are also referred to as Tridosha:

- **Space + Air = Vata**

This dosha controls movement in the body, like wind turning a windmill. It regulates breathing, blood flow and nerve signals. Even thoughts and communication are guided by vata's energy, keeping the body and mind active and balanced.

- **Fire + Water = Pitta**

This dosha can be understood as a flammable liquid fuel. It regulates metabolism, digestion, and transformation of food into nutrients, ensuring proper assimilation and vitality.

- **Water + Earth = Kapha**

This dosha is like clay or mud, providing stability and structure to the body. It supports growth, nourishes tissues, and maintains strength and resilience.

Dosha combinations are present in each cell, every tissue, every organ, and they also govern all the bodily functions. According to ancient texts, all the major building blocks of the body are formed through the interplay of doshas. The fundamental components are:

- Plasma
- Blood
- Bone Marrow
- Muscle
- Bones
- Fat
- Reproductive Tissue

The dosha arrangement in the body also plays an important role in the way we think, influencing the way we react. For a healthy mind, it is vital that the doshas are balanced. Consuming the right kind of food is important for providing the essential energy to the mind and body. When combined with a balanced lifestyle, this nourishment supports overall well-being. (See Chapter 6, 'Ayurveda—Basics'.)

Doshas are divided into three primary types: vata, pitta and kapha. While everyone possesses all three doshas, most individuals have one dominant dosha (their prakriti), followed by a secondary dosha, with the third being present in smaller proportions. In some cases, more than one dosha may be equally influential.

Dosha dominance is determined at conception and can be partially identified through personality traits and physical characteristics. However, throughout life, doshas fluctuate due to factors such as environment, lifestyle, diet and emotions. These imbalances can manifest both mentally and physically. Understanding doshas not only helps in recognizing the root causes of these imbalances but also makes their correction more effective.

VATA DOSHA

Vata is wind dominance. It collects around the area of the lower abdominals. When there is an imbalance in this dosha, it will manifest in the form of indigestion, anxiety, insomnia and flatulence. Vata is responsible for the body movement, expression of speech, circulation of blood, elimination of waste, and regulation of the immune system and nervous system. Vata dominant people have a delicate bone structure and therefore don't carry too much weight. They are generally thin and slender. Their skin is usually dry due to poor blood circulation, and their hands and feet are generally cold. They have dynamic personalities and enjoy change; however, they have less will power. They are physically attractive. Their appetite and digestion are variable. These individuals are naturally drawn to sweet, sour and salty foods.

When vata is balanced, breathing is steady and regular, appetite is healthy, and bowel function is smooth. A person feels positive, energetic and enthusiastic, with a calm mind and a steady flow of innovative ideas.

When vata is imbalanced, it can lead to body aches, weight loss, numbness, dry skin, dehydration, bloating, indigestion and insomnia. When there is a deficiency, the body feels sluggish, and the mind becomes prone to fear and anxiety. If left unbalanced, vata can contribute to conditions like osteoporosis and arthritis. Regular massages and warm baths help restore balance of the vata dosha.

There are five subtypes of vata dosha. (The subsections will sound similar to the five vayus. It should be noted that the functions of vayu and vata are different, for vayus come under the pranic energy.)

- **Prana Vata:** It is the central coordinator of all the vata, and it functions in the head, neck and chest region. Thinking, creativity, learning new information and inhalations are all governed by prana vata.
- **Udana Vata:** It governs the throat and chest region, regulating activities like sneezing, coughing and exhalations.
- **Vyana Vata:** It radiates from the heart to all over the body through the circulatory system and the skin. The beating of the heart, sweating and the sense of touch are all examples of vyana vata.
- **Samana Vata:** It works in the stomach area, governing the flow of food through the digestive tract.
- **Apana Vata:** It works in the colon and pelvic area, and governs functions such as menstruation and the expulsion of urine, semen and stool.

TIPS TO BALANCE VATA DOSHA

- Maintaining a good diet is important to keep the vata dosha in balance.
- People with vata dosha should eat small, regular meals and avoid combining too many different foods.
- Allowing sufficient time to eating and chewing will ensure that pre-existing digestive enzymes in the saliva are released, making food easier to digest.
- Meals should be predominantly warm, with cooked vegetables, as that helps subdue vata.
- People with dominant vata dosha should drink a lot of warm water.
- The meal timings should follow a consistent routine.
- All sweet fruits, such as bananas, coconut, apples, figs, grapefruit, grapes, mangos, melons, oranges, papayas, peaches, pineapples, plums, berries, cherries, apricots and avocado, will be of great helpt for people with dominant vata dosha.

- Warm spices, such as pepper, ginger and cardamom, are particularly favourable.
- Grains that are easy to digest, such as rice, oats, wheat and quinoa are recommended to avoid bloating and irregular digestion.

FOODS TO AVOID

- Avoid astringent, bitter or pungent food items.
- Raw food items are not advised for vata dosha, as it is difficult to digest.
- Sour fruits does not work for this body type.
- Lettuce, potatoes, tomatoes and raw onions are good vegetable options.
- Grains high in vata content, like millet, corn, buckwheat, split chickpeas, kidney beans, etc., should be avoided.
- Fatty foods, honey and white sugar are not suitable for vata body types.
- Stimulating drinks, like cola, coffee, black tea and any carbonated beverages, must be completely avoided. This is because they stimulate the human nervous system too much.
- Avoid cold foods, like salads, iced drinks and raw vegetables.

PITTA DOSHA

Pitta is dominated by the fire element. Pitta resides in the central region of the body. This is the heat energy of the body and manifests itself in metabolism and digestion. While fire is the dominant element, a small contribution from the water element helps maintain balance. This dosha has the power to regulate both vata and kapha dosha, playing a crucial role in digestion, metabolism and hormonal balance. Pitta also plays an important part in regulating heartbeat, body temperature, visual perception and thirst, and in maintaining dermal health. It is also responsible for liver and gut health.

Individuals with a pitta-dominant constitution are quick learners, possess a sharp intellect, and are naturally ambitious. They are born leaders, brimming with energy and strength and are more likely to be perfectionists. They generally have an aesthetic build and a medium height and weight, along with a delicate skin. People with dominant pitta dosha are charming and charismatic, with a love for attention to detail. They are able speakers and good decision makers. They love sweet- and bitter-flavoured foods, and often indulge in cold drinks.

When pitta is balanced, it promotes a healthy appetite, well-regulated hormone production, intelligence, courageous personality and a sharp eyesight.

When pitta is imbalanced, individuals are prone to become angry easily and are emotionally sensitive. They may crave the wrong foods, worsening their condition, leading to heartburn, diarrhoea and an upset stomach. Their metabolism turns hyper-acidic, causing frequent burping, excessive sweating and inflammation. Common symptoms include headaches, skin rashes, fever and high blood pressure. Workaholics are often susceptible to pitta disorders, experiencing an aversion to heat and a persistent bitter taste in the mouth.

The five subtypes of pitta dosha are as follows:

- **Alochika Pitta**: Located in the eye region, it governs both function and dysfunction of the eyes.
- **Bhrajaka Pitta:** Located in the skin, it regulates biochemical processes, influencing complexion and skin radiance.
- **Sadhaka Pitta:** Residing in the heart and brain, it governs emotional balance, contentment, intelligence and memory.
- **Pachaka Pitta:** Located in the abdomen, primarily in the small intestine, it regulates digestion by converting food into nutrients and waste.
- **Ranjaka Pitta:** Residing in the liver and spleen, it governs blood composition, supports liver functions, and facilitates nutrient distribution through the bloodstream.

TIPS TO BALANCE PITTA DOSHA

- Pitta can be adjusted with appropriate nutrition and the right kind of exercises.
- Regular meditation, adequate relaxation, with more than six hours of sleep will benefit and balance the dosha.
- It is important to consume food in moderation, avoiding overeating, as excess food can overstimulate their already strong digestion, leading to acidity and inflammation. Skipping meals is especially harmful for such individuals, as their metabolism is naturally high.
- Pitta is generally dominant during summer season, so individuals with dominant pitta dosha should focus on keeping their body cool during warmer months. Consuming cold and refreshing foods helps. Having tea with ingredients such as peppermint, rose, fennel and chamomile soothe excess heat, reduce acidity and calm the mind. Foods like leafy greens, cucumbers, coconut, and dairy products reduce internal heat and inflammation. Cooling grains like wheat, barley and basmati rice absorb excess heat and soothe acidity.
- Sweet mild spices, such as mint, dill and cinnamon are considered particularly beneficial.

FOODS TO AVOID

- Individuals with dominant pitta dosha typically have a robust digestive system and can tolerate a wide variety of foods. However, their diet should be such that it helps balance the fire element associated with pitta. To achieve this, they should avoid excessively pungent, salty, and sour flavours, as these can overstimulate gastric juices and intensify internal heat.
- They should avoid pickle, sour cream, cheese, alcohol, egg yolks, nuts, hot spices, honey, hot drinks, oily and spicy foods.
- Consumption of sour fruits like apples, grapefruit, lemons and dried fruits should be limited.
- In vegetables, consumption of garlic, radishes, tomatoes and onions should be cut down.
- Usage of almond oil, corn oil and sesame oil should be avoided.

KAPHA DOSHA

Kapha is a combination of earth and water elements. It mainly collects in the chest area. This bio-energy holds the body together by moistening the stable structure of the body. It gives substance and strength to the body. Kapha is involved in the material development of the different types of tissues. Though it primarily resides around the chest, it is also present in the abdomen and lymphatic system.

People who are characterized by kapha energy operate in a manner that is well considered and thorough. They can sometimes appear rather slow and ponderous to other people, but they have exceptional endurance and strength. Once a kapha type has a new objective in their sight, they pursue it with patience and tenacity until they have achieved a successful outcome. Eating is their great passion; consequently, kapha people have a lifelong tendency to be overweight.

Above all else, kapha personalities value inner tranquility and peace and harmony. They are also able to enjoy the little things in life; they are easily pleased and love things that are tried and tested. They find joy in a stable partnership, healthy kids and loyal friendships, for these give them satisfaction, security and personal happiness.

When kapha is balanced, it provides stability to the body by binding cells together and forming muscles, fat and bone. It also has the quality to enhance brain function, organ function and muscular and skeletal structure.

When kapha is imbalanced, the individual becomes increasingly withdrawn from life, shutting themselves off and becoming emotionally and spiritually isolated from their surroundings. It does not take long for boredom to set in. And this is most likely accompanied by food cravings and uncontrollable desire to consume sweet things, fatty foods, cheese, sausage products, etc. The result will be obvious weight gain and excessive fat in the tissues. Such people tend to undergo phases of internal withdrawal, the desire to be alone and lazy, the instinctive need to wait out periods of conflict. But once this natural regeneration phase has mutated into a typical kapha depression, the individual feels as if life is too much for them and they immerse themself completely in their own fantasy world. In this situation, they refuse any kind of emotional exchange with others, eventually becoming numb to events around them.

When kapha is in excess, it can lead to a wet cough, congestion, sluggish digestion, and an excessive desire to sleep. If not resolved, it could lead to heart problems, diabetes, high cholesterol or obesity.

The five subtypes of kapha dosha are as follows:

- **Kledaka Kapha:** It governs the chest and gastric area.
- **Bodhaka Kapha:** Located in the tongue, palate and throat, it maintains moisture and supports oral health.
- **Avalambaka Kapha**: It is found in the chest where respiration and circulation take place.
- **Tarpaka Kapha:** It is present in the area of the head and the spinal cord. It lubricates nerve tissues and enables them to carry impulses from the brain organs.
- **Shleshaka Kapha:** It is found in all joints, providing lubrication to soften friction caused by movement.

TIPS TO BALANCE KAPHA DOSHA

- To restore kapha dosha to a state of balance, a proper diet needs to be followed, along with regular physical and spiritual exercises. A well-planned active lifestyle, enriched by meaningful social connections, can be highly beneficial.
- Sleeping during the day is bad for individuals with dominant kapha dosha.
- Relying too much on a single type of meal can lead to imbalance, so a diverse diet is essential. Since such individuals tend to have a slower metabolism, their diet should focus on foods that enhance digestion and energy flow.
- Incorporate pungent and bitter-tasting foods, such as ginger, turmeric, mustard seeds and leafy greens, to counteract the dosha's moist qualities, promoting better digestion and balance.Those with dominant kapha dosha do not have an appetite in the morning and do not struggle with skipping breakfast. A warm drink of lemon and honey water is perfect to stimulate digestion first thing after waking up, as it helps prepare for subsequent meals. As a rule, such people should not eat more than three meals per day, with the main meal of the day being eaten at lunchtime because that is when the highest quality of digestive enzymes are produced.
- Lightly cooked foods or raw fruits should be given more preference.
- Those with a dominant kapha dosha often lack the natural urge to drink water, but maintaining a regular hydration schedule is essential for balance.

FOODS TO AVOID

- Too sour, salty, sweet or oily food items, or those very high in protein should be avoided, as they can aggravate the dosha with increased thirst and water retention.
- It is better to cut down on consumption of extremely sweet or sour fruits, such as pineapples, bananas, dates and custard apples.
- Extremely sweet or juicy vegetables, such as cucumbers, squash, sweet potatoes and tomatoes, should be eaten in moderation, as these increase water retention.
- Grains, such as rice, wheat and oats, should also be taken in moderation.
- Butter, coconut oil and sugar are best avoided.

ASANAS AND BREATHING FOR DOSHAS

When choosing the right yoga practice, the most crucial factor is understanding your vikruti, your current state of imbalance. In fact, this is the single most important determinant of your entire regimen. By addressing these imbalances and selecting a practice that aligns with your prakriti, your natural constitution, you can restore harmony and enjoy better health.

FOR VATA DOSHA

Anatomically, vata resides in the lower abdomen, pelvis and large intestine region of the body. People with vata constitution are most supported by yoga practices that are calming and grounding in nature, for they are usually agitated and nervous by nature. It is ideal to start the practice with calming balancing asanas.

These asanas will help release fear, worry and anxiety, and also improve physical imbalances such as irregular bowels, lower back problems and joint pains. The lower abdomen and pelvis and large intestine are the main residence of vata in the body. The asanas prescribed for vata dosha focus on compressing the lower abdomen while also strengthening the lower back to help alleviate vata imbalances.

AUTHOR'S NOTE

It should be noted that almost all the asanas under Hatha Yoga are good to maintain a balance of the doshas. It is true that some asanas are more suited to a particular dosha. People with dominant vata dosha should limit their practice of Surya Namaskara and all asanas that put excessive pressure on sensitive joints in the body. The cervicothoracic junction, which is the bony region where the neck meets the shoulders, is one of such parts. People with vata dosha tend to have weaker bones, less fatty padding, loose ligaments and more susceptibility to pain. For these reasons, some asanas like Salamba Sarvangasana and Halasana should be avoided or done with extra padding. People with vata dosha or its imbalance should not be holding asanas for a long time as it could be injurious. They are more susceptible to pain.

Primary Focus of Asanas

- Focus on postures that promote stability and grounding.
- Practise deep, calm breathing at a steady, relaxing pace.
- Hold positions for a longer duration.
- Perform a slow-paced Surya Namaskara, maintaining a 4:8 breathing ratio.
- Synchronizing breath with each movement is essential for a harmonious practice.

DISCLAIMER

Consult a qualified yoga practitioner first if you have vata-related aches and pains, especially arthritis or osteoporosis.

Yoga Practice Sequence for Vata Dosha

Standing Asanas

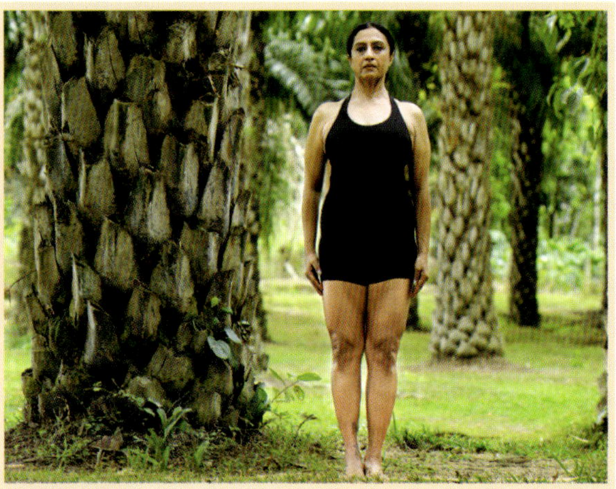

TADASANA

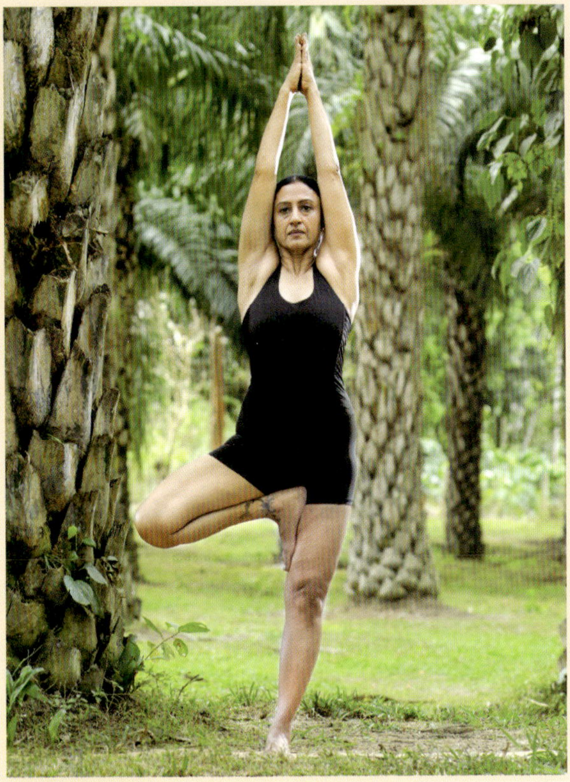

VRIKSHASANA

SURYA NAMASKARA A (5 TIMES AT A MEDIUM PACE)
(FOR REFERENCE, SEE PP. 4–5)

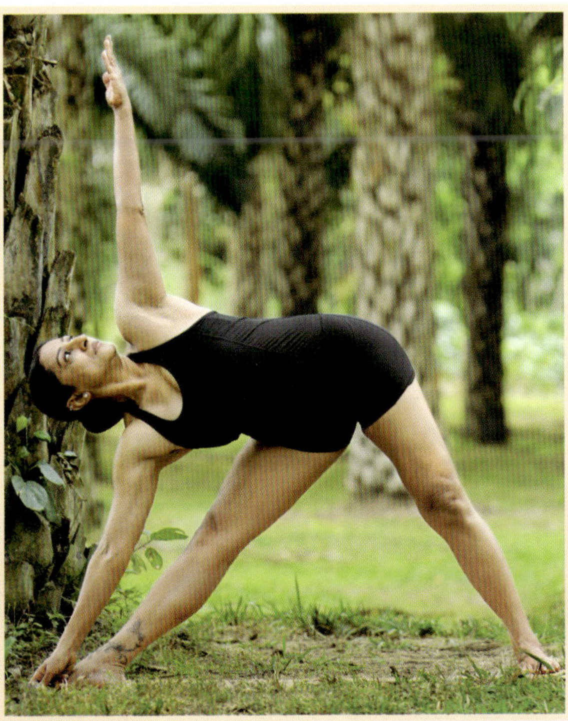

TRIKONASANA

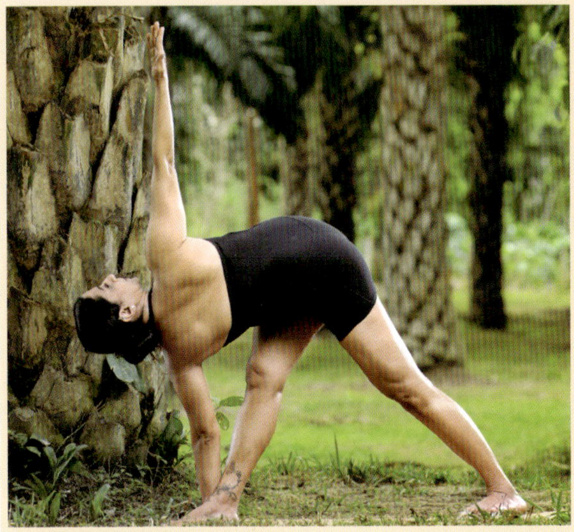

PARIVRITTI TRIKONASANA

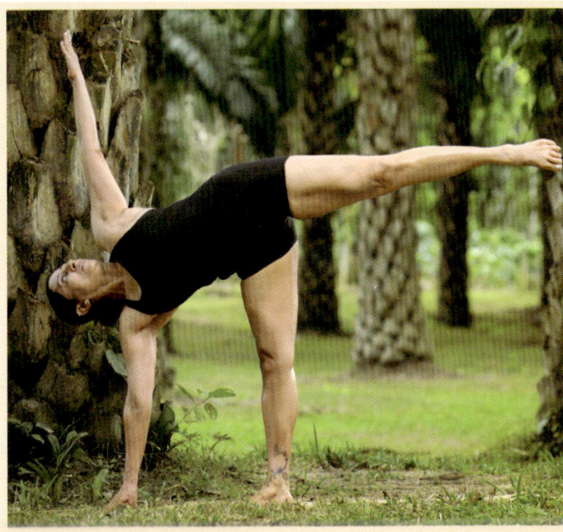

ARDHA CHANDRASANA

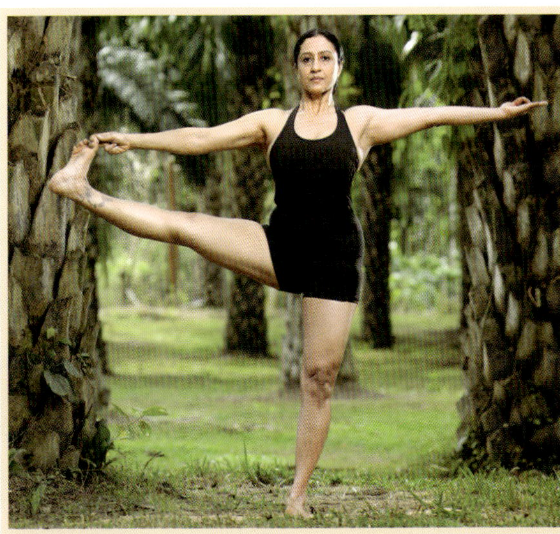

UTTHITAHASTA PADANGUSHTHASANA

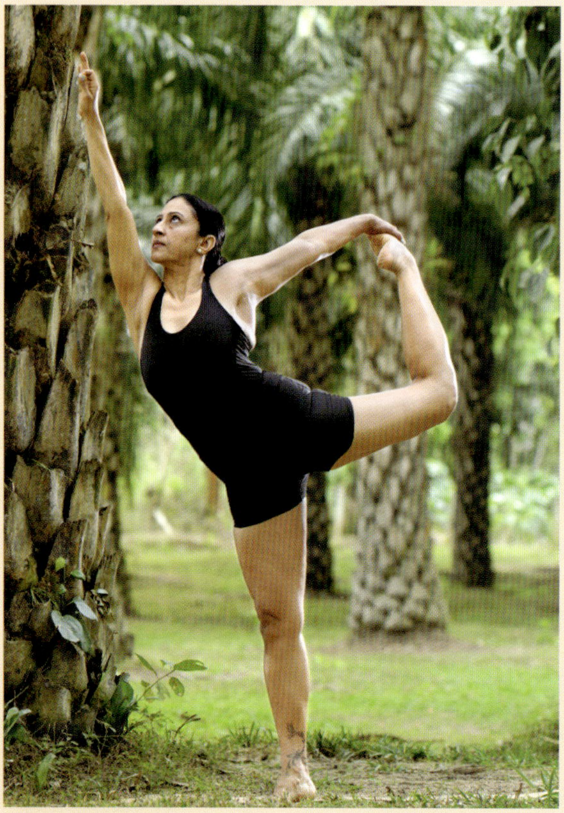
NATARAJASANA

Sitting Asanas

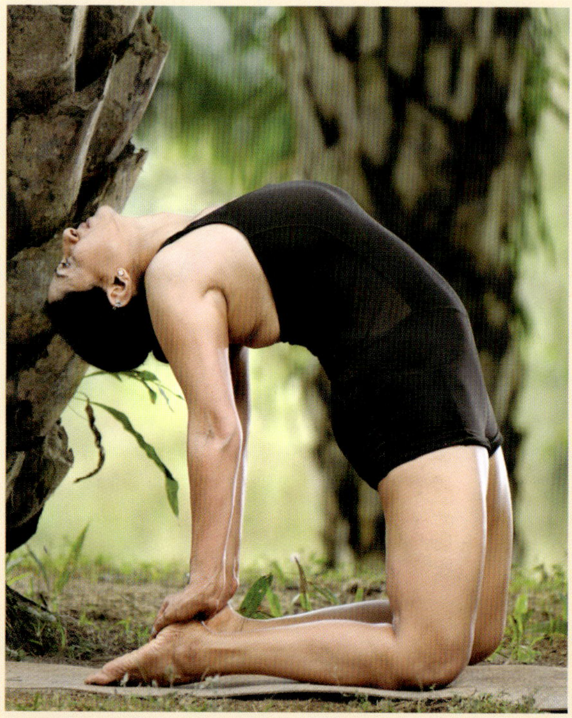
USTRASANA

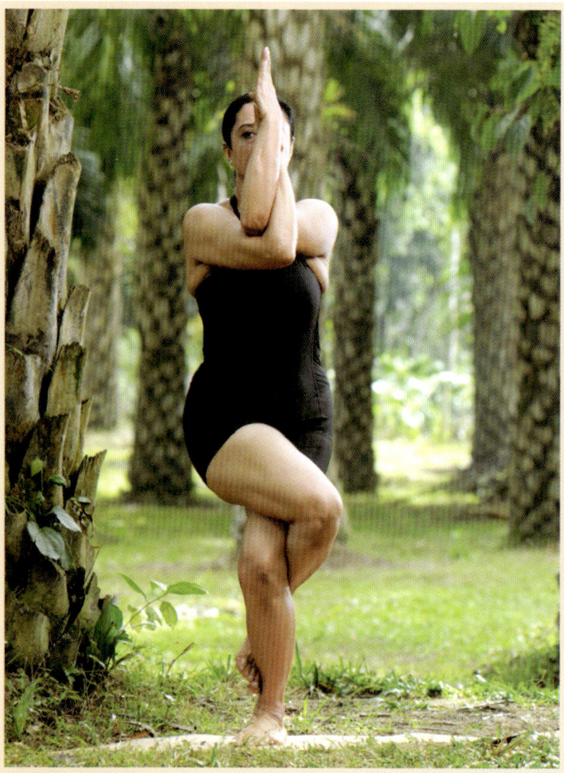
GARUDASANA

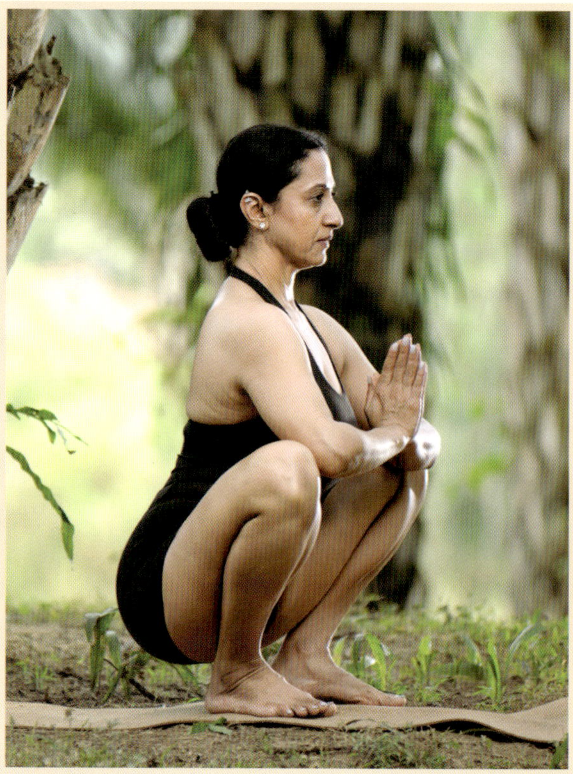
MALASANA

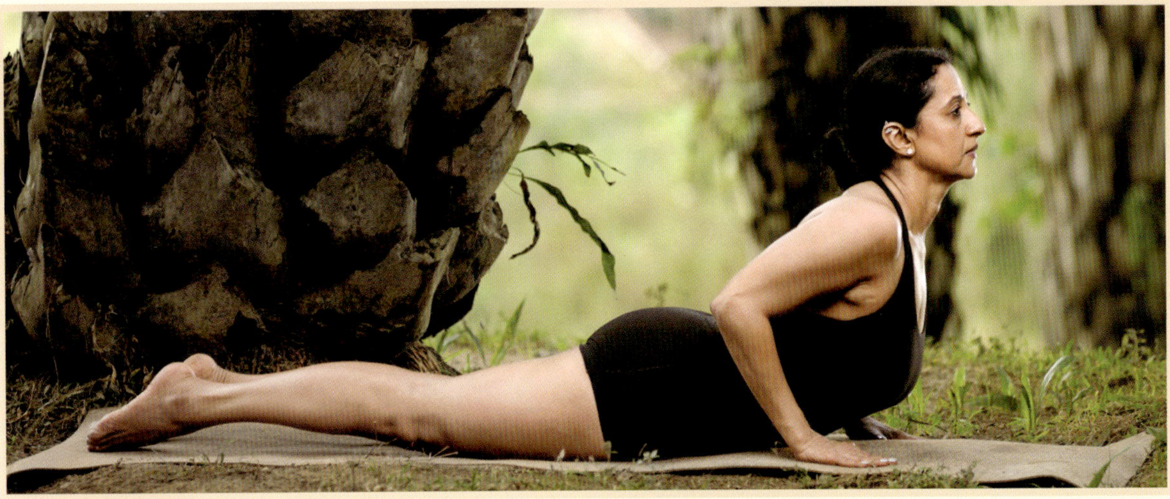

BHUJANGASANA

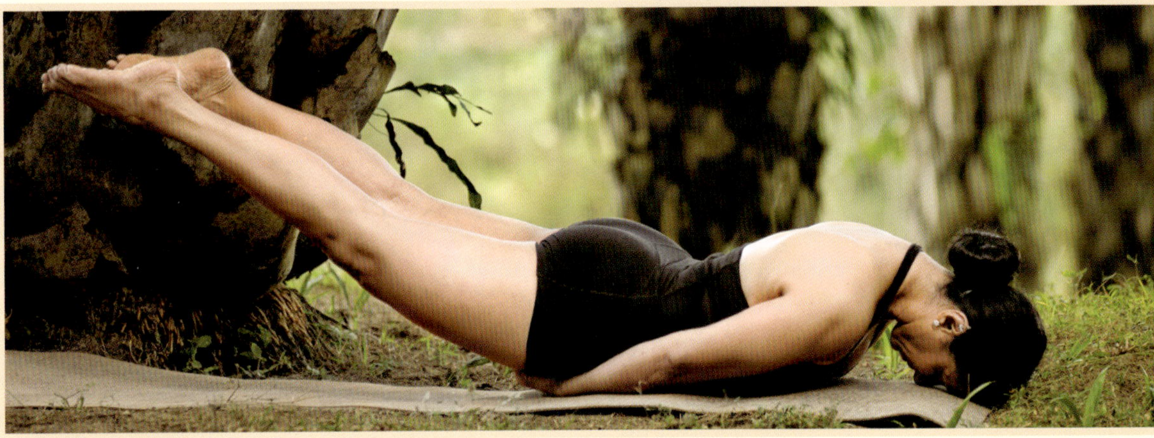

SHALABHASANA

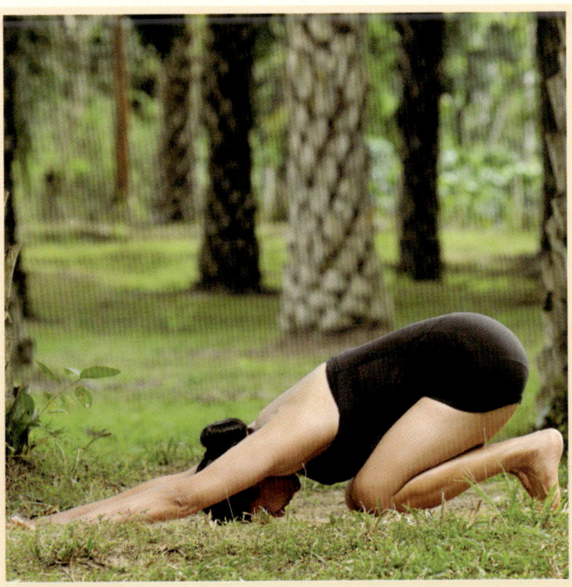

BALASANA

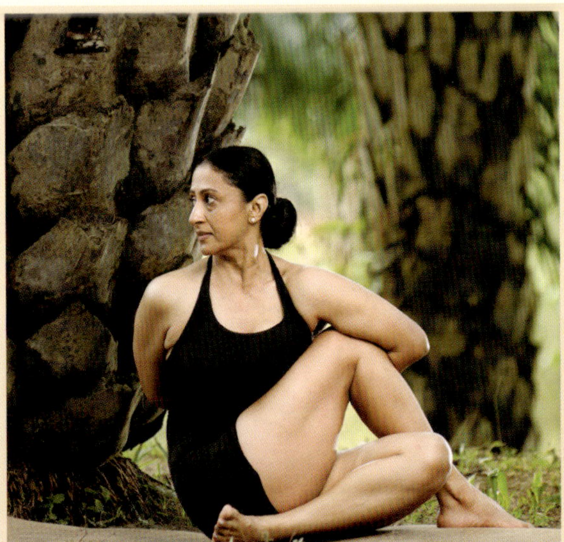

MATSYENDRASANA

Floor Asanas

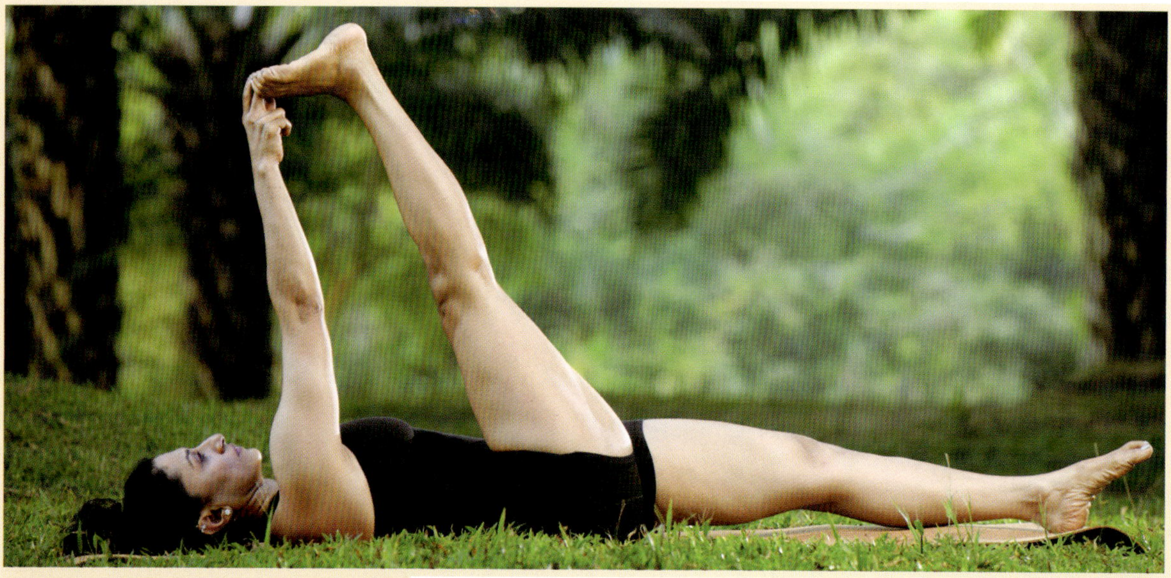

SUPTA HASTAPADANGUSHTHASANA 1

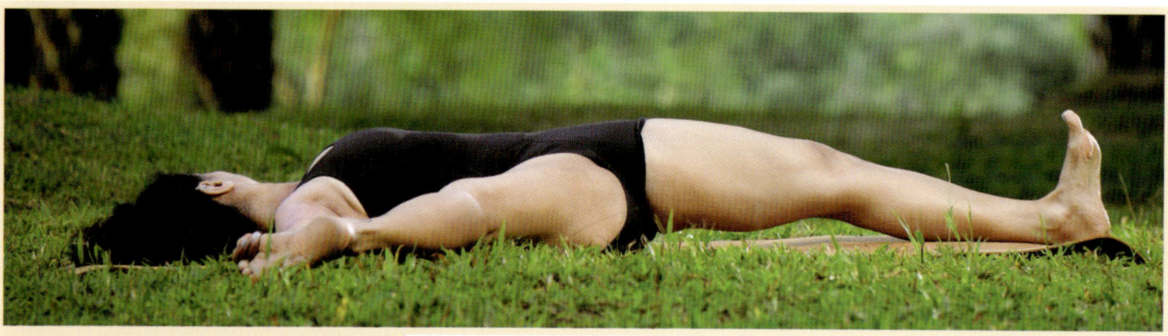

SUPTA HASTAPADANGUSHTHASANA 2

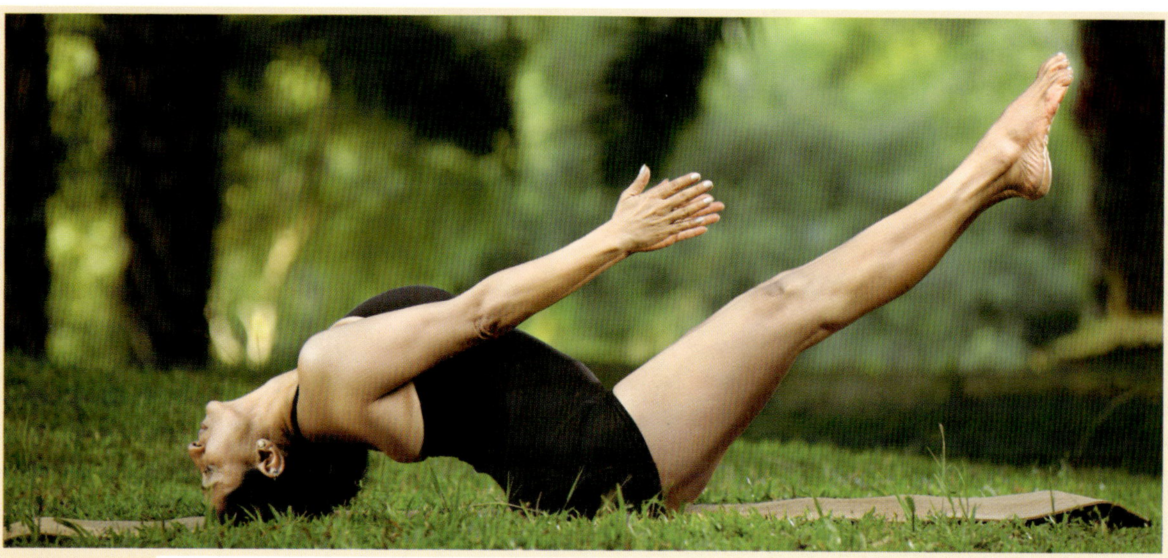

MATSYASANA

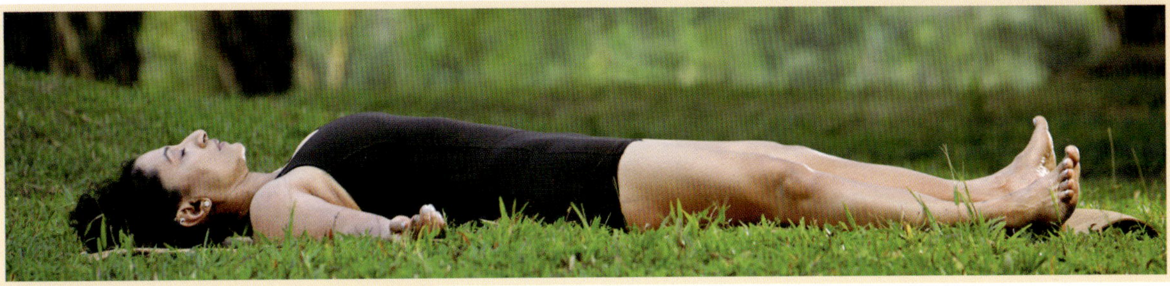

SHAVASANA (ATLEAST FOR 10 MINUTES)

Pranayama

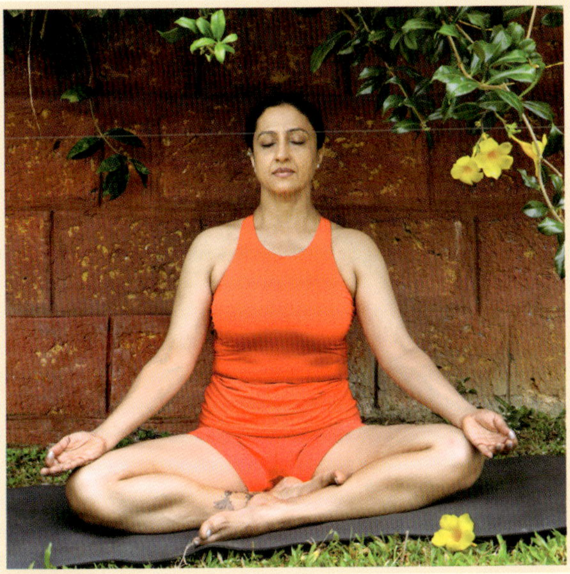

UJJAYI

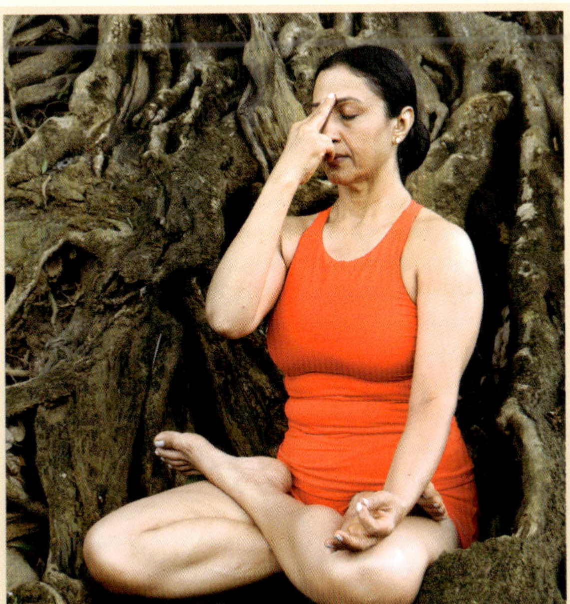

ANULOM VILOM

Mudra

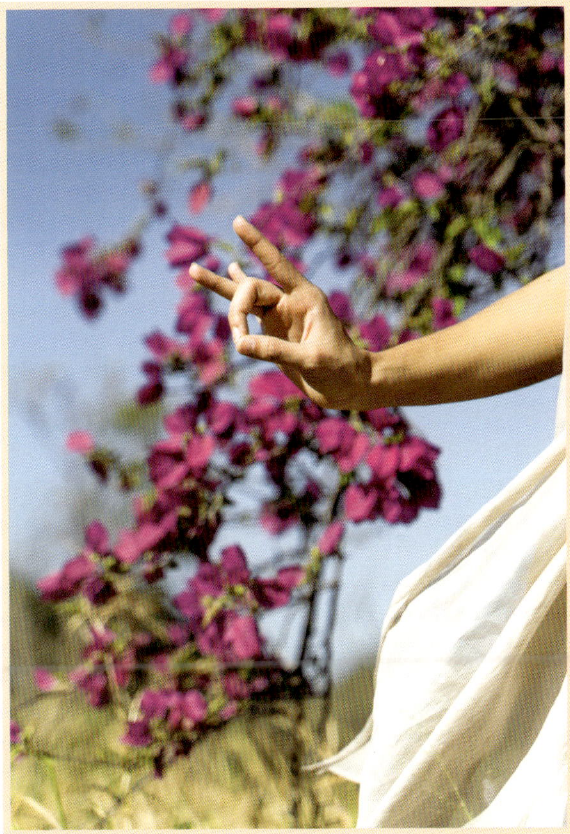

AKASHA MUDRA

Hold Akasha Mudra for 15 minutes. It is okay to split it across morning, afternoon and night.

FOR PITTA DOSHA

Anatomically, pitta resides in the middle section of the body around the solar plexus, near the small intestine.

The best asanas for pitta are those that are calming and do not heat the body excessively.

Those with an imbalanced pitta tend to be more assertive and intense. Calming poses help in easing the emotions of anger and resentment. By alleviating pitta, these asanas help control ulcers, hyperacidity, diarrhoea, etc.

Primary Focus of Asanas

- The postures placing gentle pressure on the navel area or the solar plexus are beneficial.
- It also covers small intestines where the pitta resides.
- The asanas also directly affect the liver and the spleen, and help regulate the strength of the digestive fire.

Yoga Practice Sequence for Pitta Dosha

Standing Asanas

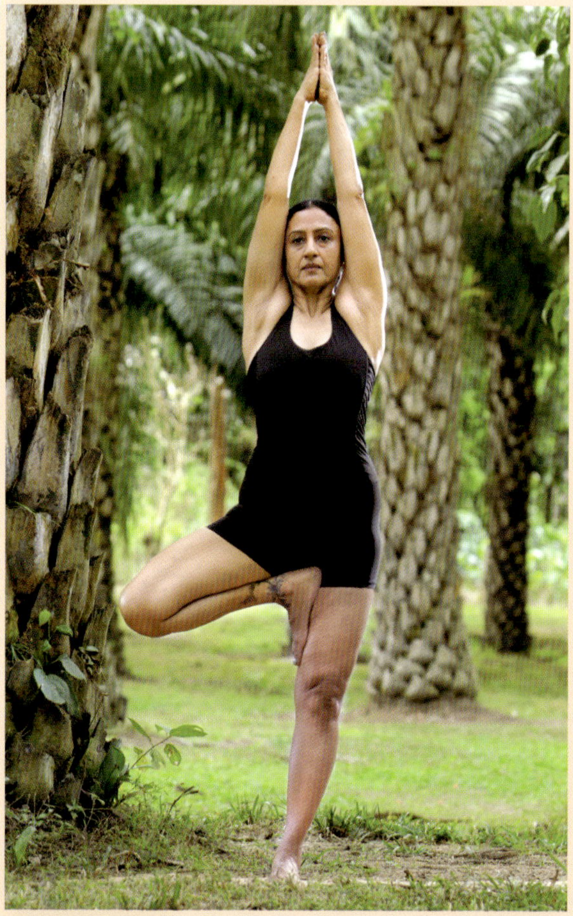

VRIKSHASANA

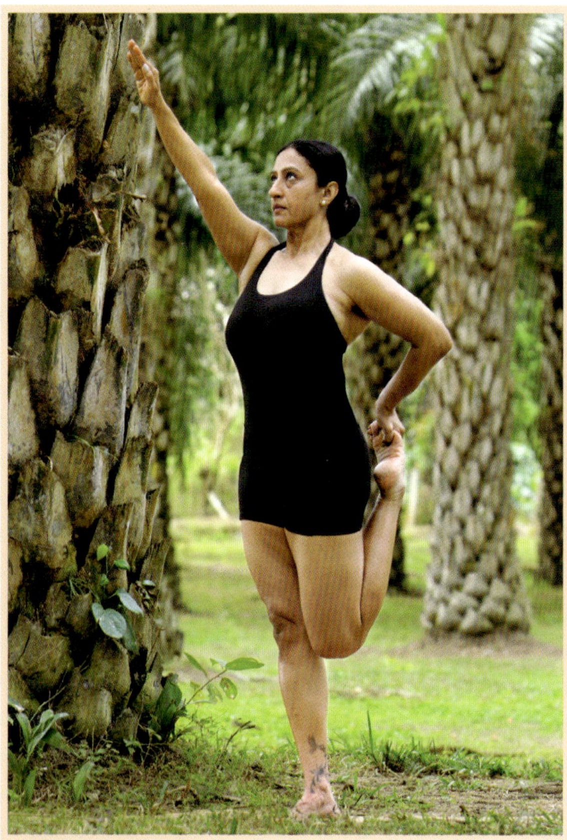

SANTULANASANA

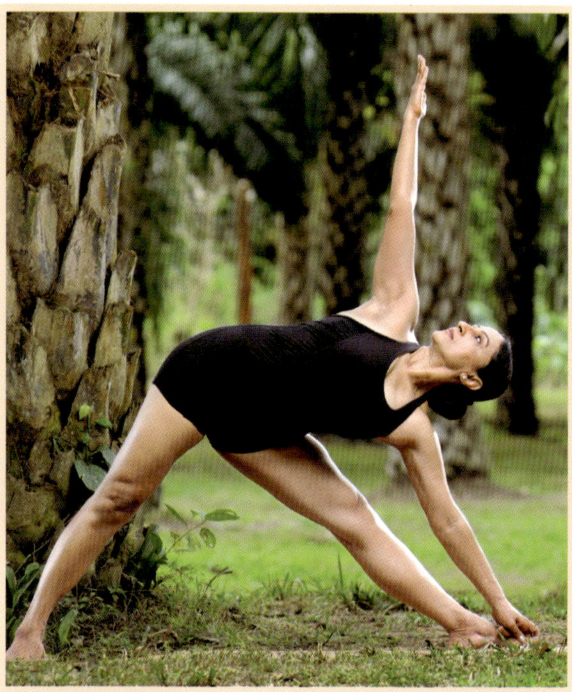

TRIKONASANA

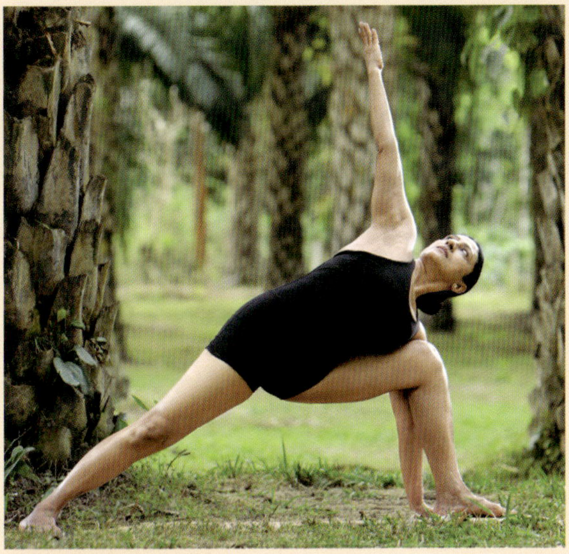

PARSHVAKONASANA

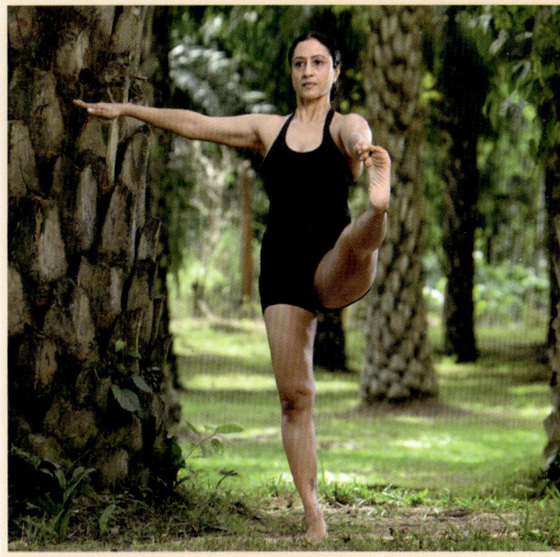

HASTA PADANGUSHTHASANA 2

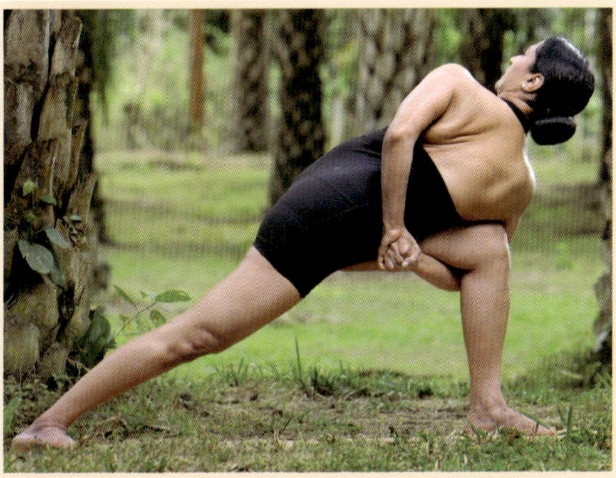

PARIVRITTI PARSHVAKONASANA BANDA MUDRA

Sitting Asanas

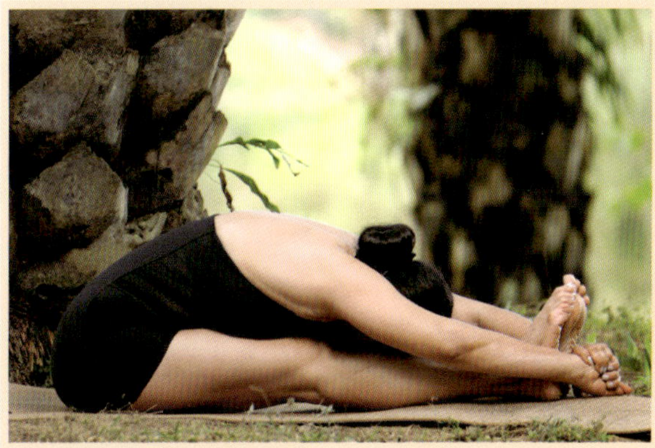

PASCHIMOTTANASANA

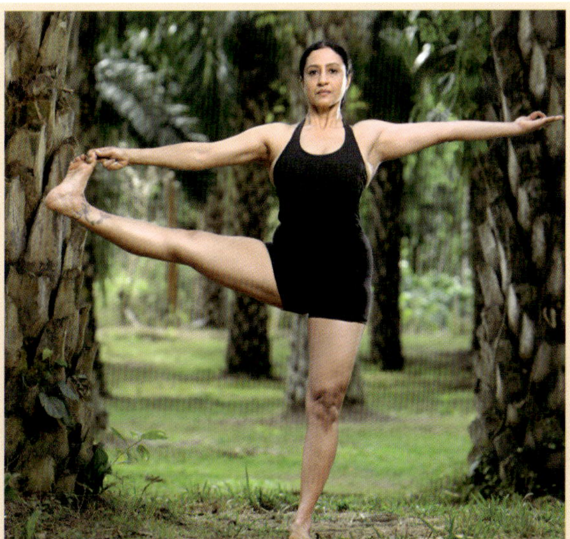

HASTA PADANGUSHTHASANA 1

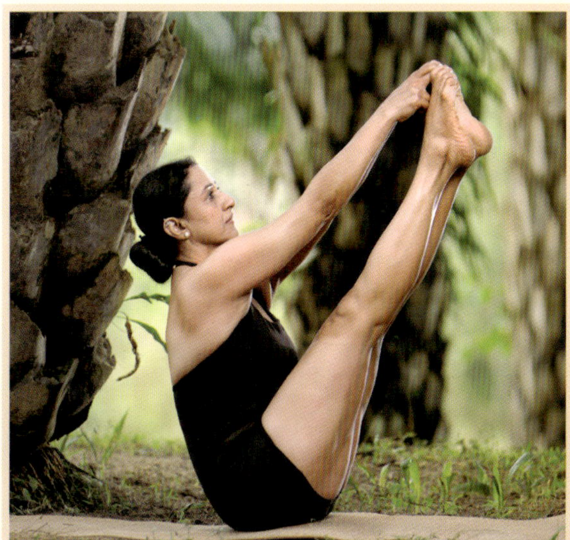

SAMPURNA NAVASANA

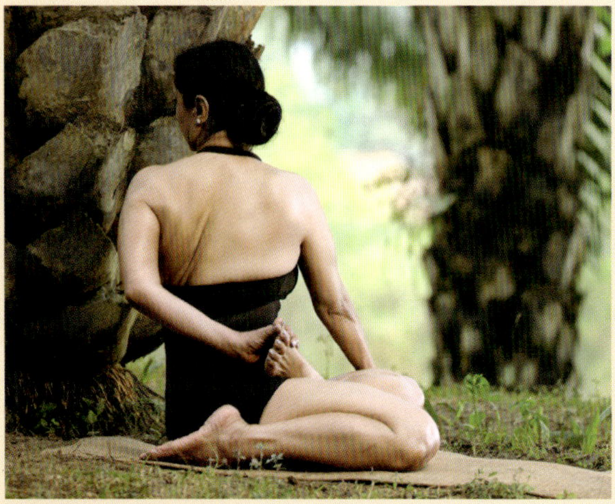

BHARADWAJASANA

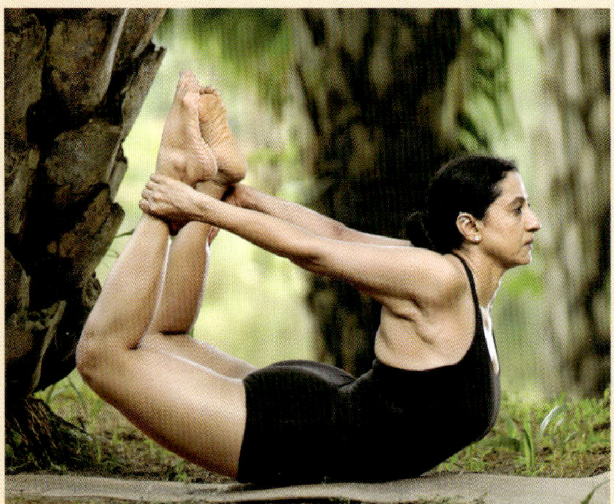

DHAURASANA

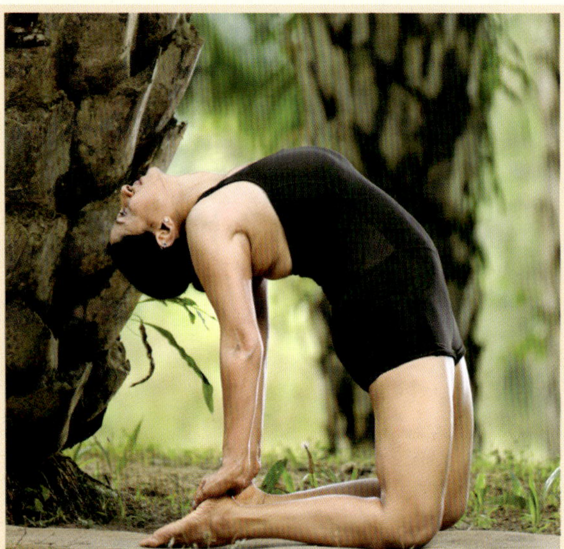

USHTRASANA

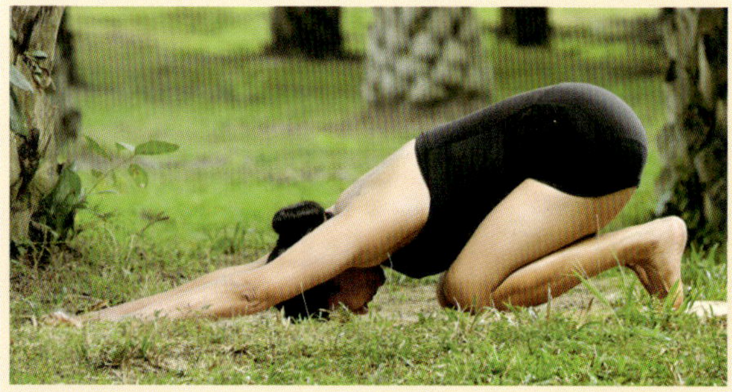

BALASANA

Floor Asanas

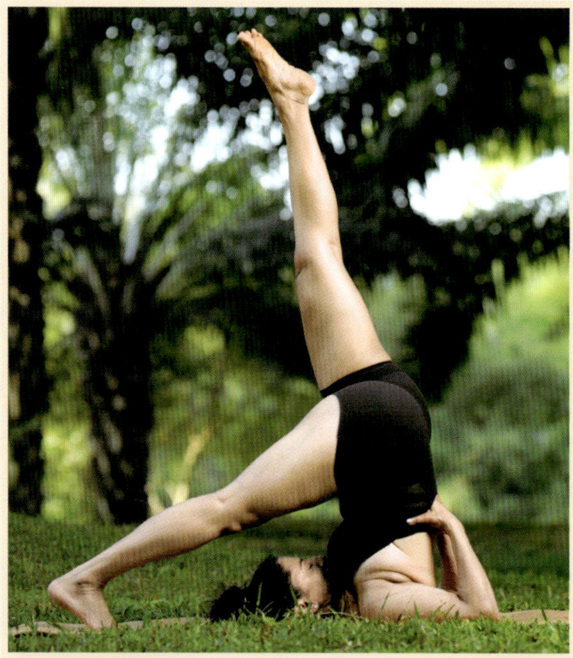

SARVANGASANA

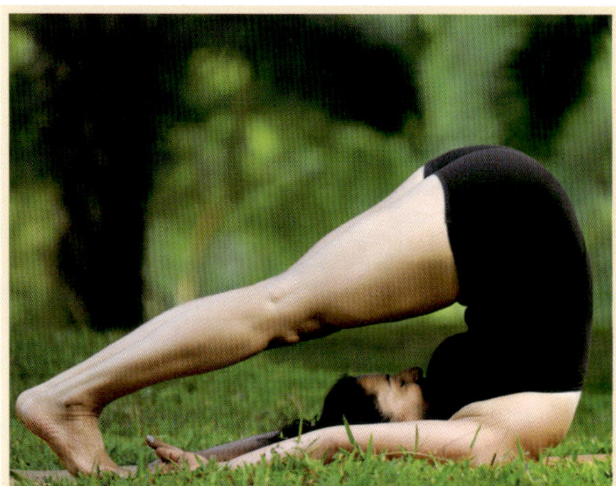

HALASANA 1

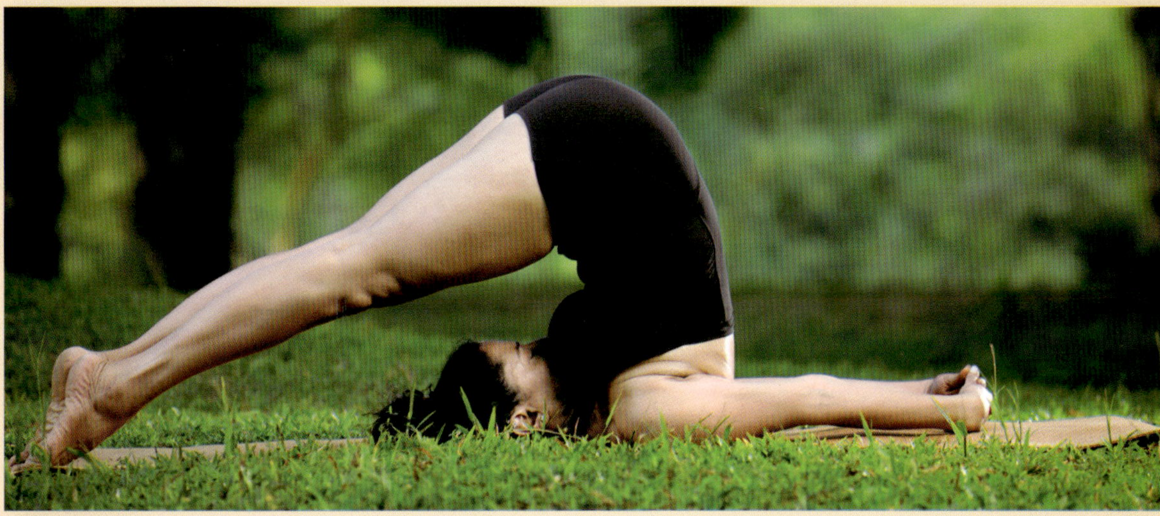

HALASANA 2

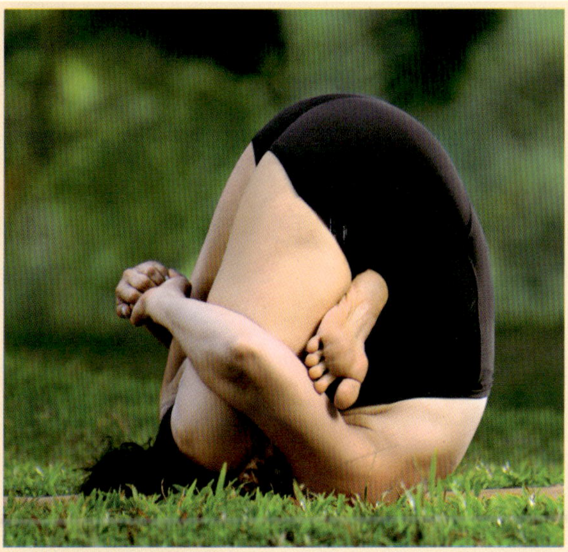

GARBHA PINDASANA

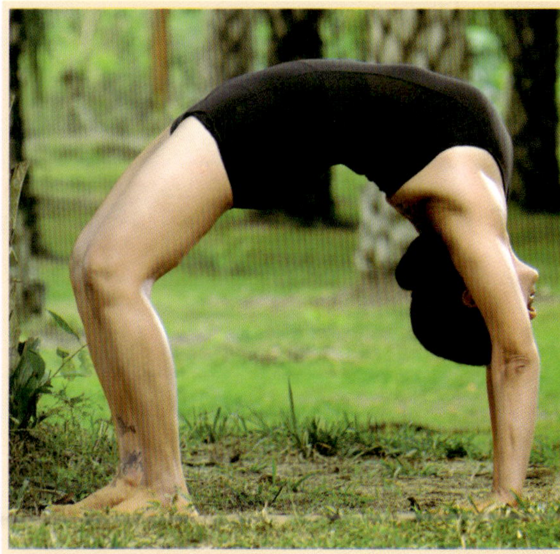

URDDHWA DHANURASANA

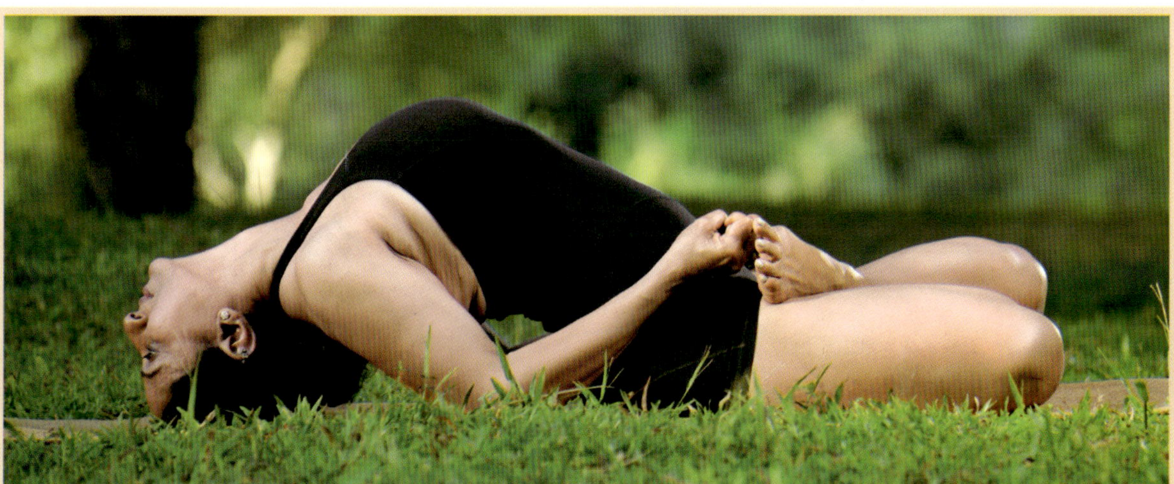

MATSYASANA 1

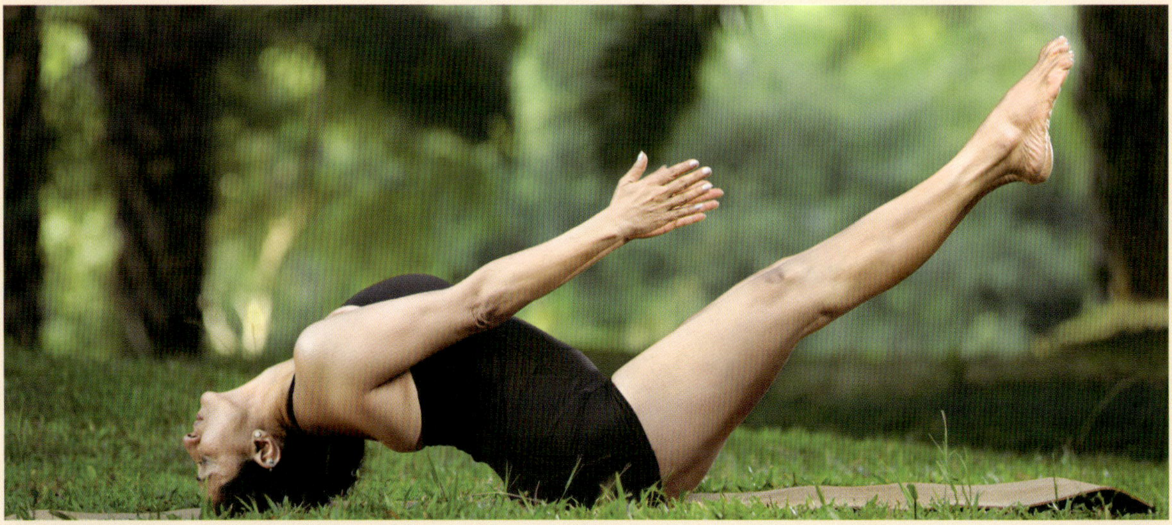

MATSYASANA 2

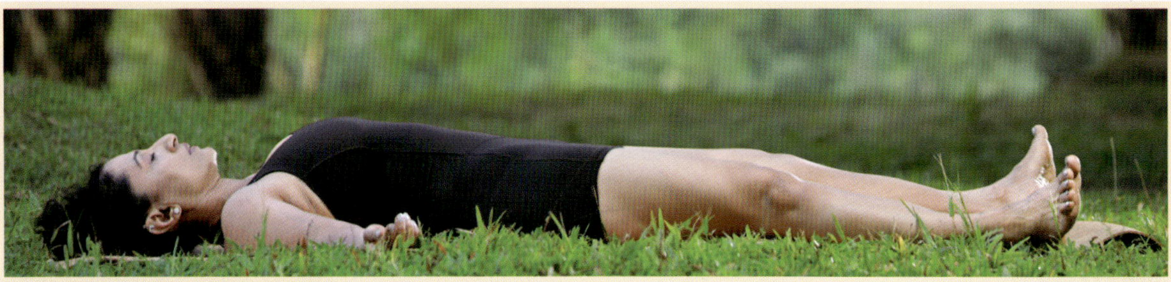

SHAVASANA (FOR 10 MINUTES)

Pranayama

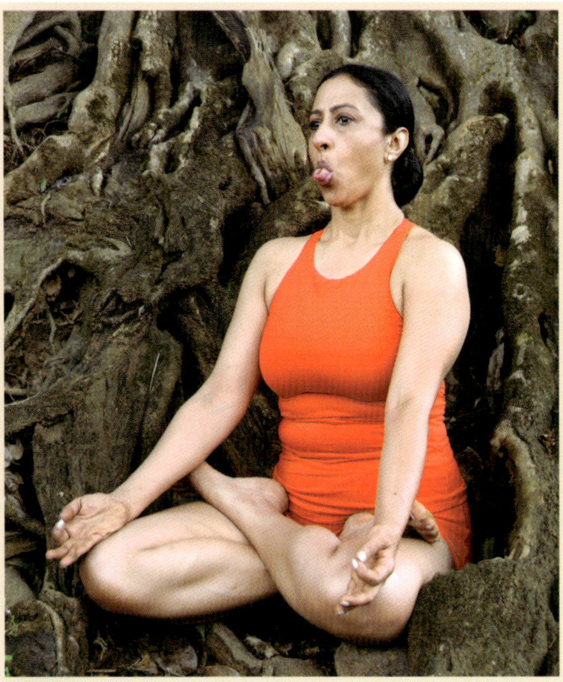

SITALI

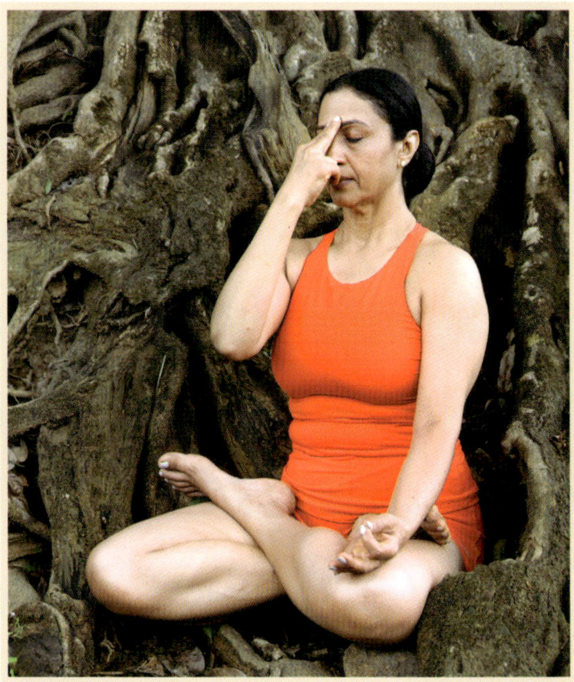

ANULOM VILOM

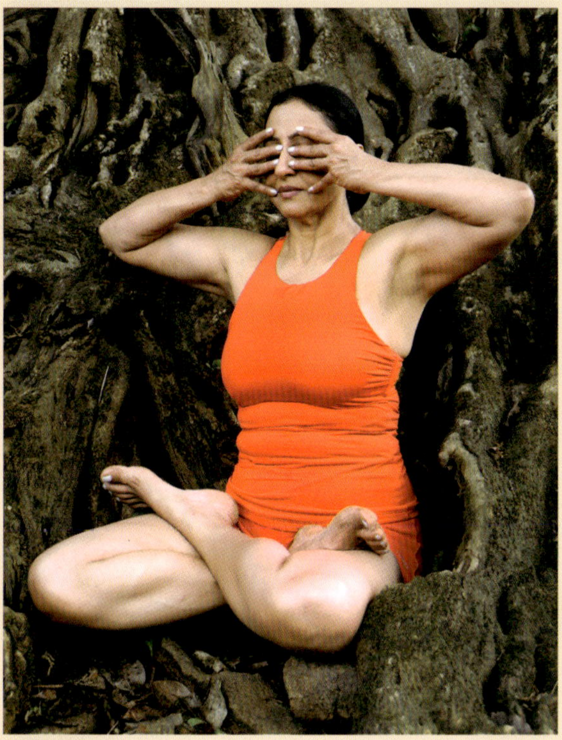

BHRAMARI

Mudra

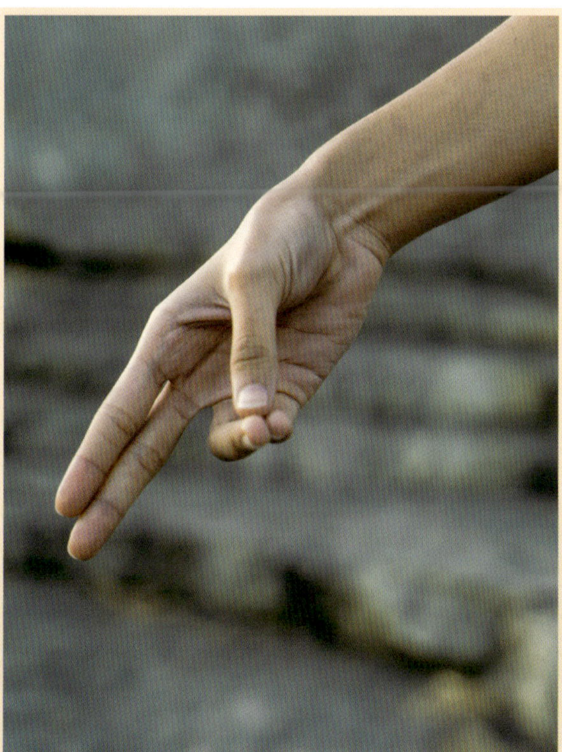

PRANA MUDRA

Hold the Prana Mudra for 15 minutes, which can be distributed into five minutes in the morning, five in the evening and five at night. This mudra can be practised any time to calm the discomfort caused by excess pitta.

FOR KAPHA DOSHA

Kapha primarily accumulates in the stomach and chest, where it manifests as mucus. Thus the asana sequence should focus on both preventing and treating respiratory congestive conditions, such as bronchitis, pneumonia and asthma.

When kapha is elevated, the body may experience dampness, heaviness, lethargy and dullness in the eyes.

Primary Focus of Asanas

- Light, stimulating and strengthening asana performed at a medium pace with powerful ujjayi breathing is ideal.
- A strong vinyasa will balance the kapha efficiently.
- The place of practice should be slightly warm. Outdoor yoga is not suitable for kapha dosha.
- Practising asanas in groups proves to be beneficial for individuals with higher kapha dosha as it can inspire and motivate to keep up with a group.
- A combination of strengthening and balancing asanas is good.
- Such individuals highly benefit from standing asanas.

Yoga Practice Sequence for Hatha Kapha Dosha

Standing Asanas

SURYA NAMASKARA A (3 ROUNDS) (FOR REFERENCE, SEE PP. 4–5)

SURYA NAMASKARA B (3 ROUNDS) (FOR REFERENCE, SEE PP. 6–8)

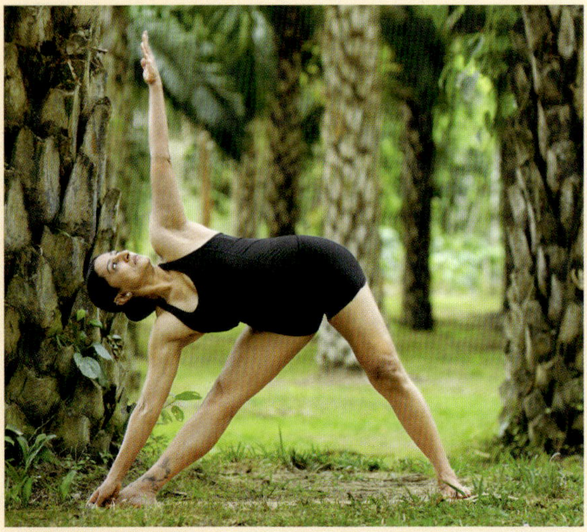

TRIKONASANA 1

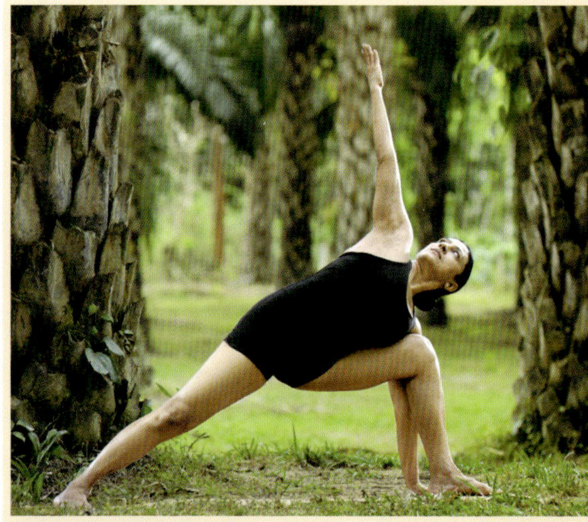

PARSHVAKONASANA

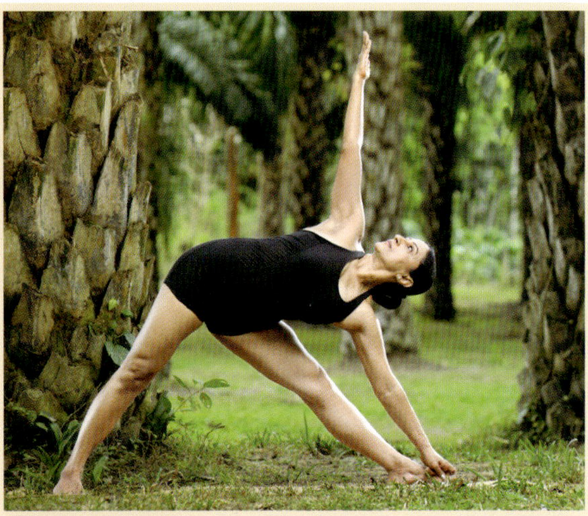

TRIKONASANA 2

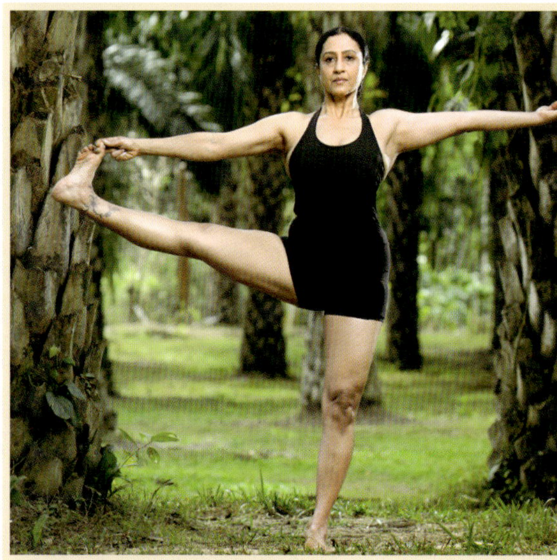

HASTAPADANGUSHTHASANA 1

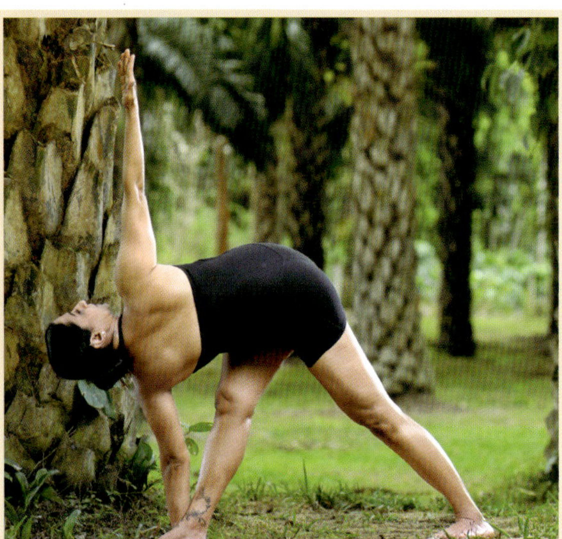

PARIVRITTI TRIKONASANA

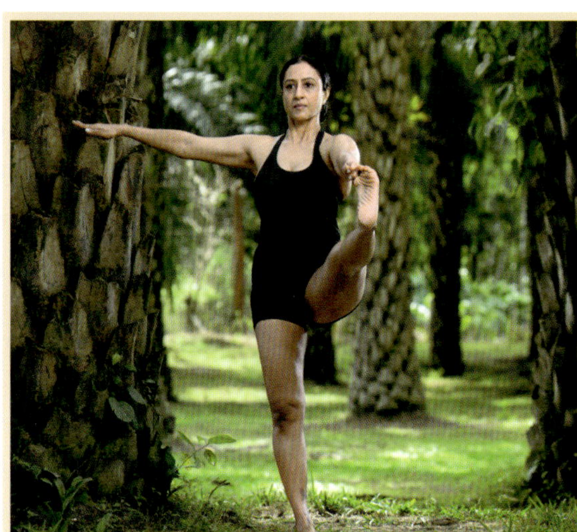

HASTAPADANGUSHTHASANA 2

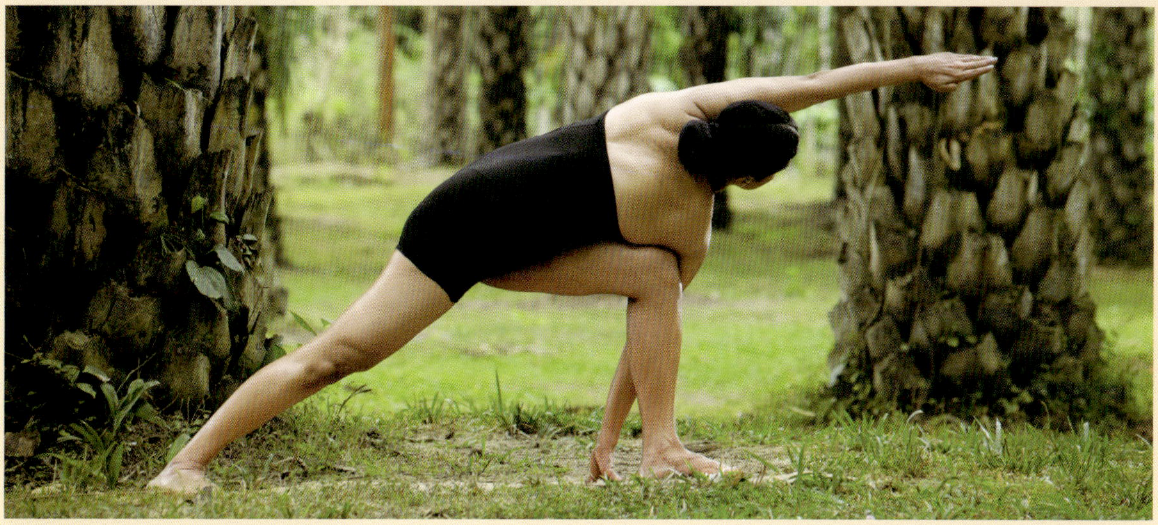

PARIVRITTI PARSHVAKONASANA

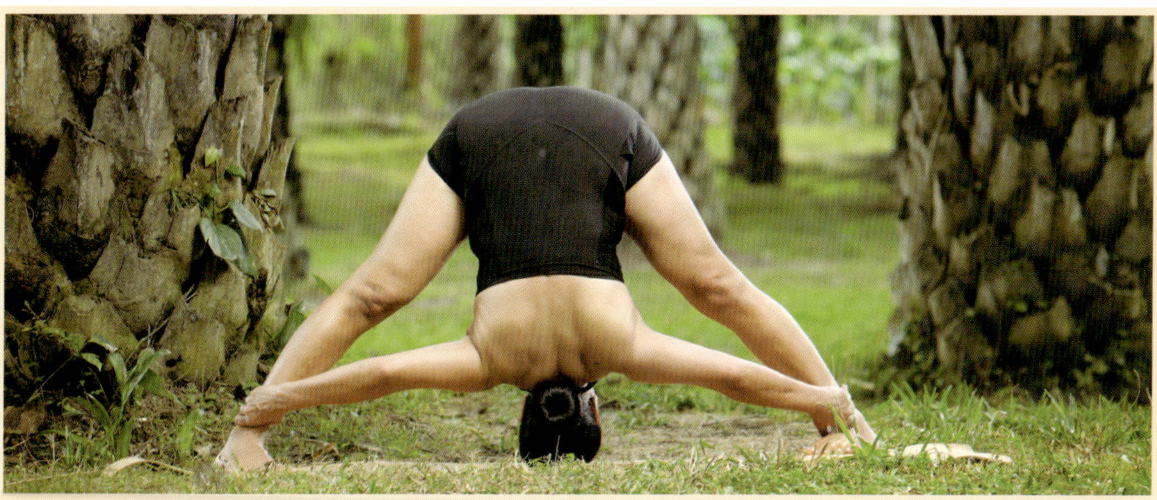

PRASARITA PADOTTANASANA

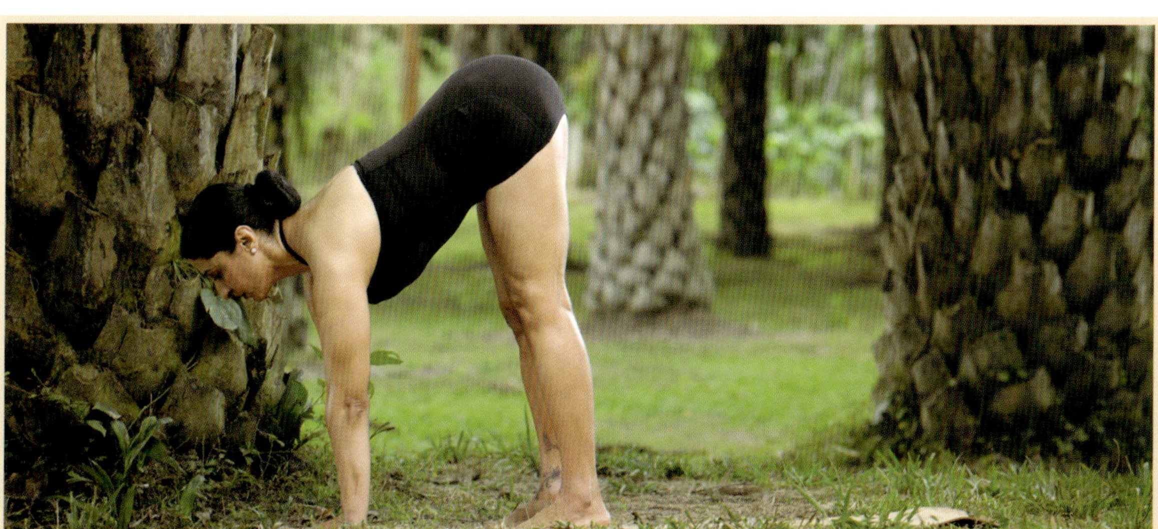

CHATUSHPADASANA

Sitting Asanas

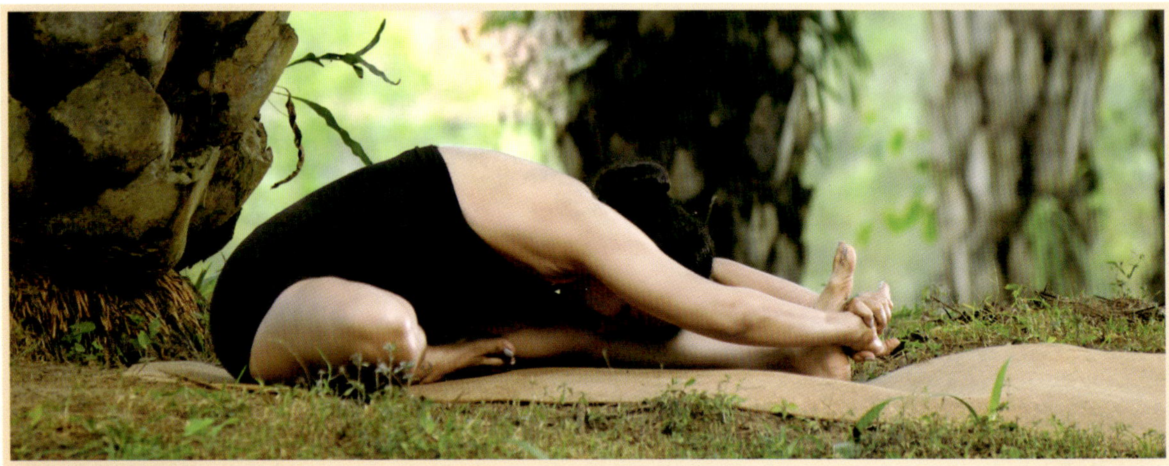

JANU SHIRASANA

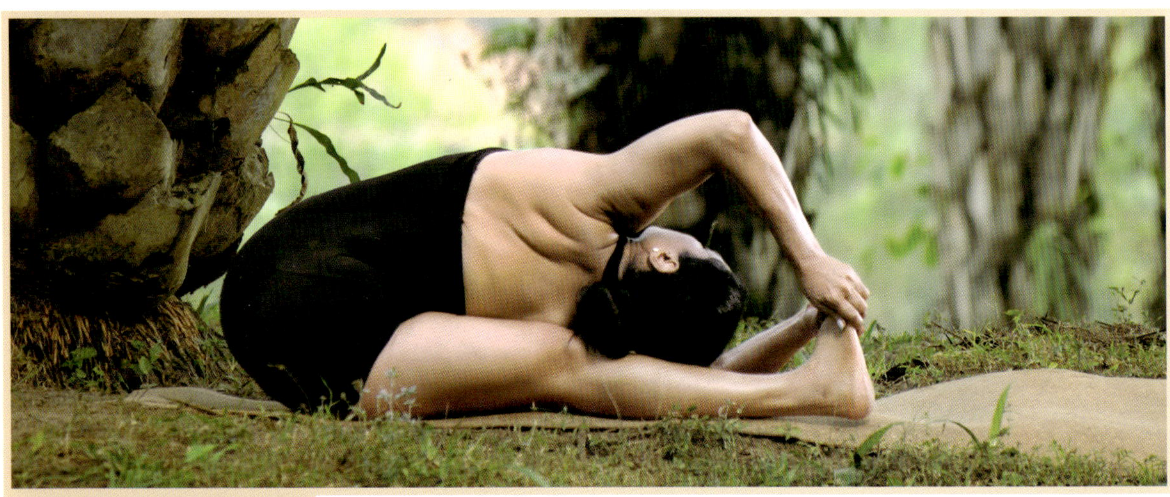

PARIVRITTI JANUSHIRASANA

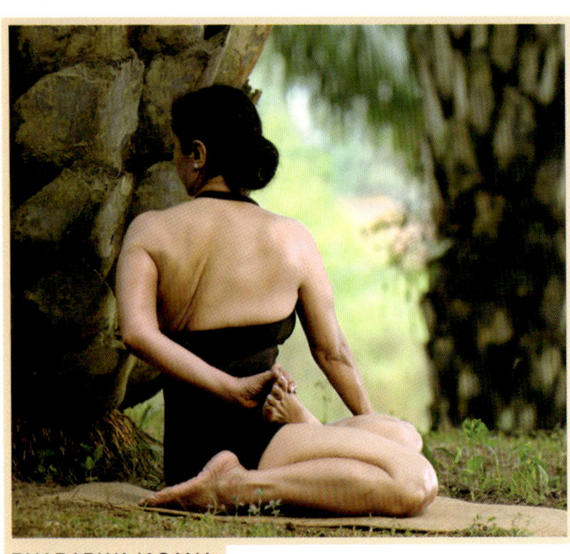

BHARADWAJASANA

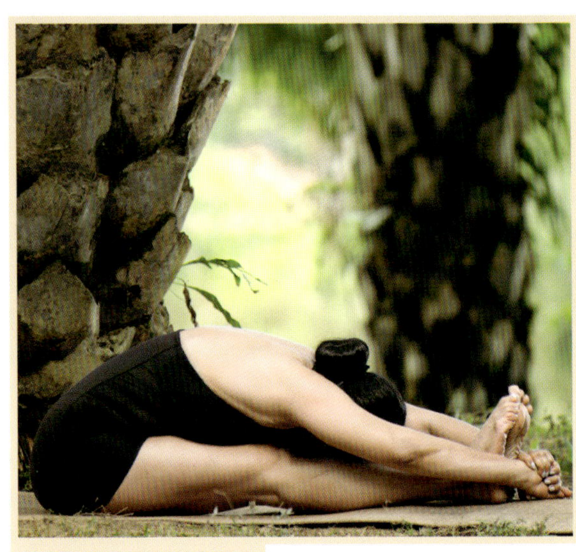

PASCHIMOTTANASANA

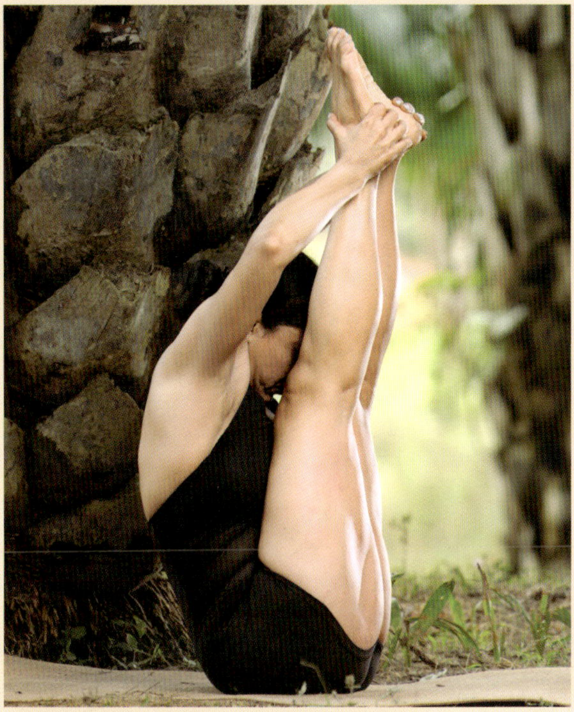

URDDHWAPADA PASCHIMOTTANASANA

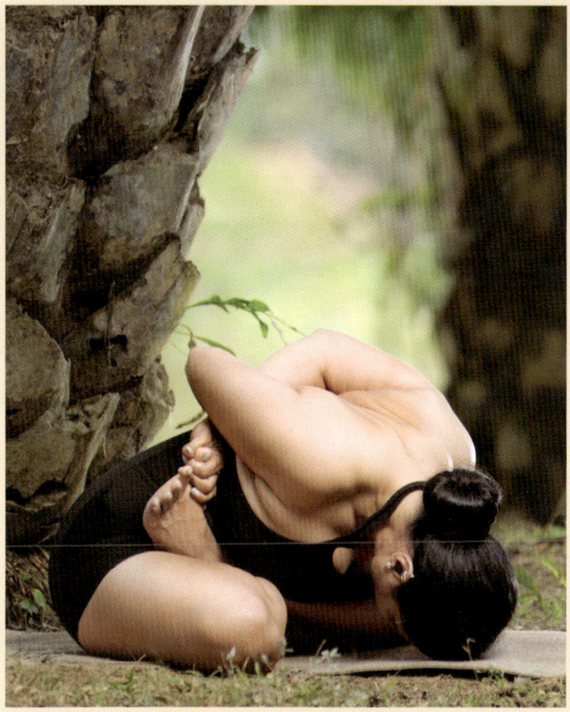

BADHAPADMA PASCHIMOTTANASANA

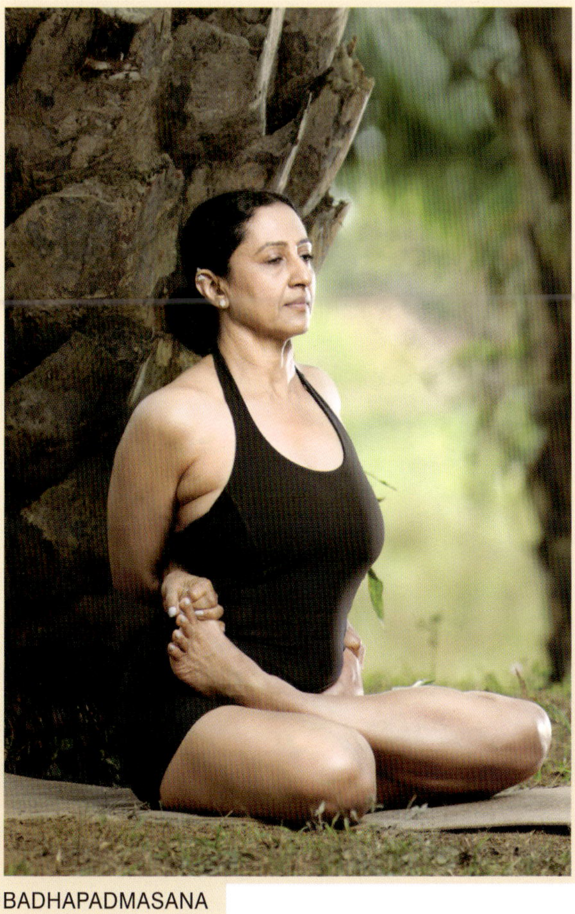

BADHAPADMASANA

Floor Asanas

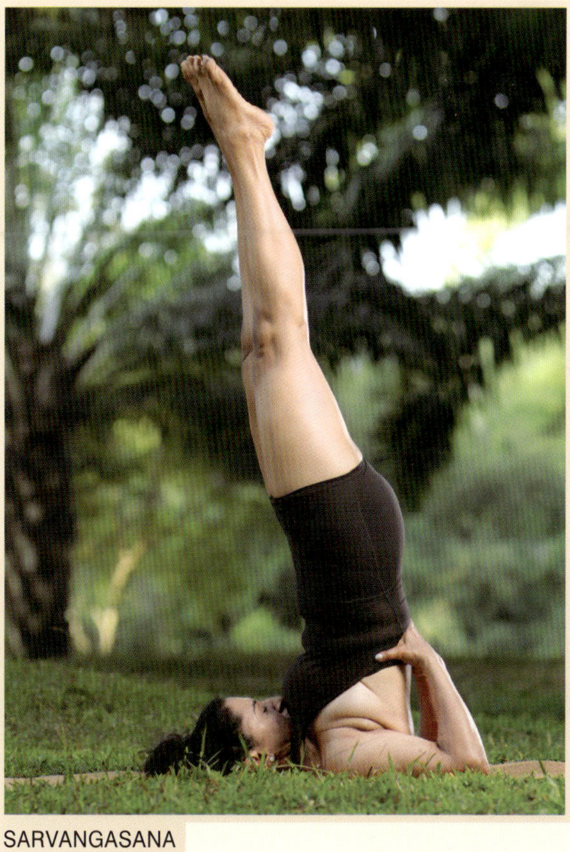

SARVANGASANA

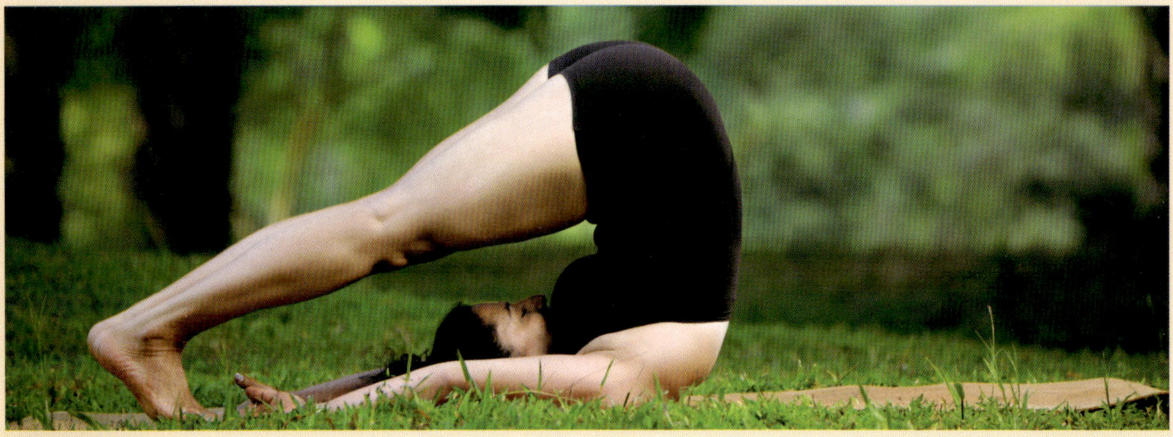

HALASANA 1

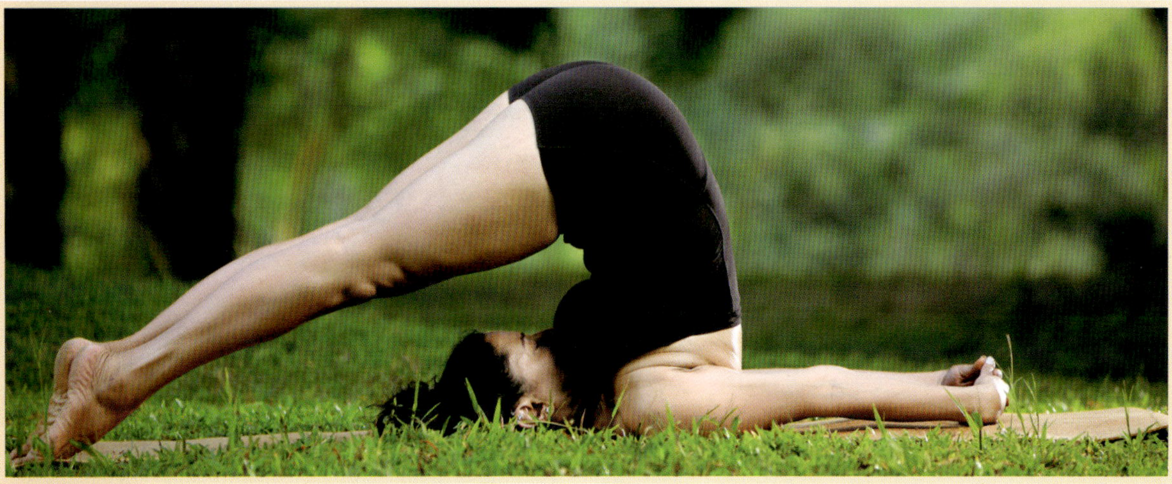

HALASANA 2

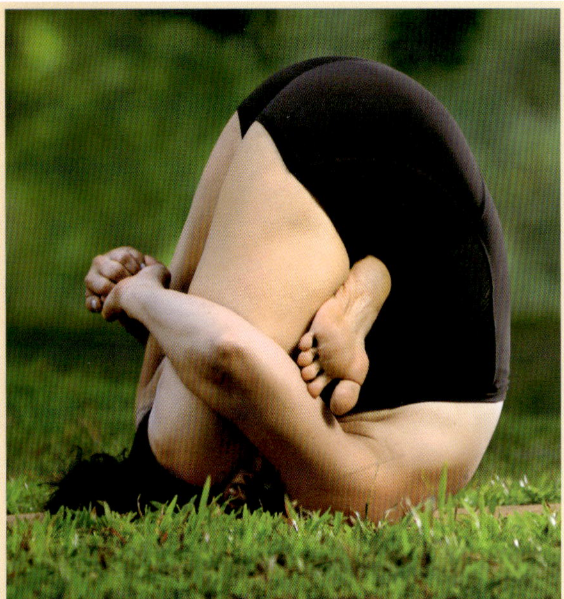

GARBHA PINDASANA

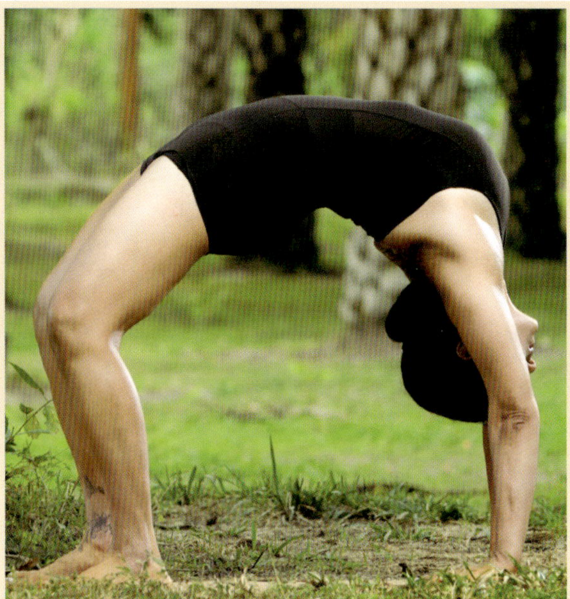

URDDHWA DHANURASANA

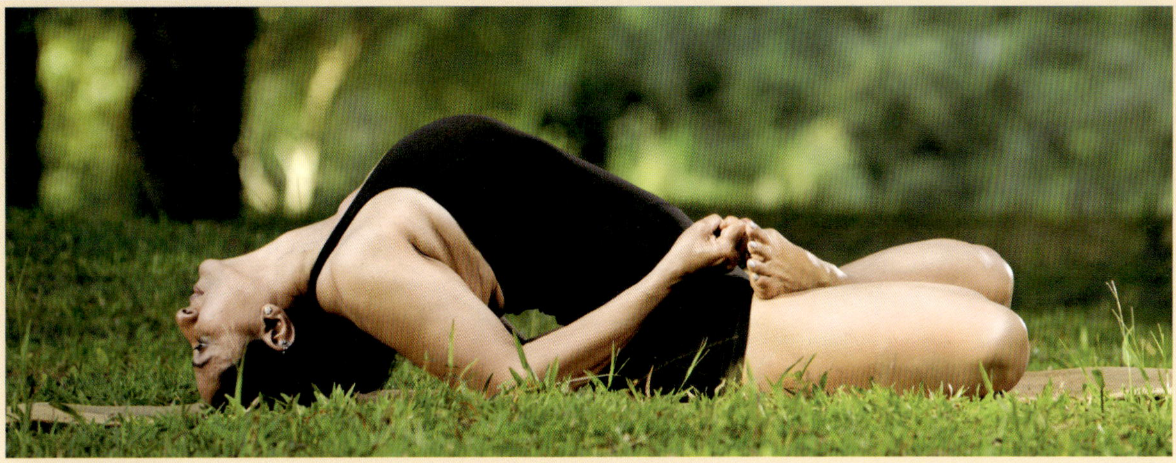

MATSYASANA 1

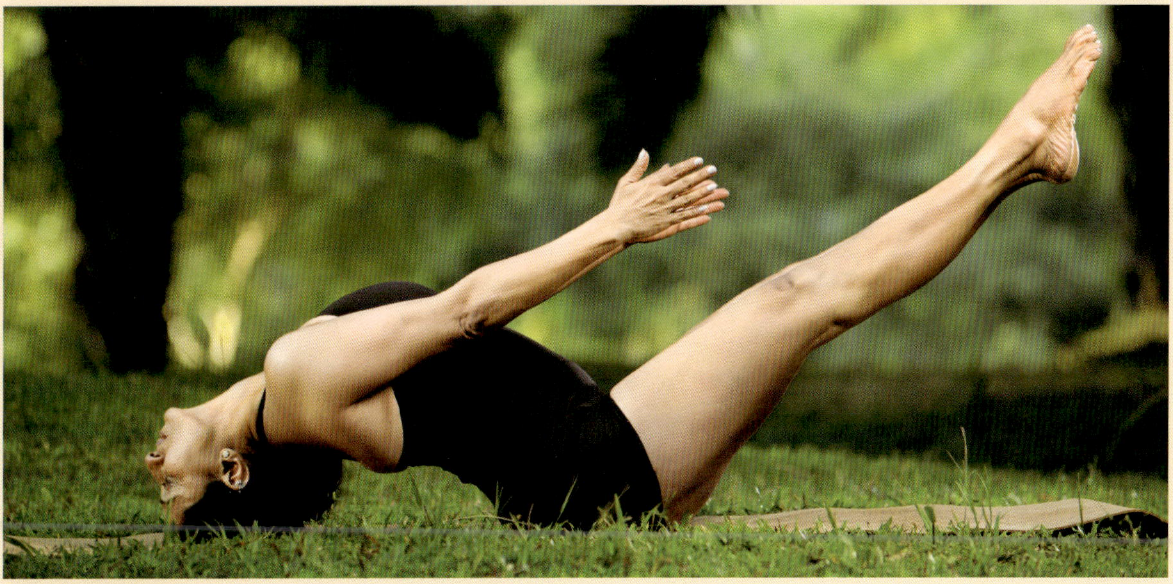

MATSYASANA 2

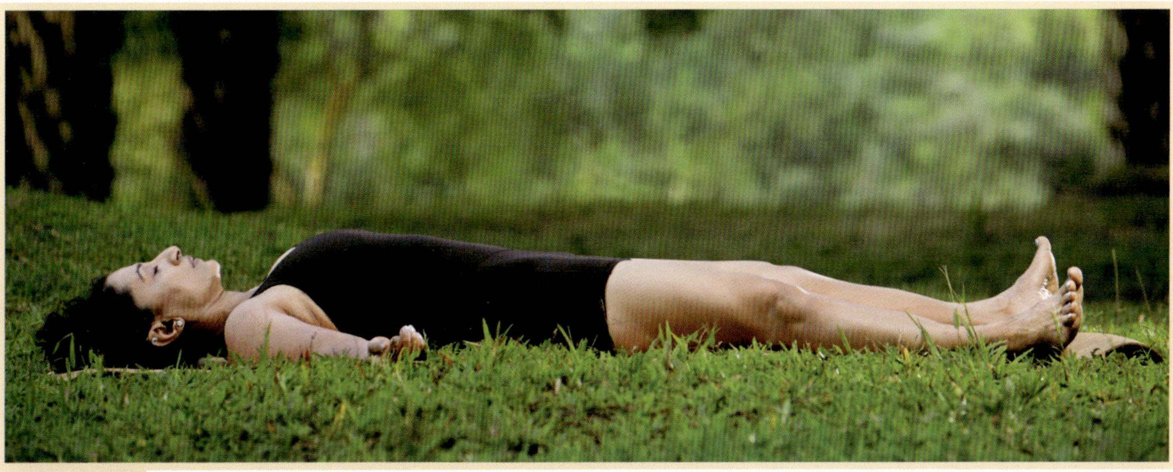

SHAVASANA

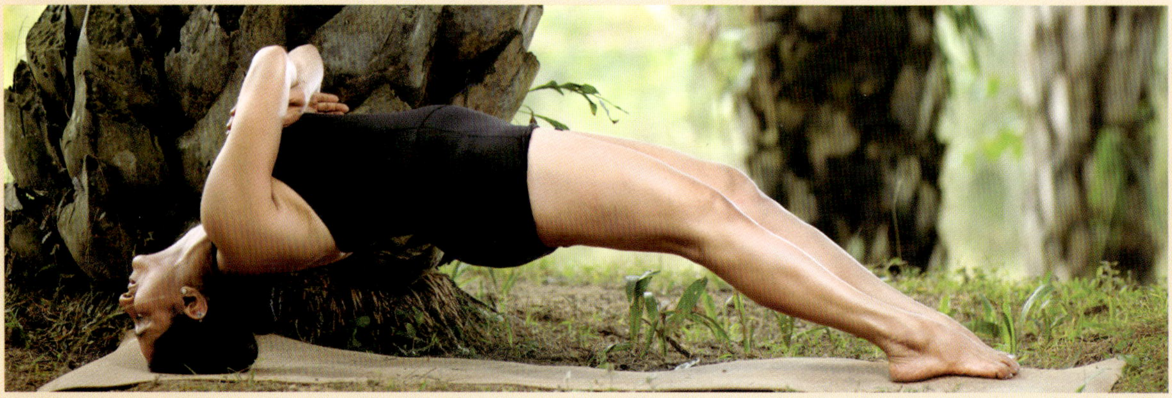

SETUBANDHASNA

Pranayama

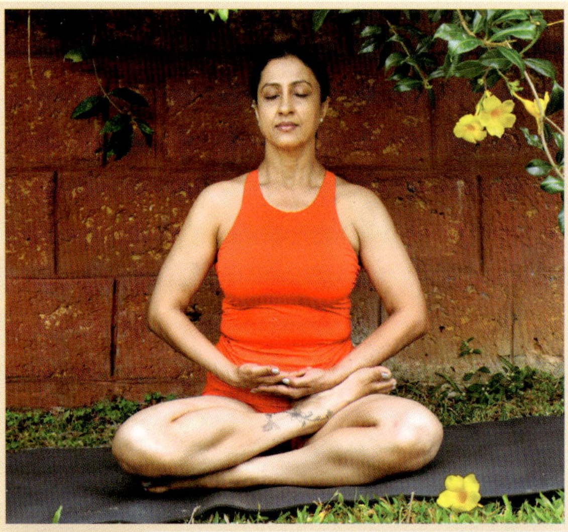

KAPALBHATI

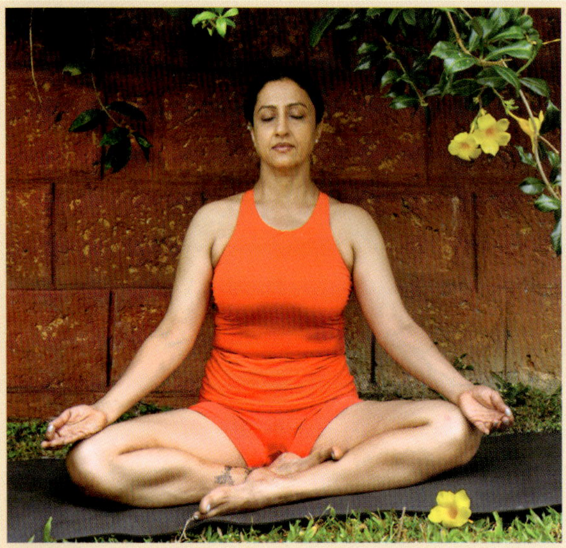

UJJAYI

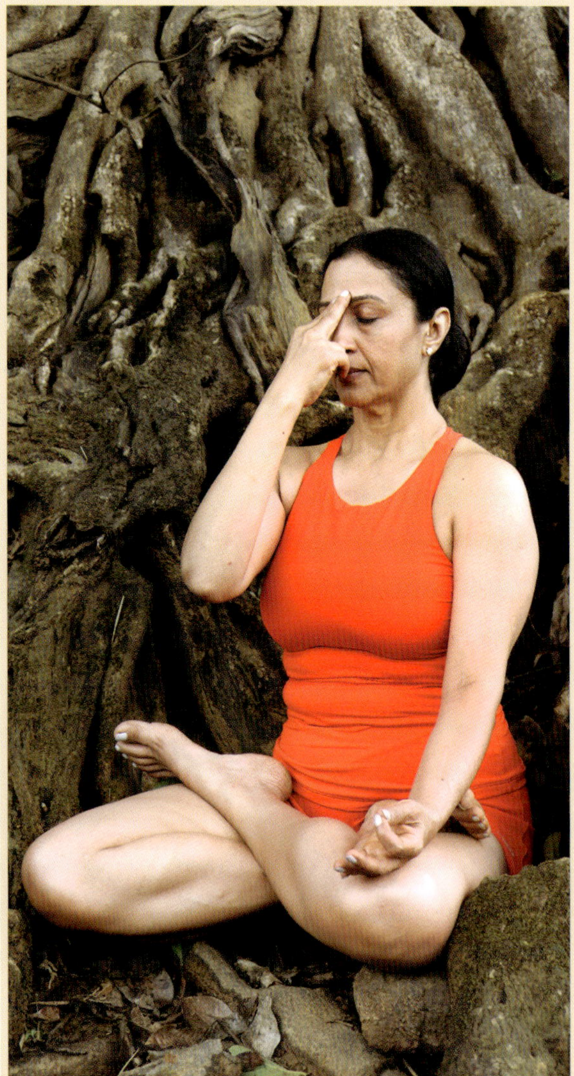

ANULOM VILOM (WITH ANTAR KUMBHAKA AND BAHYA KUMBHAKA)

Mudra

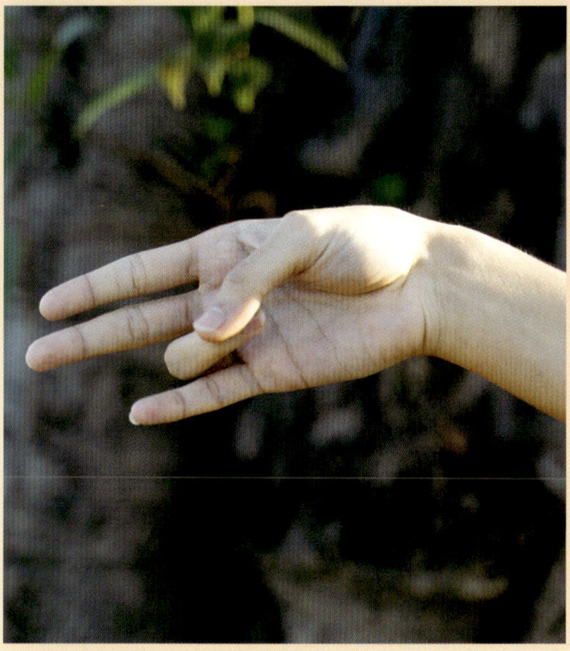

SURYA MUDRA/ AGNI MUDRA

This mudra is held by bending the ring finger and pressing the thumb on it. Hold this mudra for 10 to 15 seconds, after a gap of two hours post meals.

INFLUENCE OF TIME ON DOSHAS

People of all doshas can benefit from Surya Namaskara when it is practised during kapha-dominant hours (6.00–10.00 a.m. and p.m.), provided there is no serious pitta or vata imbalance. People with dominant kapha dosha should perform several repetitions of the sun salutation. Those with vata dominance should practise Surya Namaskara in moderation, holding and being mindful of every pose. Individuals with high pitta dosha should limit their practice of Surya Namaskara, as it can generate excessive heat.

People with kapha dominance generally benefit from all forms of stretching and movement. They tend to have weak lungs and kidneys, thus asanas that place excessive pressure on chest and the lower abdomen should be avoided, especially if the kapha dosha is highly imbalanced. For example, if the practitioner is experiencing severe diarrhoea, it is better to avoid asanas that compress the lower abdomen, like Dhanurasana.

AGE

Throughout different stages of life, the influence of doshas shifts naturally:

- From birth to puberty, our bodies are more affected by kapha.
- From puberty to the time of retirement, the influence of pitta increases.
- In the years that follow, vata takes dominance.

SEASONS

- Cold and damp season increases kapha.
- Warm season increases pitta.
- Cold and dry season increases vata.

HOURS

- Kapha increases between 6.00 a.m. and 10.00 am as well as 6.00 p.m. to 10.00 p.m., regardless of one's prakriti.
- Pitta increases between 10.00 a.m. to 2.00 p.m. and 10.00 p.m. to 2.00 a.m.
- Vata is high between 2.00 p.m. and 6.00 p.m.

FOR ASANA PRACTICE

- Practising yoga before 6.00 a.m., with a focus on quiet and gentle asanas, is ideal.
- After 6.00 a.m., more demanding and challenging asanas can be incorporated.
- Between 12.00 noon and 5.30 p.m., only relaxing kriyas and Shavasana are recommended.

It is important to set up a yoga lifestyle, depending on the unique prakriti of each individual. This is an Ayurvedic path to balance the doshas and enhancing sattva guna.

A SIMPLE TEST TO KNOW YOUR DOSHA

1. **Which of these describe your physical frame best?**

   V: Small

   P: Medium

   K: Large

2. **Do you put on weight easily?**

   V: Not easily (but feel bloated at times)

   P: No

   K: Yes (body feels heavy)

3. **How is your weight usually?**

   V: Average

   P: Rather low

   K: High

4. **How do you describe your physical activity?**

   V: Active (cannot stand still, always on the move)

   P: Very active (athletic and goal-oriented)

   K: Rather inert (slow and easy)

5. **What is your personality?**

   V: Outgoing, talkative, casual

   P: In control, ambitious, intense

   K: Reserved, laid back, concerned

6. **What is your emotional situation when you are worried?**

   V: Anxious and scared

   P: Angry and stressed

   K: Withdrawn and depressed

7. **How are your dreams?**

   V: Multiple, quick, fearful

   P : Often about conflicts, emotional

   K: Slow, romantic, long

8. **How do you adapt to weather changes?**

   V: Easily feel cold

   P: Intolerant of heat

   K: Uncomfortable in humidity

9. **How is your appetite?**

   V: Frequently hungry

   P: Cannot skip meals at meal time

   K: Never feel very hungry

10. **How often do you feel thirsty?**

    V: Variable

    P: Need water regularly

    K: Don't need water much

11. **Taste preference?**

    V: Normal

    P: Spicy

    K: Cold food

12. **Which of these traits sounds more like you?**

    V: Intuitive

    P: Reactive

    K: Non-judgemental

13. **Any of these sounds more like you?**

    V: Restless

    P: Irritable

    K: Calm

14. **Does any of these describe how you talk?**

    V: Fast and a lot

    P: Sharp and concise

    K: Slow and calm

15. **How is your memory?**

    V: I have a great memory

    P: I learn quickly and forget quickly

    K: It takes me a while to memorize but once I do, I don't forget

16. **Does any of these describe your personality?**

    V: Creative, joyful and introspective

    P: Competitive, perceptive and efficient

    K: Responsible, nurturing and sensitive

17. **Do you identify with any of these traits?**

    V: Stubborn

    P: Jealous

    K: Indecisive

18. **Which of these describe your skin?**

    V: Dry

    P: Oily

    K: Normal

19. **Which of these describe your hair?**

    V: Straight and fine

    P: Thick and lustrous

    K: Dry and curly

20. **Which of these describe your eyes?**

    V: Small

    P: Meidum

    K: Large

Identifying your dosha is a key step in maintaining balance and overall health. Understanding its functions and potential imbalances allows for a quicker, more effective response to health concerns. When you recognize your innate tendencies, making nourishing lifestyle choices becomes easier.

Good health depends on the equilibrium of the doshas, while their imbalance can lead to various disorders. By staying aware of the three doshas, you can detect disturbances early and restore harmony in the body and mind.

SUBTLE FORMS OF TRIDOSHA

Vata, pitta and kapha are collectively known as tridosha. When these three are in balance, they maintain optimal health and well-being. It is essential to understand that doshas are universal principles governing all living organisms, each playing a vital role in regulating specific physical functions.

Beyond the body, tridosha also influences subtle energy movements that shape the mind. When out of balance, they can disrupt the three fundamental mental energies—ojas, tejas and prana. These energies exist in both physical and mental realms and are deeply interconnected, with prana and tejas being rooted in ojas.

OJAS

Ojas is often referred to as the fountain of youth. In Ayurveda, it provides strength to the body in both physical and mental terms. It is governed by kapha dosha. There is no particular definition for ojas, but it can be understood as the vital energy that sustains the body's seven essential tissues called the Sapta Dhatus (explained in Chapter 6). Ojas is considered to be the purest energy in the universe, omnipresent as consciousness, and with pure and healthy thoughts and positive feeling in every situation. It also governs intelligence, longevity and memory.

If our ojas is weak, our health, vitality and spirits also diminish.

When Ojas Is Strong

- Calm and attractive personality
- Sparkling eyes
- Good physical strength
- Ample energy
- Alert sense organs
- No aches and pains
- Robust health and immunity
- A sense of lightness in the body and mind
- Clarity in thoughts and steady focus
- Ample vitality
- Creativity
- A profound sense of well-being
- Feeling happy and joyful in all circumstances

When Ojas Is Weak

- Dry skin
- Cold hands and feet

- Week sense organs (sensitivity to light and sound)
- Depression and/or feelings of loneliness
- Muscle pain and/or joint pain
- Bodily heaviness
- Impaired bodily functions
- Frequent drowsiness and/or fatigue
- A tendency to get sick frequently
- Mental confusion or fuzziness
- Lack of focus
- A consistent negative attitude
- Anxiety

Diet to Follow

Avocados, bananas, dates, figs, sweet potatoes, yam, turnips, leafy greens, zucchini, nuts (especially almonds), tofu and wholegrains.

Tips for Healthy Ojas

- Getting ample sleep
- Being outdoors, surrounded by nature
- Opting for selfless service and volunteering in community service
- Having healthy, fresh and organic food
- Being in the company of good friends

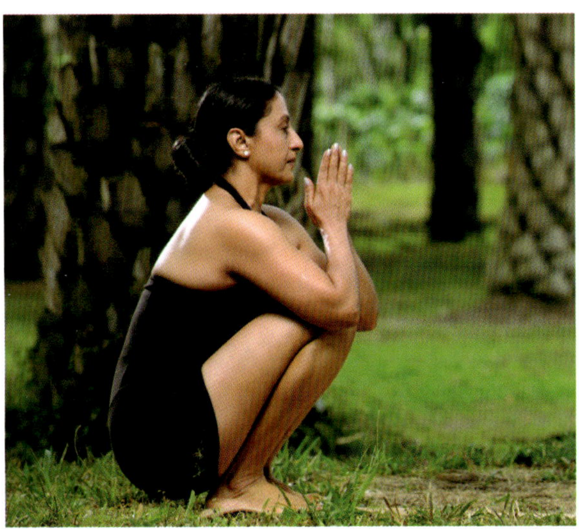

AUTHOR'S NOTE

Ojas is strong with proper nutrition which results in perfect digestion and metabolism. *Ama* is the opposite of Ojas where the toxic residue of undigested food, undigested thoughts and negative emotion creates a poison in the mind and body. Overexertion, improper diet, lack of routine, excessive emotional reaction (like anger, grief, worry, anxiety, fear) are all causes for ama in the body and mind.

TEJAS

Tejas is the element of Agni in the body. It is often defined as 'Inner Radiance', 'Inner power', etc., which are necessary for spiritual growth. It is governed by pitta dosha. It is responsible for intelligence, discernment, self-discipline, enthusiasm, reasoning, focus and clarity. Tejas is the force behind any transformation goals. It relates to the individual's inner fire, which can be used to gain spiritual benefits from yoga or any other type of meditation exercise, as well as guides our development and enhances our perception of the world.

When Tejas Is Strong

- Uncluttered and disciplined mind
- Healthy glowing skin
- Brilliance in both mind and body
- Personality exuberating trust and compassion
- Clear perception of the world
- Dilution of mental fog
- Fearless aura

When Tejas Is Weak

- Cold and dry skin
- Poor decision-making skill
- Slow movement
- Lack of passion
- Confusion

Diet to Follow

Ayurveda suggests some methods to maintain strong Tejas in the body. The most important way to keep the Tejas bright is nutritious food. Too much intake of the wrong kind of food or lack of attention to what is being eaten decreases Tejas. A steady commitment to a daily routine is the only way to keep the Agni balanced.

- Include spices like ginger, pepper, cardamom, cinnamon
- Chew a small piece of ginger with some lemon juice and salt sprinkled helps build tejas.
- Bitter ghee is good to increase tejas without increasing pitta.

Tips for Healthy Tejas

- Enforce positive thinking
- Meditate
- Chant mantras
- Practise awareness in thoughts, words and action
- Avoid gossip, excessive talking, negative talk, etc.

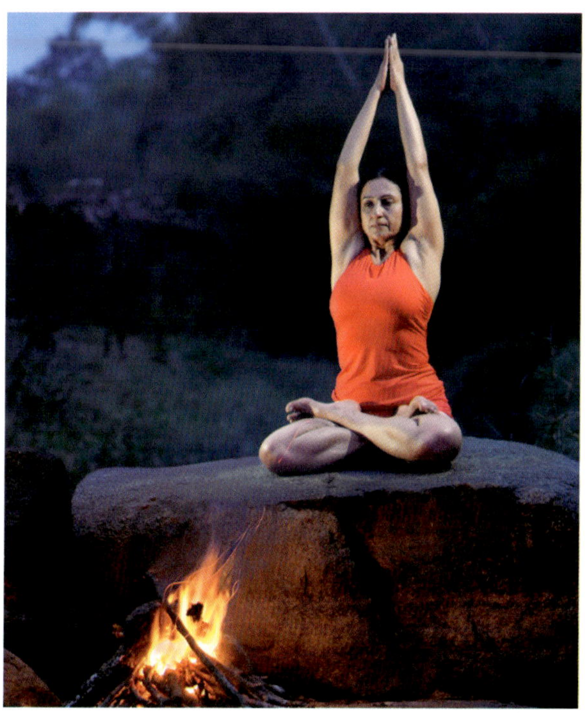

PRANA

Prana is the vital force that binds and animates ojas and tejas—the subtle essences of immunity and inner radiance. When the intake of prana is inadequate or disturbed, both ojas and tejas begin to wane.

It encompasses respiration, oxygenation, and circulation—the movements that sustain life itself. Prana acts as the bridge between body, mind and consciousness, flowing invisibly but powerfully through every breath we take.

Prana governs the very spark of life. In yoga, the practice of pranayama is a means to harness, refine and elevate this vital energy—awakening awareness and nourishing the entire being.

Tips for Enhancing Prana Flow

Ujjayi

Also known as diaphragmatic or victorious breath, ujjayi involves a full, conscious inhalation that engages and lifts the diaphragm. The breath is drawn in with a distinct sound, resonating from the hollow of the throat—often compared to the gentle hiss of ocean waves.

On exhalation, the body softens and relaxes as the breath flows out smoothly, accompanied by a soothing, wave-like sound. This rhythmic, audible breath calms the mind while energizing the body. There are various techniques to cultivate and refine the practice of Ujjayi, each deepening awareness and control over the breath.

Nadi Shodhana

It's a yogic breathing technique aimed at clearing and balancing the subtle energy pathways (nadis) in the body—especially the two main ones: ida and pingala. It helps calm the nervous system and reduces stress. It involves inhaling from one nostril, exhaling through the other, and then reversing the cycle.

Mentioned below are a few easy-to-follow methods to work on Nadi Shodhana:

- Anulom Vilom
- Shakti Chalana
- Surya Bhedana
- Chandra Bhedana

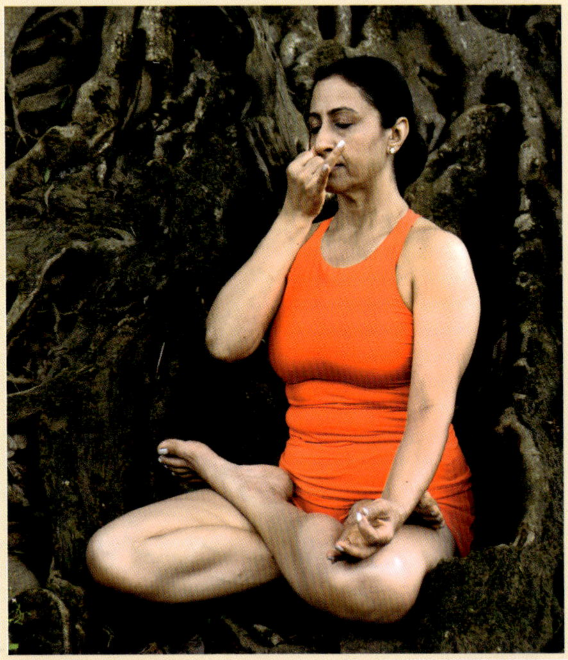

ANULOM VILOM 1

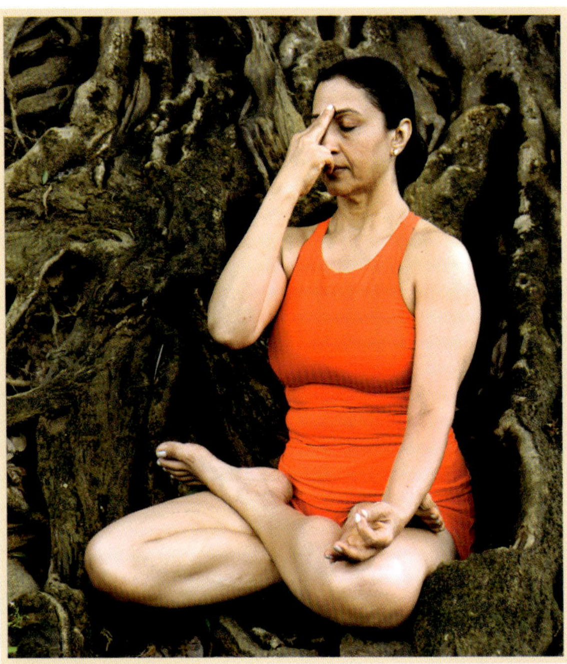

ANULOM VILOM 2

Bhastrika

Bhastrika Pranayama comes from the Sanskrit word 'bhastra', meaning bellows—like the kind blacksmiths use to fan flames. Just like a bellows pumps air into fire, Bhastrika pumps prana (life force) into your body with forceful, rhythmic breaths that awaken energy, burn toxins, and ignite inner heat.

Sit tall, spine straight, hands on knees. Inhale deeply and forcefully through the nose. Exhale just as powerfully through the nose. Both inhalation and exhalation are active, vigorous and equal in force. Breath is rapid, but controlled—like blowing air in and out quickly and strongly.

Sitali

It's a yogic breathing technique designed to lower body heat, calm the mind, and soothe the nervous system.

Sit comfortably with your spine straight and shoulders relaxed. Stick your tongue out and curl the sides upward to form a tube. Inhale slowly through the curled tongue (or teeth), drawing in cool air. Close the mouth and exhale through the nose, slowly and smoothly.

Kapalbhati

It's a cleansing breathing technique meant to detoxify, energize and illuminate both body and mind. Sit in a comfortable meditative posture, spine straight . Take a deep breath in. Begin forceful exhalations by snapping the abdomen inward, as if you're trying to blow something out of your nose with energy. Let the inhalation happen naturally in between each pump.

AUTHOR'S NOTE

The balance of prana, tejas and ojas supports both physical and emotional well-being, as they are deeply interconnected. Adjusting lifestyle and diet to maintain this harmony enhances overall health and quality of life over time.

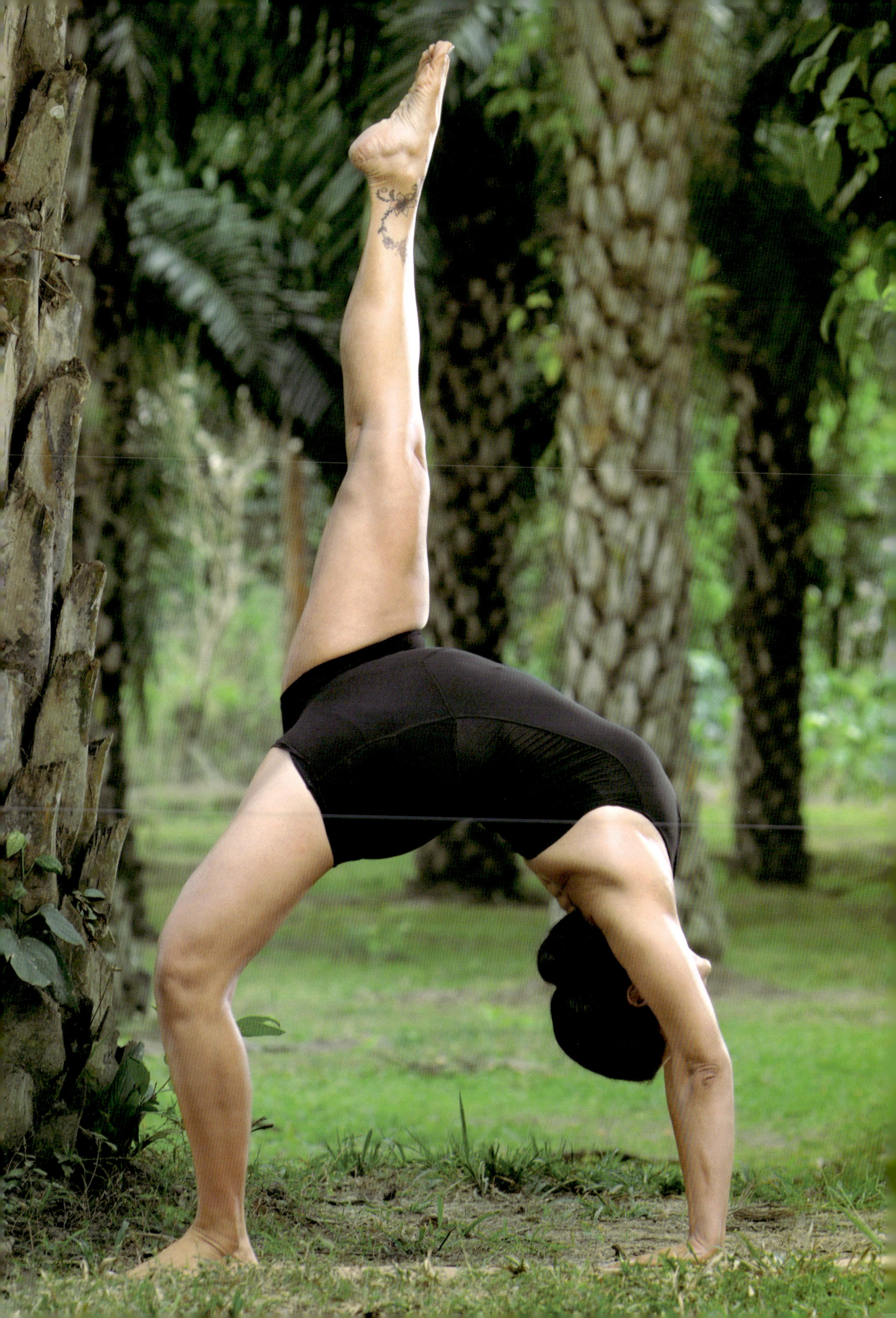

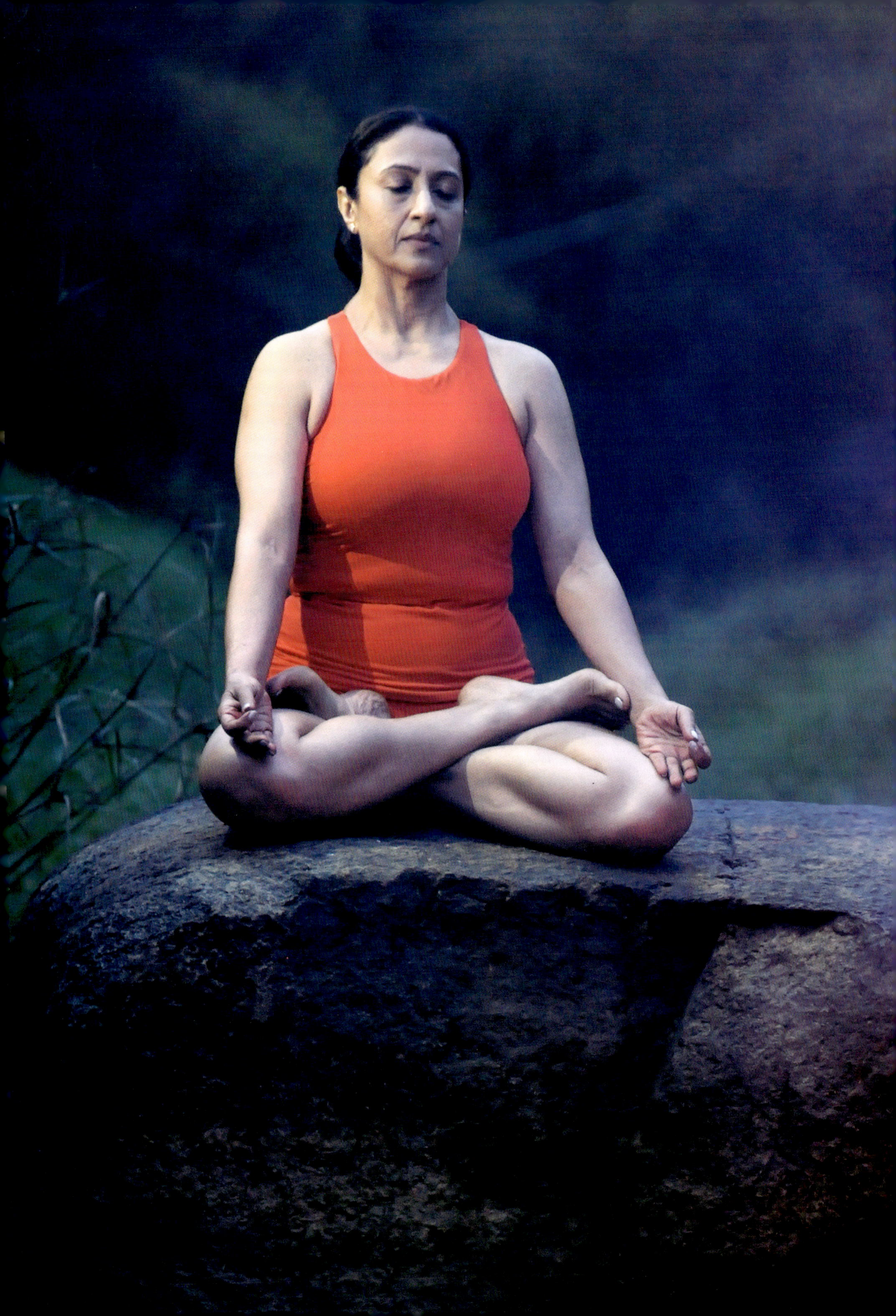

CHAPTER 6

AYURVEDA: BASICS

Ayurveda and yoga both originate from ancient Vedic philosophy and share a common understanding of health. While yoga aims to connect the individual self with the universal self, Ayurveda supports this journey by promoting yogic practices for physical, mental and spiritual well-being.

The origins of Ayurveda are considered divine knowledge. The word *ayus* means 'lifespan', while veda signifies 'sacred knowledge'. The ancient texts of Ayurveda contain therapeutic and healing wisdom in the form of shlokas. References to healing plants can be found across the Rig Veda, Sama Veda, Yajur Veda and Atharva Veda.

Ayurveda is the collective wisdom of ancient rishis and healers, eventually evolving into a structured medical science. Its foundational texts include *Charaka Samhita* (focuses on medicine and internal healing); *Sushruta Samhita* (covers the art and science of surgery); and *Ashtanga Hridaya* (a significant reference text integrating key Ayurvedic principles). These texts continue to guide Ayurvedic practices.

In Ayurveda, the Sapta Dhatus (seven bodily tissues) form the foundation of the human body. They are responsible for growth, development and overall well-being. These dhatus (as listed below) are nourished by food and undergo transformation through metabolic processes.

- *Rasa* (plasma/lymph): Provides nutrition and hydration to the body
- *Meda* (fat tissue): Maintains lubrication and energy storage
- *Rakta* (blood): Governs oxygenation, circulation and vitality
- *Asthi* (bone tissue): Gives structural support and strength to the body
- *Majja* (bone marrow and nervous tissue): Responsible for nerve function and immunity
- *Mamsa* (muscle tissue): Supports movement and strength
- *Shukra* (reproductive tissue): Essential for reproduction and vitality

In Ayurveda, optimal health is not just about nutrition and tissue formation but also about proper elimination, or *trimala*. The trimala constitutes essential by-products of metabolism; their proper elimination is crucial for maintaining dosha balance, digestion and overall well-being. Trimala includes:

- *Purisha*
- *Mutra*
- *Sweda*

Trimala is formed as a by-product of the body's metabolic and digestive processes. According to Ayurveda, an imbalance in the tridosha disrupts waste elimination, leading to toxin accumulation. This toxic buildup is known as ama—an undigested substance that clogs bodily channels. Other severe form of toxicity is *saama*.

AUTHOR'S NOTE

Ama is a toxic by-product of undigested food, disrupting the tridosha and trimala. It first manifests as digestive issues and, if or when not eliminated, spreads through the body, impairing various physiological functions.

When ama mixes with the doshas, dhatus and trimala, it creates a more severe, disease-causing state known as saama. This condition leads to inflammation, blockages and chronic illnesses.

Once the body successfully eliminates ama through digestion, detoxification or purification therapies, it reaches the state of nirama—restoring health and balance.

AYURVEDA AND DOSHA

Doshas form the foundation of Ayurvedic treatment:

- Vata dosha regulates cellular functions, electrolyte balance and waste elimination. Its imbalance increases dryness.
- Pitta dosha governs body temperature, optic nerve coordination and hunger and thirst regulation. It is aggravated by heat.
- Kapha dosha provides joint lubrication, and is influenced by sweat and fatty foods.

FOOD

Ayurveda does not focus on calories, fat or protein content but on how food influences consciousness and emotions. It views nourishment as a transformative force that affects both mind and body.

According to Ayurveda, the body is composed of five elements, as explained in Chapter 5: Prakriti and Dosha.

- **Prithvi:** Represented by bones, teeth and nails, these solid structures provide stability and support.
- **Jal:** Present throughout the body in the form of blood, lymph and other fluids, it ensures hydration and fluidity.
- **Agni:** This is the digestive energy residing in the belly.
- **Vayu:** This is the propelling force within the body, also centred in the belly.
- **Akasha:** This is the vast openness within the body that allows movement and interaction between elements.

FOOD AND LIFESTYLE

Ayurveda recommends that traditional foods, passed down through generations, are the best way to maintain prakriti in the body. The composition of food, along with the methods of preparation and consumption, plays a crucial role in well-being. Ayurveda also emphasizes the importance of timing, seasonal suitability and even the posture maintained while eating, as these factors influence digestion and overall health.

- **Seasonal food:** Eating according to the season keeps the body healthy and free from discomfort and disease. Food helps the body acclimatize with the changes in the

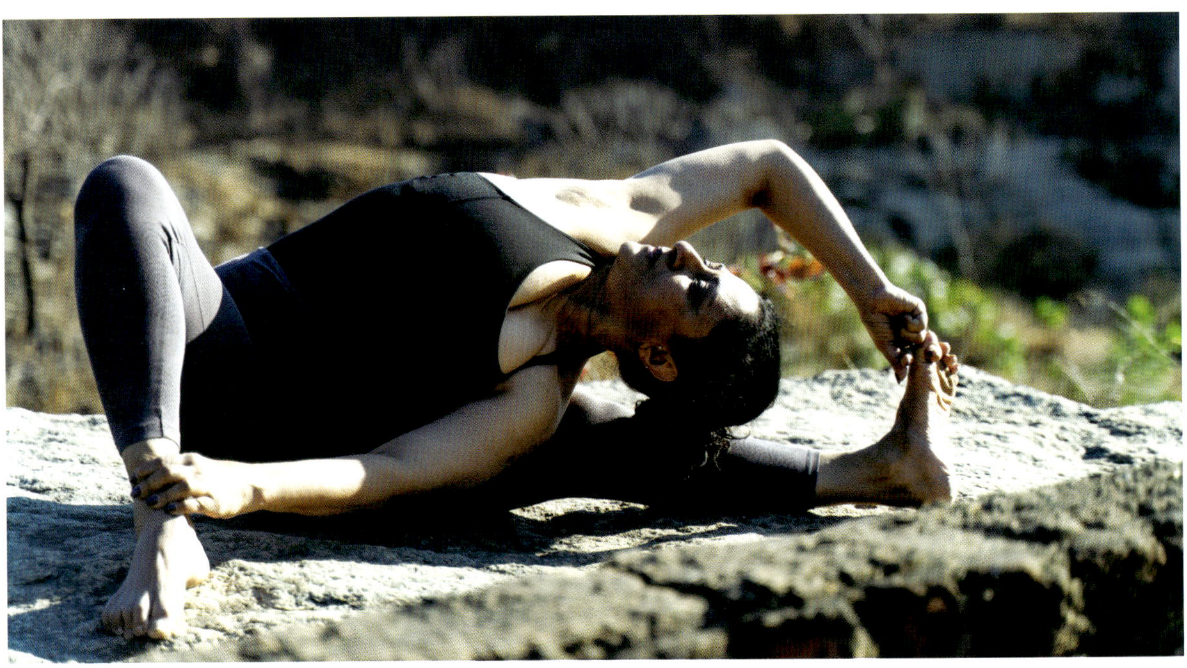

environment. Each season comes with its salient features and that has a direct impact on the body, especially the digestive system.

- **Eating food at the right time of the day:** To ensure proper digestion, it is important to eat food at the right time. The digestive system is at its peak functioning during the early hours of the day and it diminishes by the end of the day. Be mindful of what you consume during the day and have a light dinner preferably before 7.30 p.m. Help yourself to a glass of warm turmeric milk if you feel hungry before bedtime.
- **Food combinations:** It is important to be mindful of the combination of foods, as the digestive system is delicate. Certain combinations can affect the gut health and leave one feeling bloated.
- **Balanced diet:** A balanced diet is necessary for proper body growth and development. A balanced diet helps replenish the body with necessary nutrients, vitamins, amino acids, minerals, fat and carbohydrates for general well-being.

How Much and What to Eat

- **Vata:** Consuming five to six meals in small quantities throughout the day will be ideal. Sweet, salty, sour foods suit this body type.
- **Pitta:** Eating on time is important and so is not skipping breakfast. Three meals a day will be ideal. Sweet and bitter foods suit this body type. Spicy foods should be either consumed in moderation or completely avoided.
- **Kapha:** Having two meals a day, with a light breakfast, is sufficient. Spicy, bitter and astringent food items suit this body type. Cold food can be consumed in moderation or completely avoided.

In general, all body types should have only three-dish meal at a time. If the number of ingredients exceed, the body will have to produce different juices and acids to digest it. Raw foods has high pranic energy and is thus difficult to digest; Ayruveda recommends cooked food to help ease digestion.

Ideally, fruits should be consumed at least an hour before a meal or two hours after to optimize digestion and nutrient absorption. After lunch, lying on the right side for 30 minutes can aid digestion.

Beneficial Food Habits

- Having home-cooked nutritious food with locally grown ingredients is best for the body.
- Drinking warm water after 15 minutes of meals is ideal.
- For optimal digestion, eat in moderation, filling only half your stomach.
- Onion and garlic are heavy to digest, which can divert the body's energy towards processing the food and make it harder to maintain focus during practice of yoga.
- Food should be lukewarm. Consuming extremely hot food can overstimulate digestion, increasing inner heat and promoting a rajasik state.
- Freshly prepared food starts to lose its vitality and becomes harder to digest if the food is not consumed within three hours.
- Frozen food undergoes prolonged storage periods and low temperatures, all of which reduces its vitality, freshness and nutritional potency, making it heavier to digest and less nourishing for the body.
- Different cooking methods support dosha balance. Boiling and steaming suit Vata, adding warmth and moisture. Stir-frying and sautéing work for Pitta, preserving nutrients without excess heat. Grilling, roasting and baking help Kapha by reducing heaviness.
- Avoid eating cold foods/drinks, as they can weaken digestive fire.
- Avoid consuming alcohol, tea or coffee with meals, as these interfere with the digestive process.

- Avoid reheating food too many times; every time the food is reheated, it becomes more toxic.

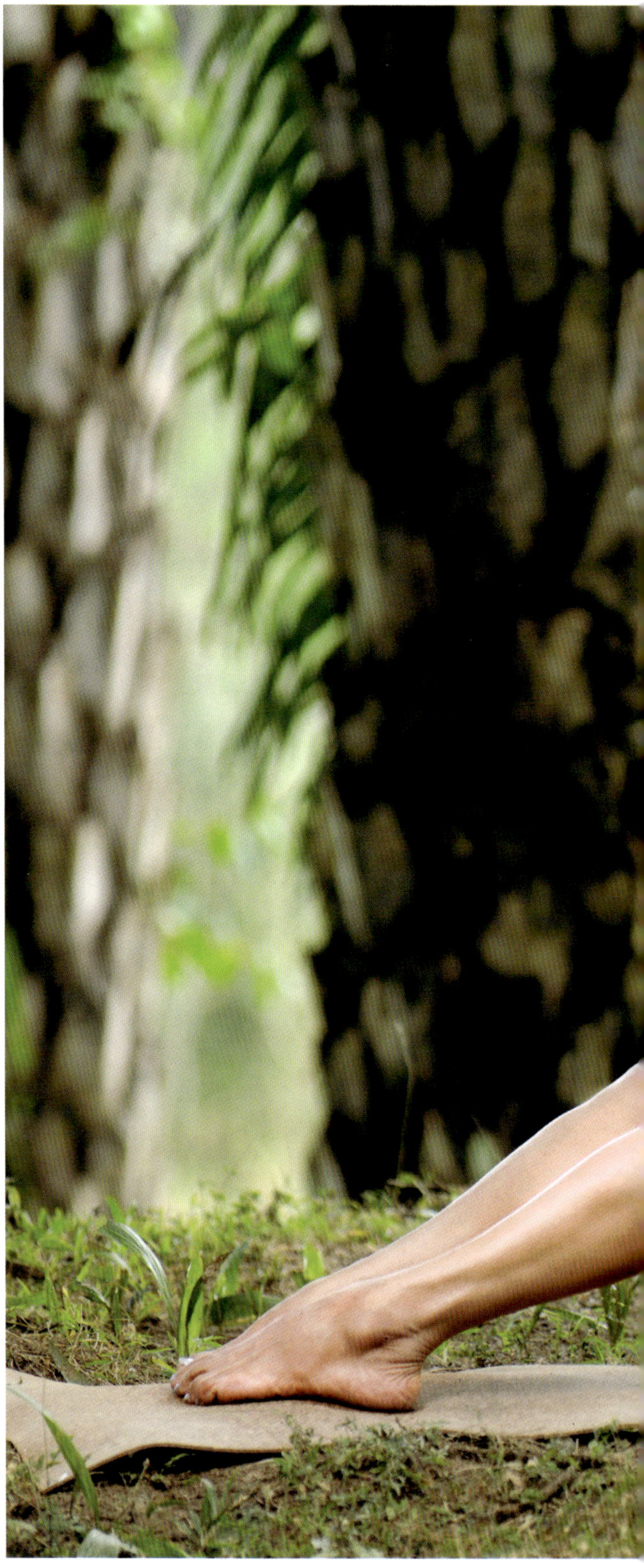

UNDERSTANDING RASA

In Ayurveda, rasa is a fundamental concept that goes beyond just taste—it represents the essence of food, medicine, and even life experiences. While being mindful of the food habits that should be avoided, it should also be known how each rasa has specific effects on the body and mind, influencing digestion, doshas and overall well-being.

- Sweet: Grains, wholewheat pasta, bread, sweet potatoes, yam, all starchy vegetables, carrots, pumpkins, avocados, all meats, eggs, soya bean, cashew, walnuts, almonds, milk butter
- Salty: Soya sauce, pickled and salted preserved foods
- Sour: Citrus fruits, tomatoes, yoghurt, fermented and/or pickled foods, vinegar
- Pungent/spicy : Chillies, ginger, black pepper, onions, garlic, cinnamon
- Bitter: Grape fruit, bitter melon, most leafy vegetables
- Astringent: Cauliflower, broccoli, mushrooms, olives, cabbages, asparagus, olive oil, legumes.

AUTHOR'S NOTE

The best way to plan a healthy diet is to consult an Ayurvedic doctor who can recommend foods after analysing your dosha.

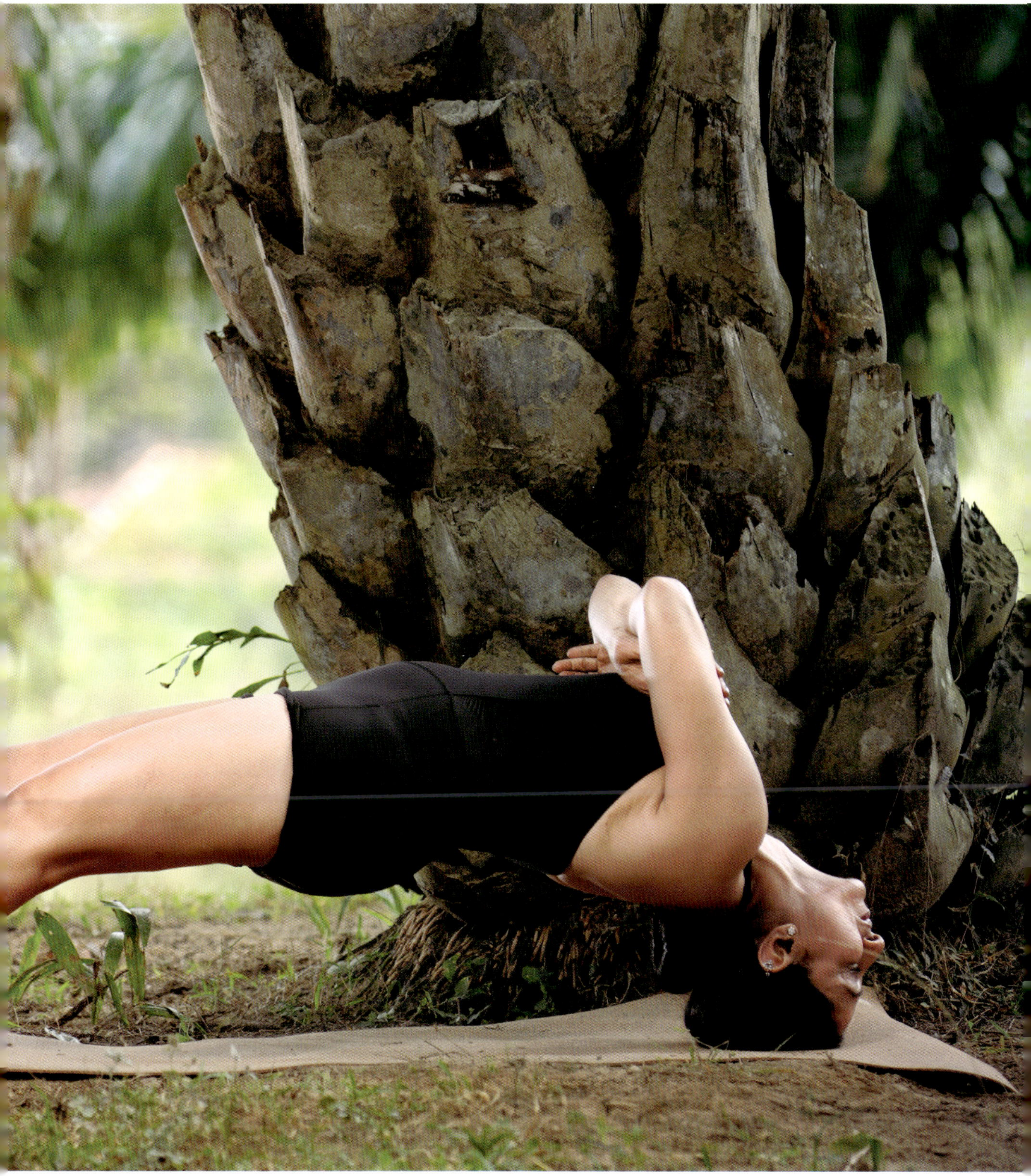

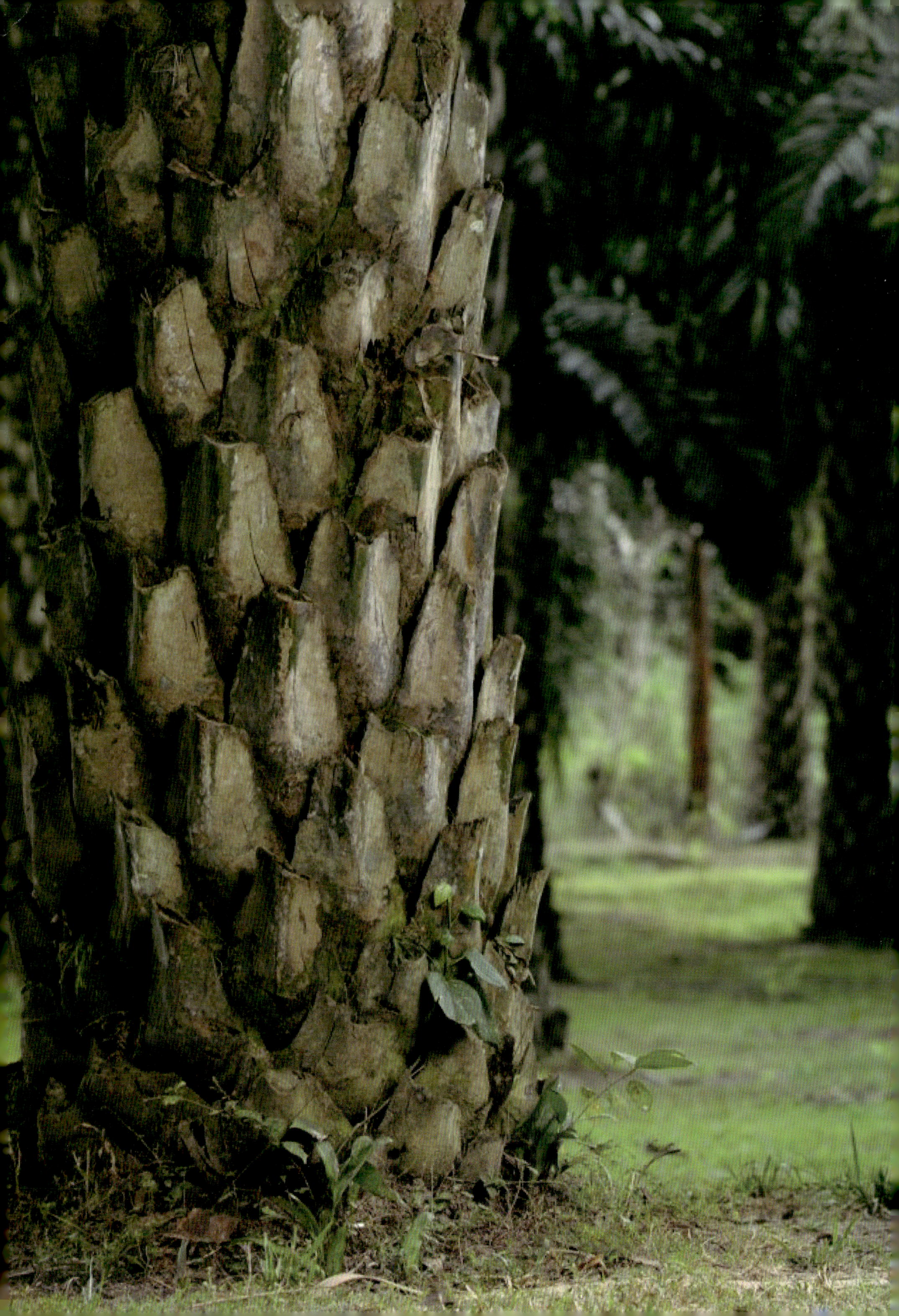

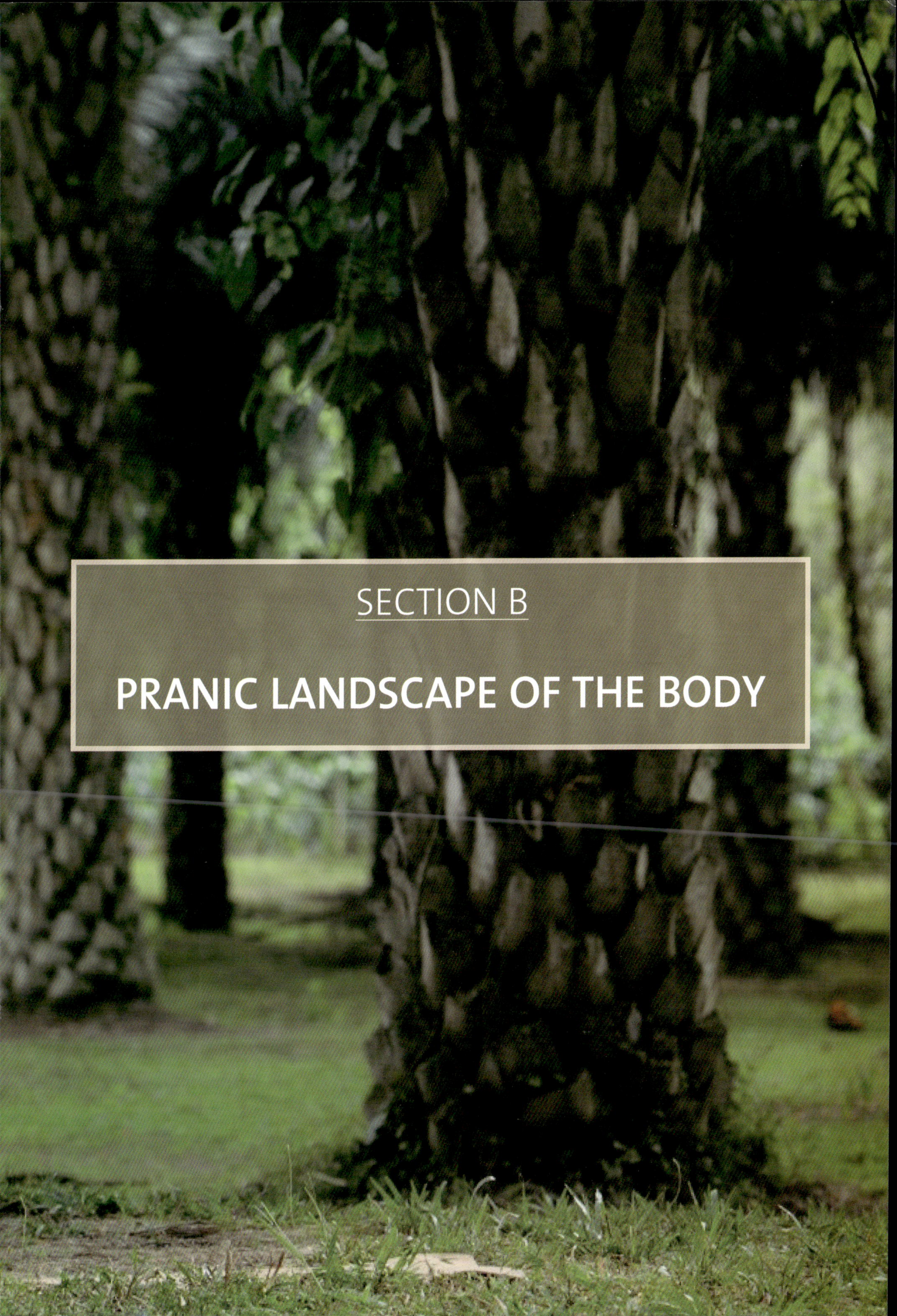

SECTION B

PRANIC LANDSCAPE OF THE BODY

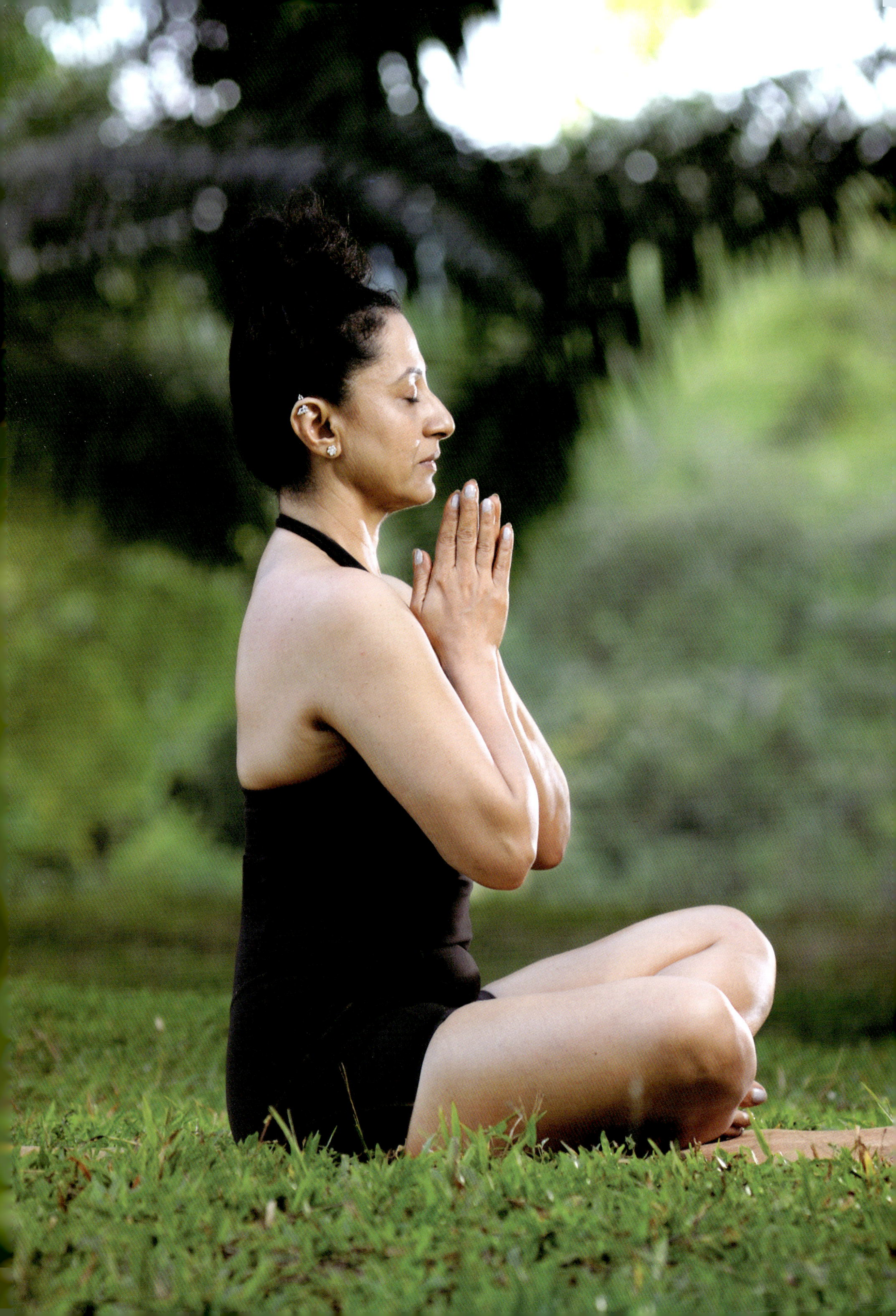

CHAPTER 7

SUKSHMA SHARIRA

In yoga and Vedantic philosophy, the sukshma sharira, or the subtle body, is the bridge between the gross physical body and the causal body. It consists of pranamaya kosha, manomaya kosha and vijnanamaya kosha.

Yoga plays a vital role in purifying, strengthening and harmonizing the sukshma sharira. It cultivates deep awareness and keen observation, allowing practitioners to connect with and understand their bodies from within. The prescribed way to achieve this is by observing the flow of breath and its interactions with the internal scene of the body. Two main opposing energies are at play during the process of breathing: prana (the inward moving air) and apana (outward moving air). These are the foundation for all the life force that exists in the universe.

The word *prana* was first found in *Chhandogya Upanishad*. It was further studied and developed in the texts of Ayurveda and Hatha Yoga. This energy is flowing around us and inside us. Breath is considered as the most subtle force of prana. It plays a crucial role in regulating physical functions like respiration, cellular growth, circulation, digestion, reproduction, etc. Prana energy is also responsible for thoughts and emotions. Prana comes into the body not only by breath but also by the food we eat.

Within the context of yoga asanas, it is important to synchronize breathing along with the movement of the body. While building a posture, different parts of the body are engaged with a focus on both stability and fluidity. Asanas create new positions and spaces for prana to flow, expanding both body and mind, promoting health, and enhancing alertness. The knowledge of how this sensitive life force moves helps accelerate the body's inborn ability to heal and stay healthy.

VAYUS OF THE PRANIC BODY

Vayu is the force that moves prana, or life energy, through the pranamaya kosha, or pranic body. In yogic tradition, there are five primary vayus, each responsible for regulating everything from respiration and digestion to circulation and mental clarity.

- Prana Vayu
- Apana Vayu
- Samana Vayu
- Udana Vayu
- Vyana Vayu

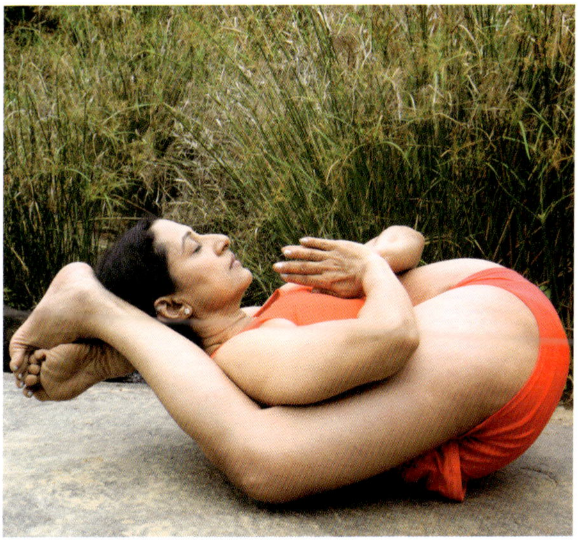

PRANA VAYU

Prana is drawn from everything we consume—air, food, water, sunlight, and even space. When the body efficiently absorbs these universal elements, it generates prana, the most essential energy for life.

Imagine prana as an invisible power source, and the nadis, or the energy channels, as the wiring system that carries it throughout the body.

Physical Level

- Prana vayu resides in the chest region.
- It is the energy moving inwards.
- It governs breathing and absorption, enabling us to take in air, food, sensory experiences and thoughts.
- It generates energy, motivation and vitality.
- The organs that are activated by prana vayu are heart and lungs.

Subtle Level

- Prana vayu influences emotions by receiving sensory input, transmitting it to the brain, and generating a mental response.
- It gives heightened sensitivity both to the external senses and inner awareness.
- It allows clarity to see the world in all its possibilities.

Spiritual Level

- The prana vayu calms, stabilizes and balances the mind. Mastering this prana is like controlling the senses like a charioteer controls the horse. When prana vayu is not strong on a spiritual level, the person feels lost and distracted.

Imbalanced Prana Vayu

- When the prana vayu is faulty, the person suffers from cravings, with increased tendencies of falling prey to bad habits.
- On a physical level, ailments like chest infections, common cold, low energy, flu, bronchitis, etc., are indications of a weak prana vayu.
- On a mental level, when prana vayu is strong, tasks requiring mental and emotional stability do not seem tough. When weak, the body and mind feel tired.
- On a spiritual level, weak prana vayu leads to lethargy and lack of clarity.

Asana Practice to Increase the Power of the Prana Vayu

The Hatha Yoga practices mentioned below will help enhance the balance and function of prana vayu. The asanas targeted here supports the intake of prana and helps maximize the effectiveness of the pranayama by strengthening, aligning and activating the upper body.

- Most of the asanas target expanding of the chest to enable deep breathing.
- The asanas to be held in a comfortable stretch for five breaths.
- Focus on the inhalation while keeping the mind calm and stress-free.
- Overstretching can limit the natural flow of breath.

Standing Asanas

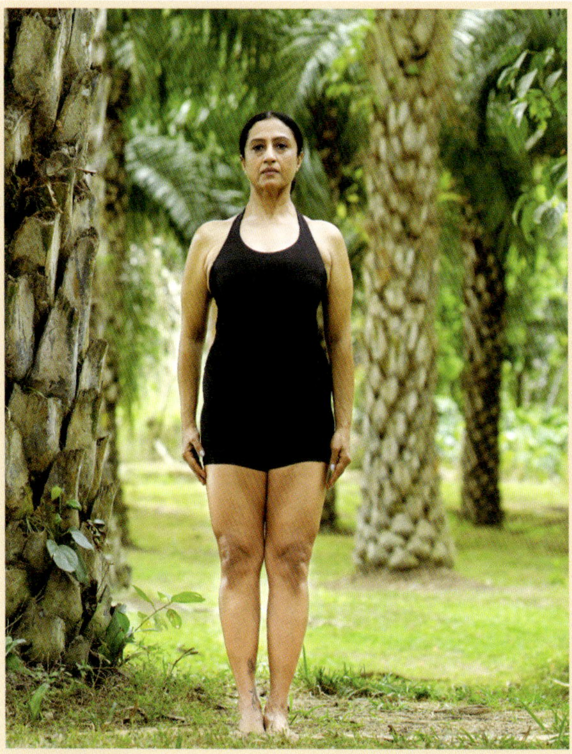

TADASANA

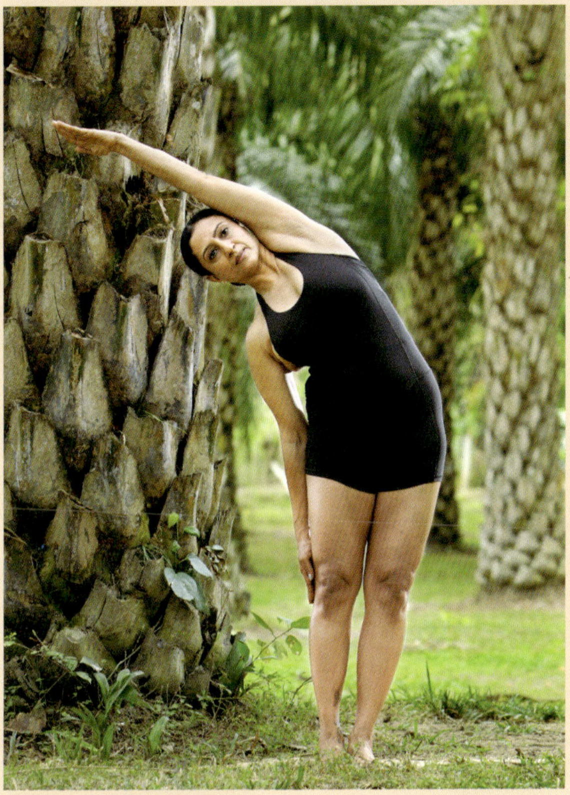

ARDHAKATI TADASANA

SURYA NAMASKARA A (FOR REFERENCE, SEE PP. 4–5)

SURYA NAMASKARA B (FOR REFERENCE, SEE PP. 6–8)

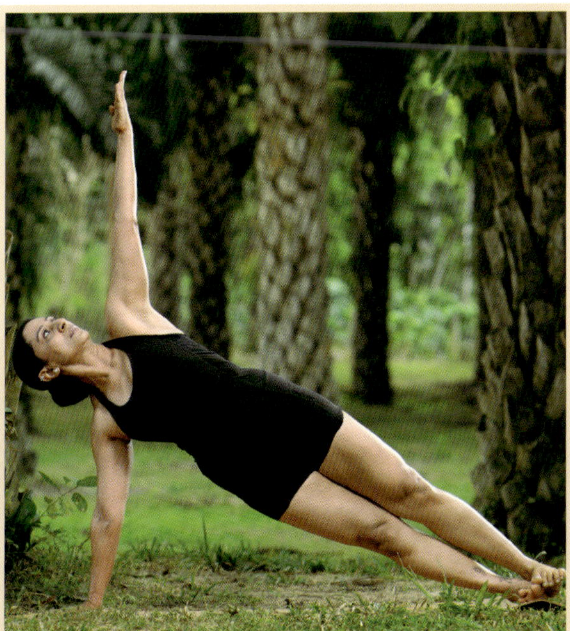

VASHISHTHASANA

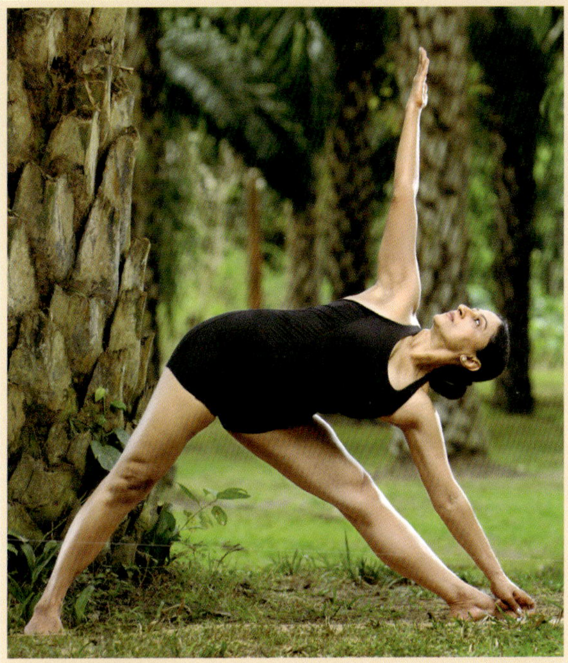

TRIKONASANA

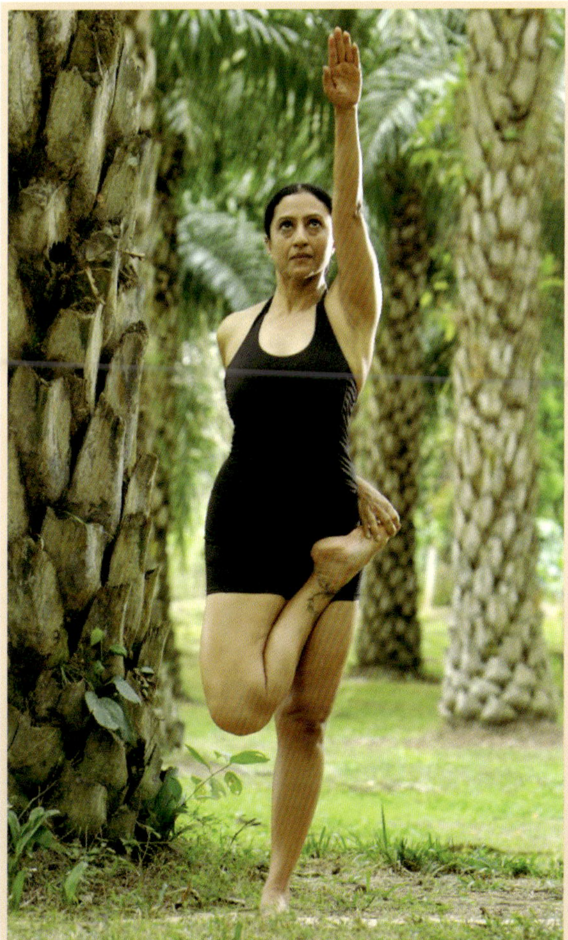

EKAPADA PADMASANA

Sitting Asanas

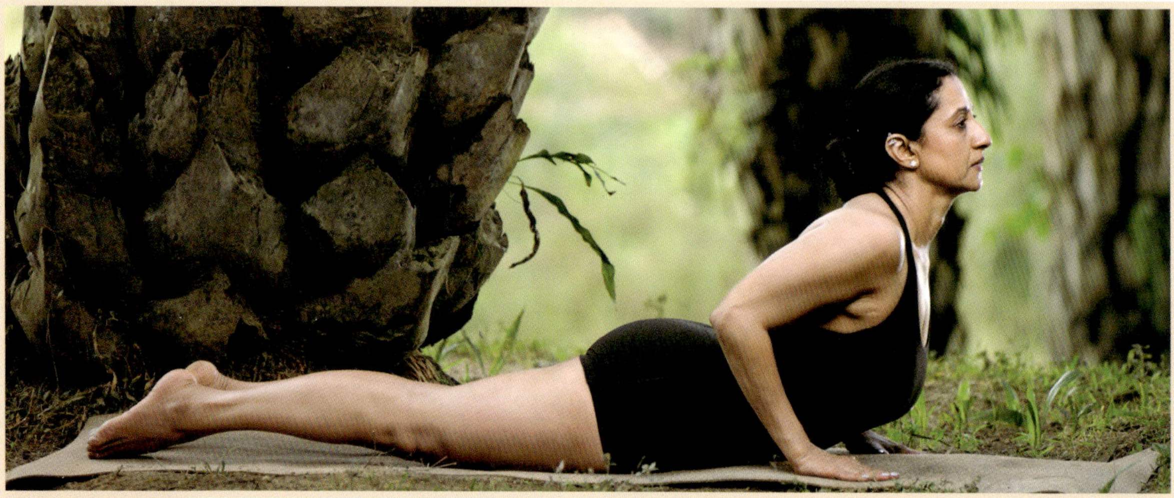
BHUJANGASANA

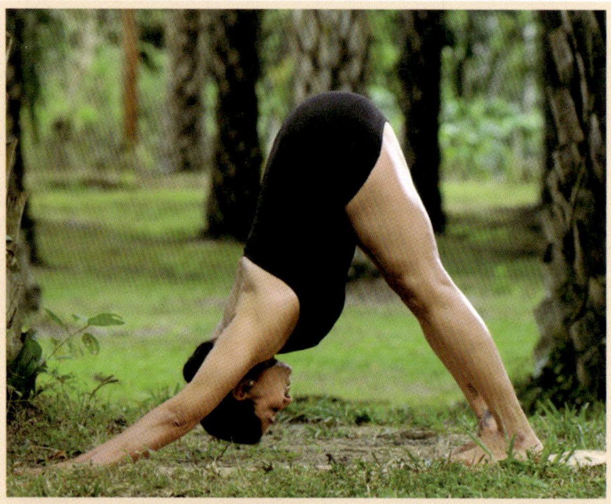
ADHO MUKHA SVANASANA

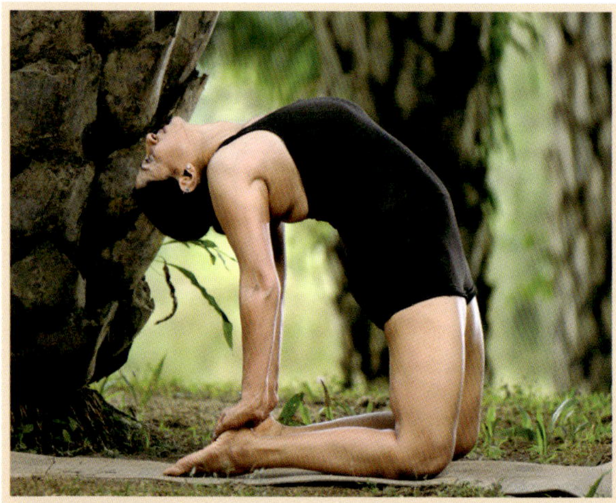
USHTRASANA

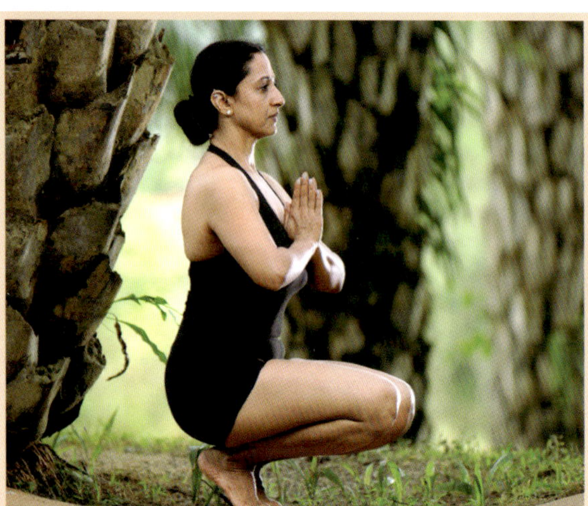
BHADRASANA

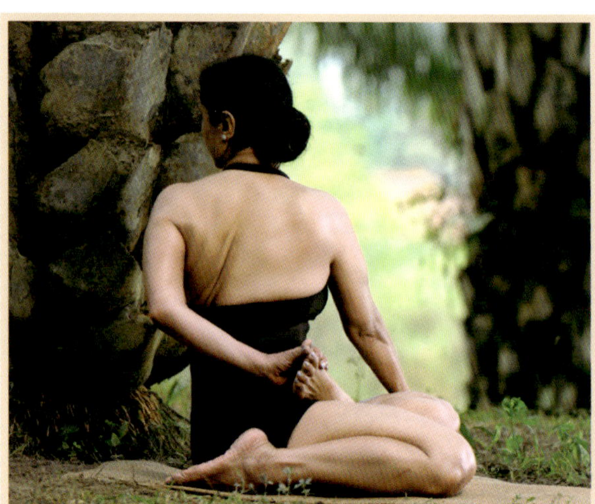
BHARADWAJASANA

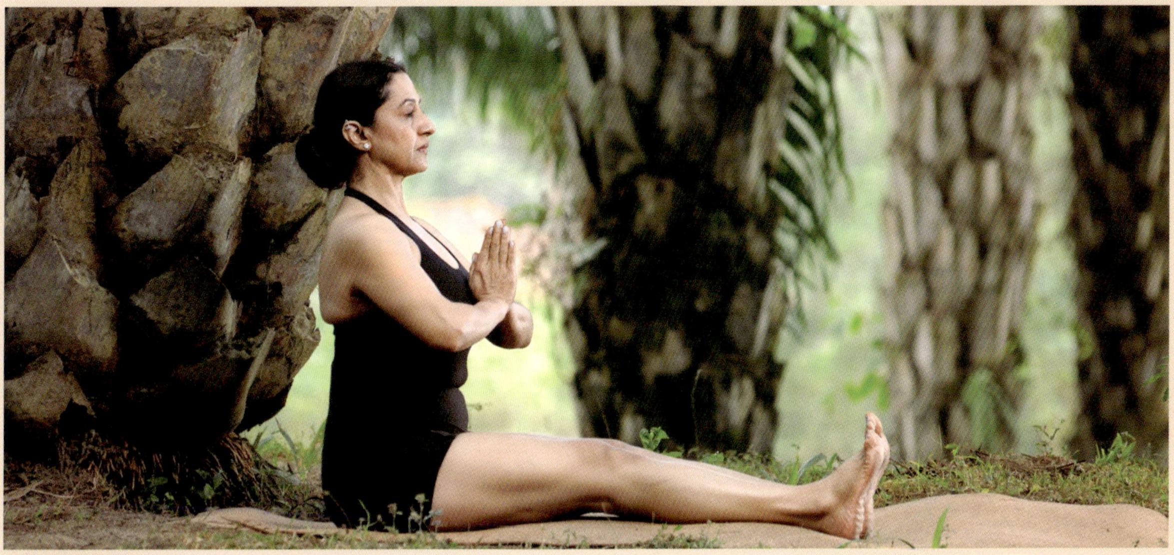

DANDASANA

Floor Asanas

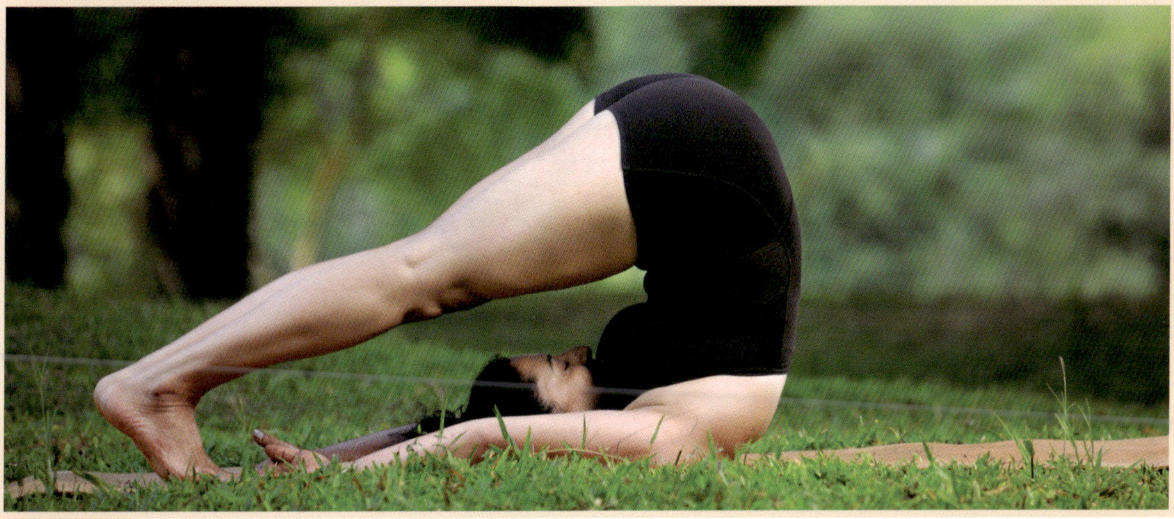

HALASANA

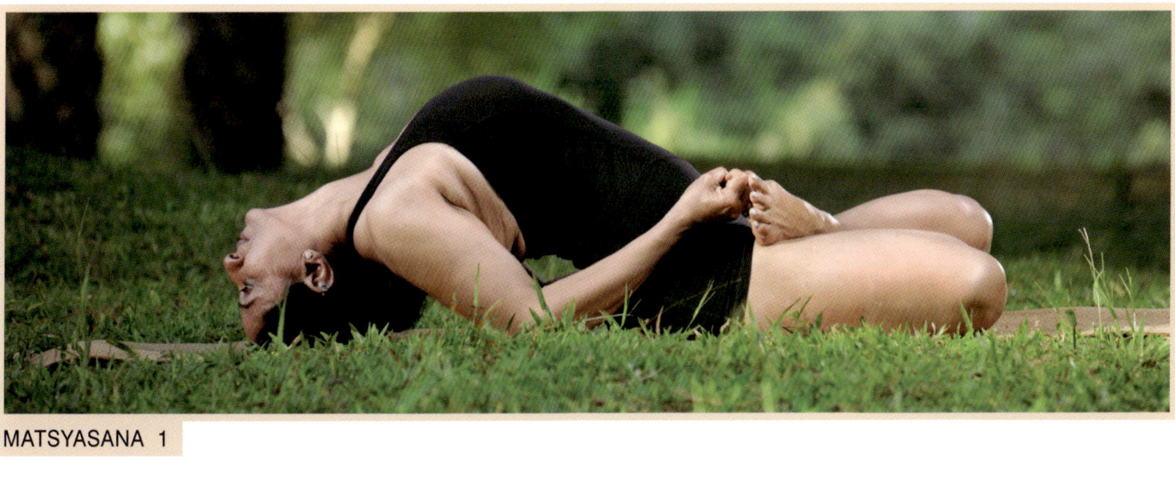

MATSYASANA 1

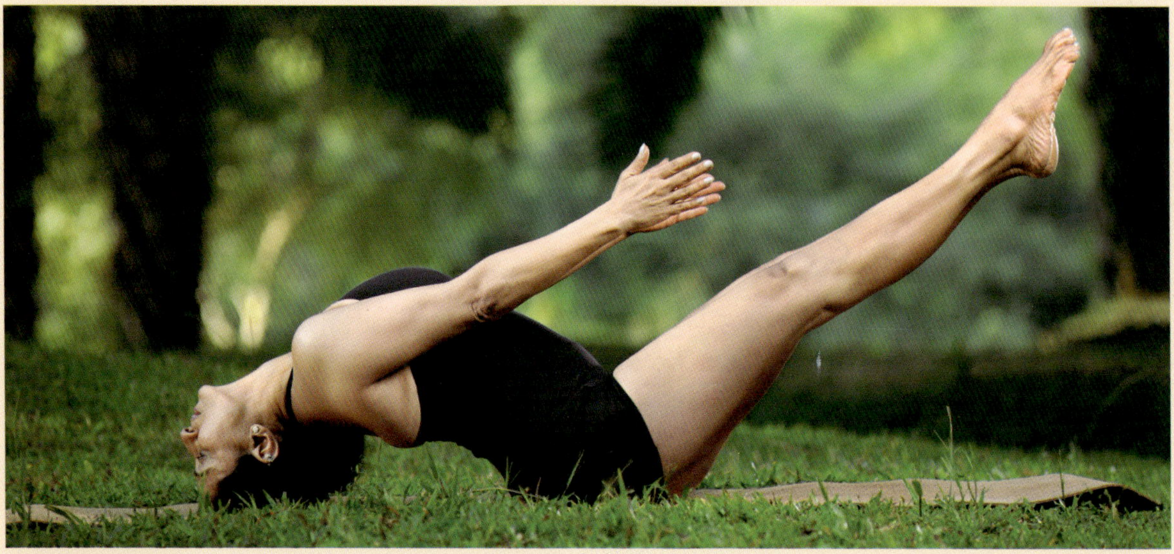

MATSYASANA 2

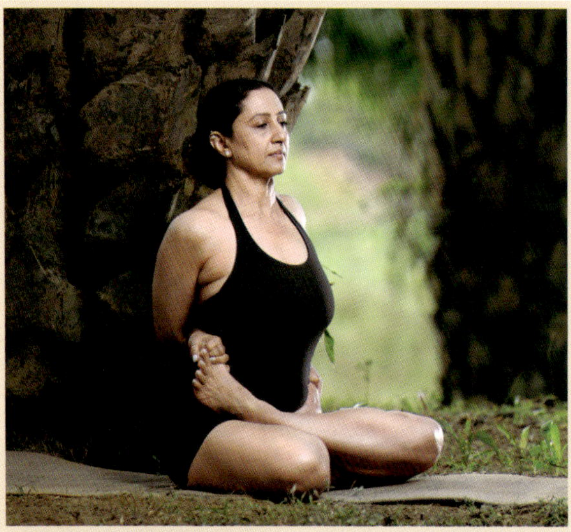

BADDHA PADMASANA 1

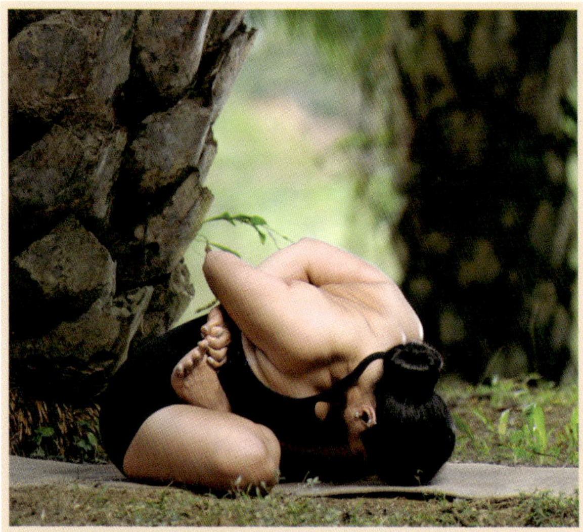

BADDHA PADMASANA 2

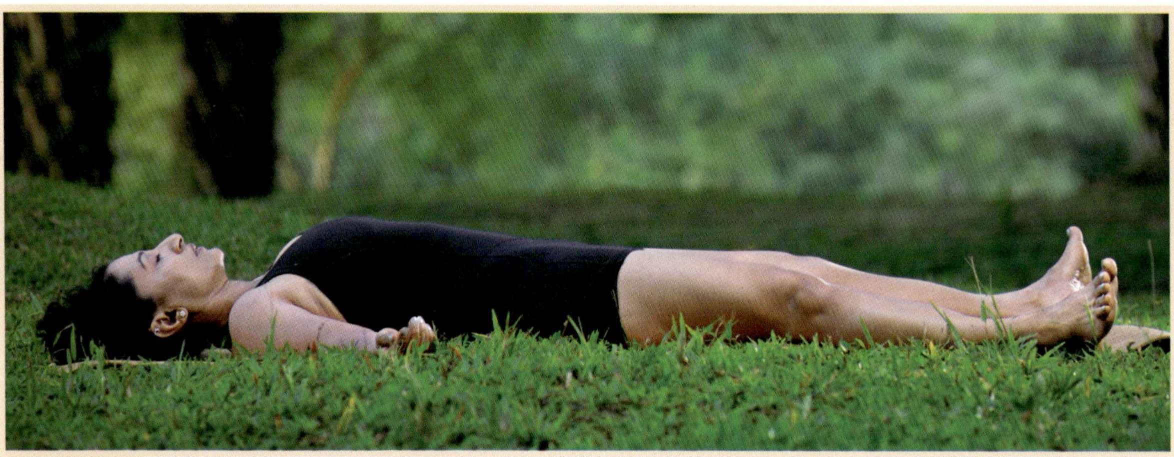

SHAVASANA

Pranayama

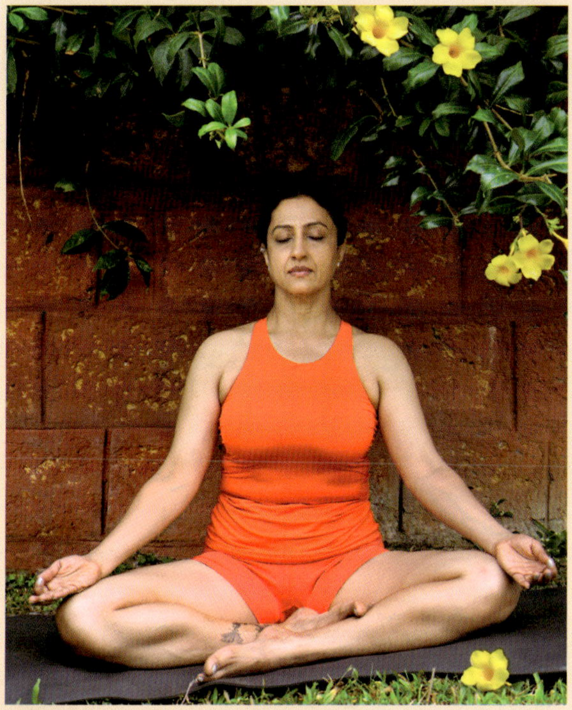

UJJAYI (WITH ANTAR KUMBHAKA)

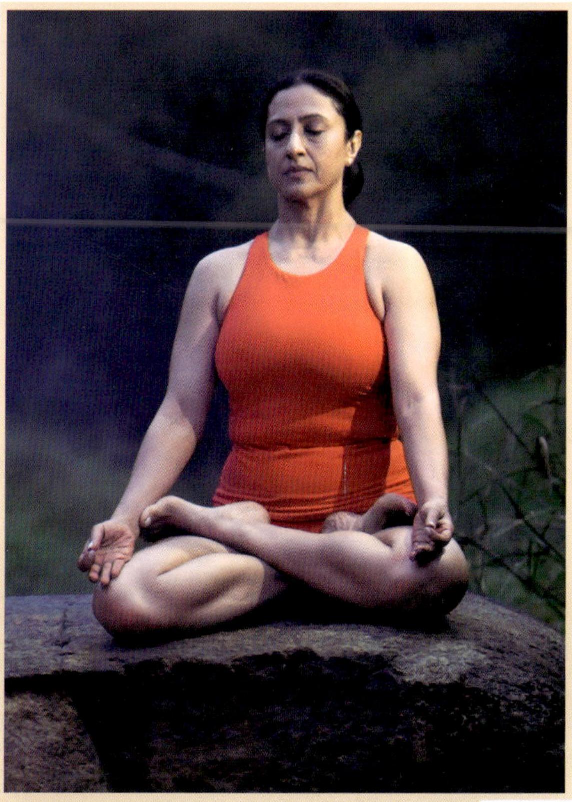

BHASTRIK (RAPID AND STRONG INHALATION AND EXHALATION)

Mudra

Hold Prana Mudra in both hands and visualize a vast, open space filled with fresh air—such as a meadow, seashore, or endless sky—expanding infinitely around you.

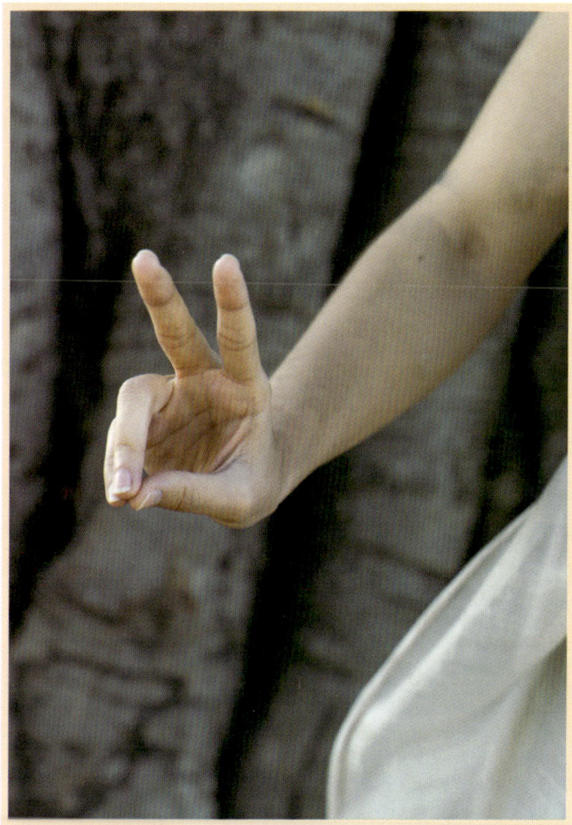

PRANA MUDRA

APANA VAYU

Apana vayu is situated in the region below the navel, close to the pelvic floor, and its energies pervade the lower abdomen. It directs the downward-flowing energy, nourishing the organs of digestion, reproduction, menstruation and elimination.

Apana vayu governs the elimination process in the body, like elimination of carbon dioxide, carbon monoxide, urine, sweat, stool, etc. It provides energy for kidneys, intestines and genitals. It activates all the waste disposal units of the body and governs the outward flow of energy in the body.

Physical Level

- Apana vayu supports the immune system by continuously cleansing the body, eliminating toxins, and removing harmful elements.
- It resides in the Muladhara Chakra. It provides grounding and stability, creating a strong foundation for a healthy body and a positive mindset.

Subtle Level

- Apana vayu has the power to eliminate the unwanted impressions that the mind creates from day-to-day circumstances and experiences.
- A strong apana vayu enhances physical strength, supports a healthy body by efficiently eliminating toxins, and fosters a positive mindset.
- Once a calm mind is established, focus follows next.

Spiritual Level

- Apana vayu is responsible to release waste and stagnant energy from the body. It has the power to release the energy which no longer serves, and to make space for new energy which is crucial for spiritual growth.

Imbalanced Apana Vayu

- When the apana vayu is weak, the body will face pain and discomfort due to air lock and excess vata dosha.
- When the apana vayu is overactive, the body suffers indigestion in the form of frequent urination or diarrhoea.

Yoga Sequence to Increase the Power of Apana Vayu

A structured Hatha Yoga practice helps regulate and direct apana vayu. The asanas in this sequence activate apana yayu in the pelvis, allowing it to move freely and be redistributed throughout the body.

The engagement of apana vayu is linked to Mula Bandha. Physically, Mula Bandha is a gentle activation of the lower belly, but it should not be confused with simply tightening the sphincter muscles. Instead, it is a subtle yet controlled lift that supports energy flow, helping to conserve and redirect apana vayu effectively. If practised regularly, it is possible to redirect this energy to access deeper and higher planes of awareness.

Focusing on asanas that target and compress lower abdomen is effective for apana vayu.

- The asanas should start with standing poses.
- The asanas mentioned in the mini-sequence mainly target pelvic alignment.
- Standing asanas energize the pelvic floor along with legs that root the pose to the ground, directing apana vayu into the construction and geometry of the asanas.
- Sitting asanas stabilize the apana vayu, engaging it at a deeper level.
- Forward-bending asanas and backward-bending asanas performed in a combination release apana vayu and allows smooth flow of energy from the root up to the spine.
- While performing each asana, actively engage the legs, then the pelvic floor, and finally the lower belly. This alignment helps channel and maximize the energy of apana vayu.

MULA BANDHA

Mula Bandha is the activation of an internal energy lock (bandha). Many people think it is simply clenching the sphincter muscle, but it actually involves lifting and engaging the entire pelvic floor, including the urogenital muscles and anal sphincters.

At a muscular level, Mula Bandha feels like a gentle lift in the lower belly rather than just squeezing the sphincter. This subtle hold helps energy move freely, conserving and redirecting apana vayu. With regular practice, it can enhance awareness and deepen concentration.

To properly control apana vayu, another gentle lock deep in the lower belly should be engaged. This prevents excessive clenching and allows energy to flow smoothly.

Do not practise Mula Bandha during menstruation. It is also to be avoided when suffering from indigestion.

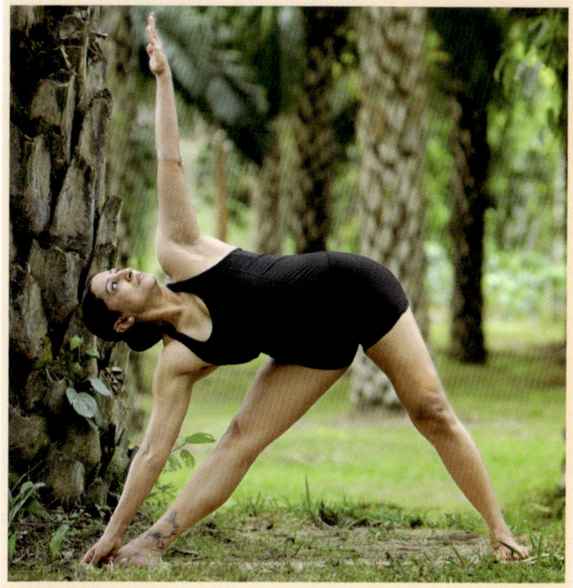

TRIKONASANA

Standing Asanas

SURYA NAMASKARA A (FOR REFERENCE, SEE PP. 4–5)

SURYA NAMASKARA B (FOR REFERENCE, SEE PP. 6–8)

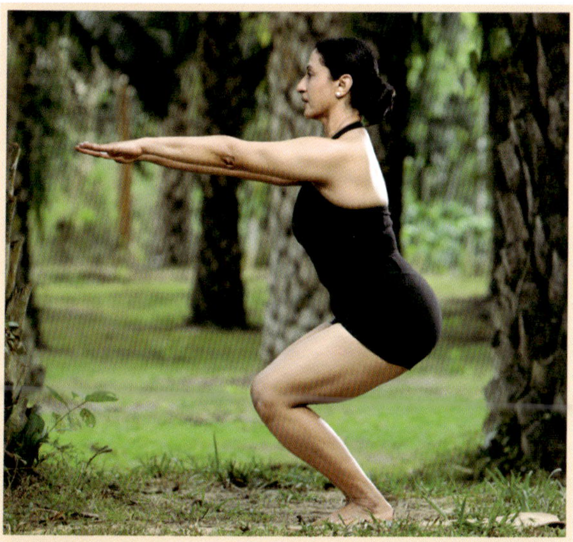

UTKATTASANA

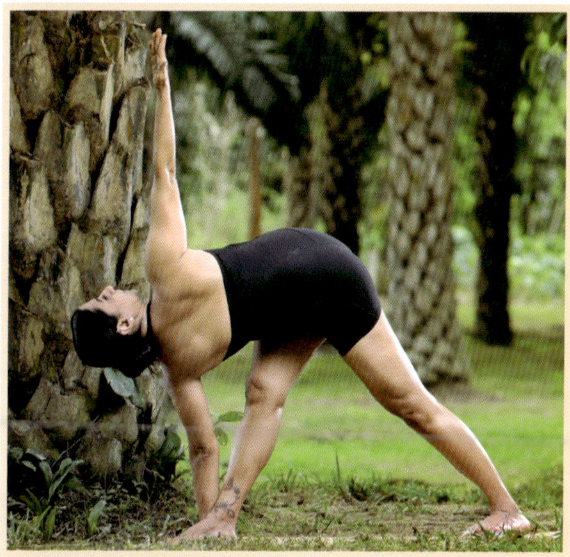

PARIVRITI TRIKONASANA

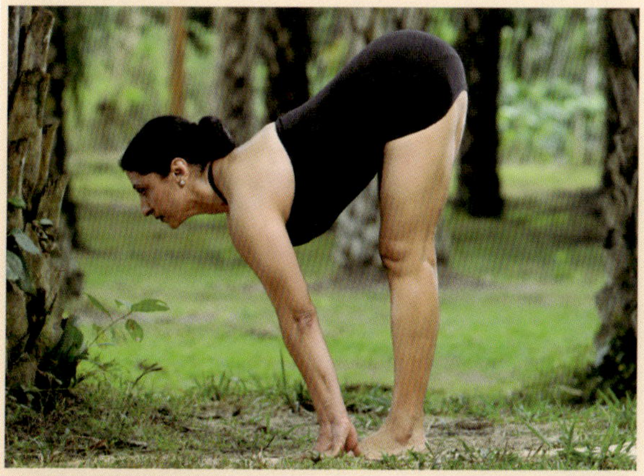

HASTAPADASANA

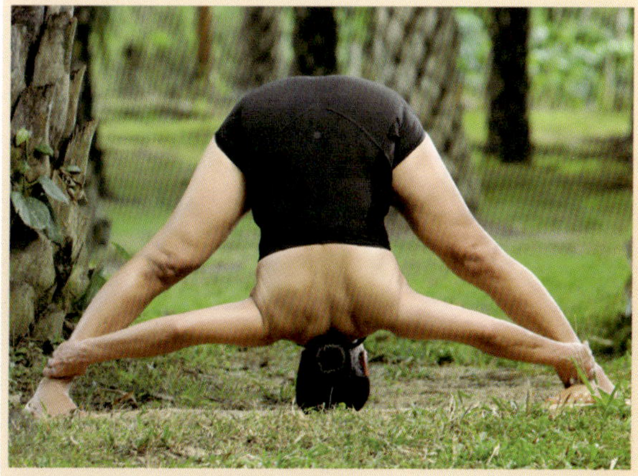

PRASARITA PADOTTANASANA

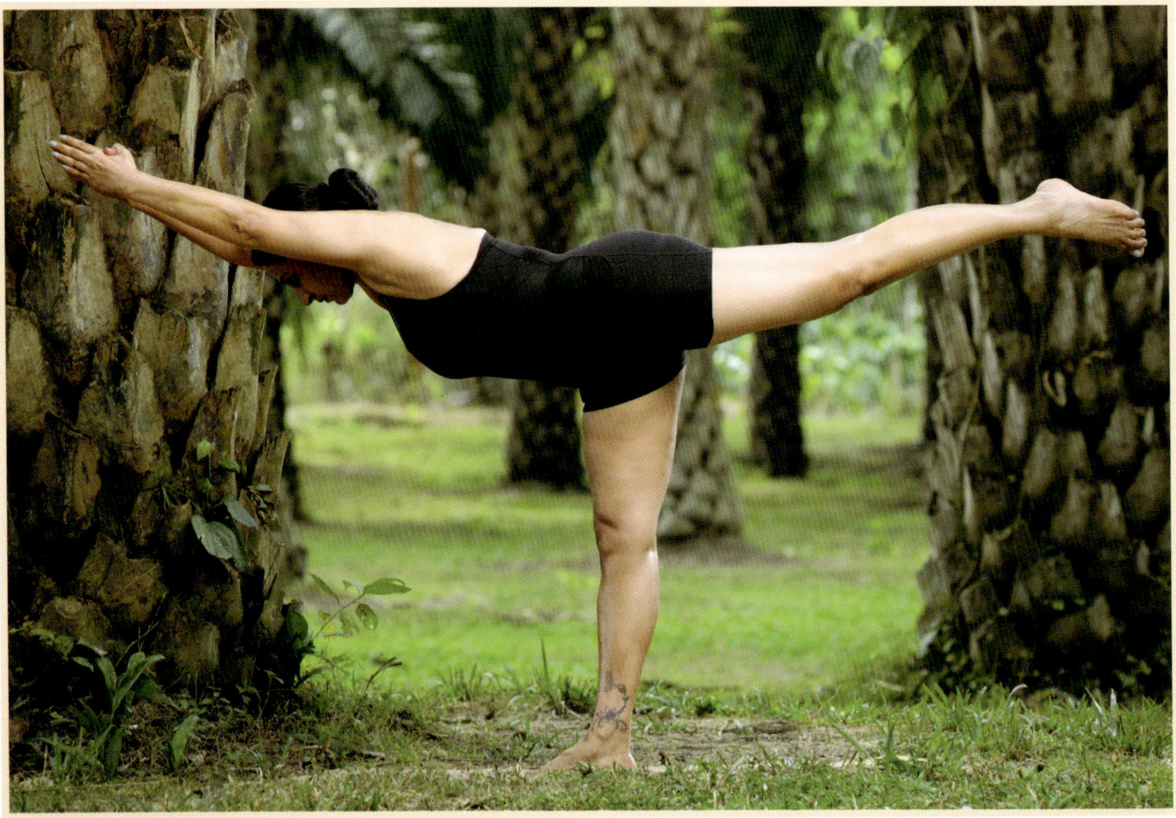

VEERABHADRASANA

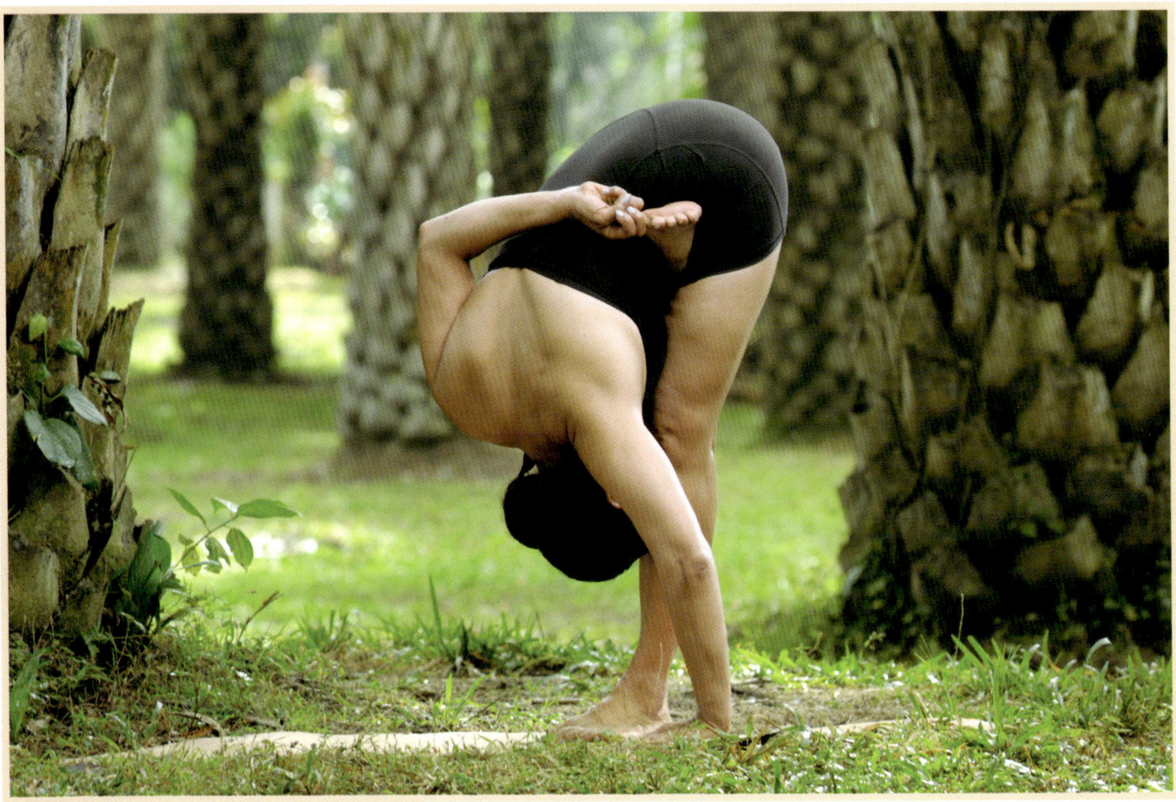

BADDHA PADMA PADANGUSHTHASANA

Sitting Asanas

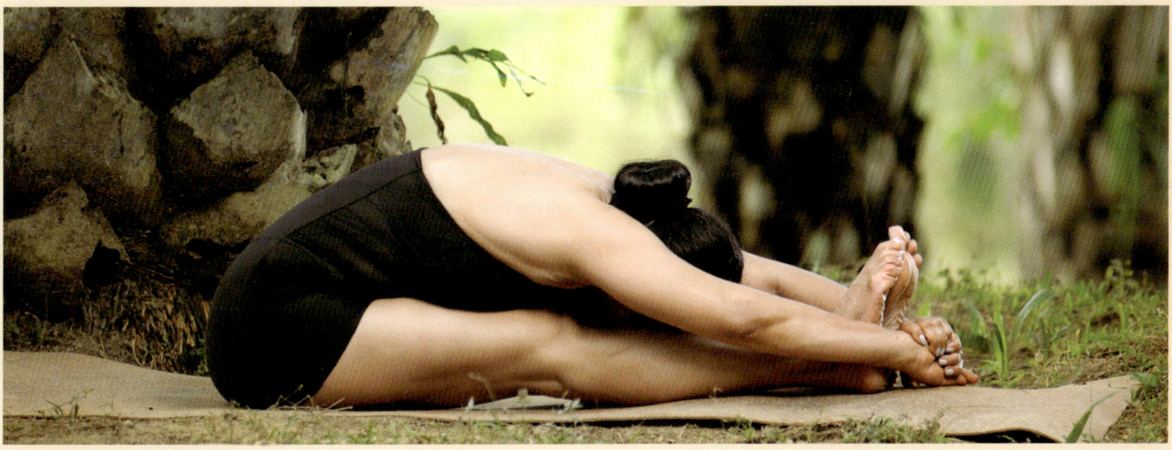

PASCHIMOTTANASANA

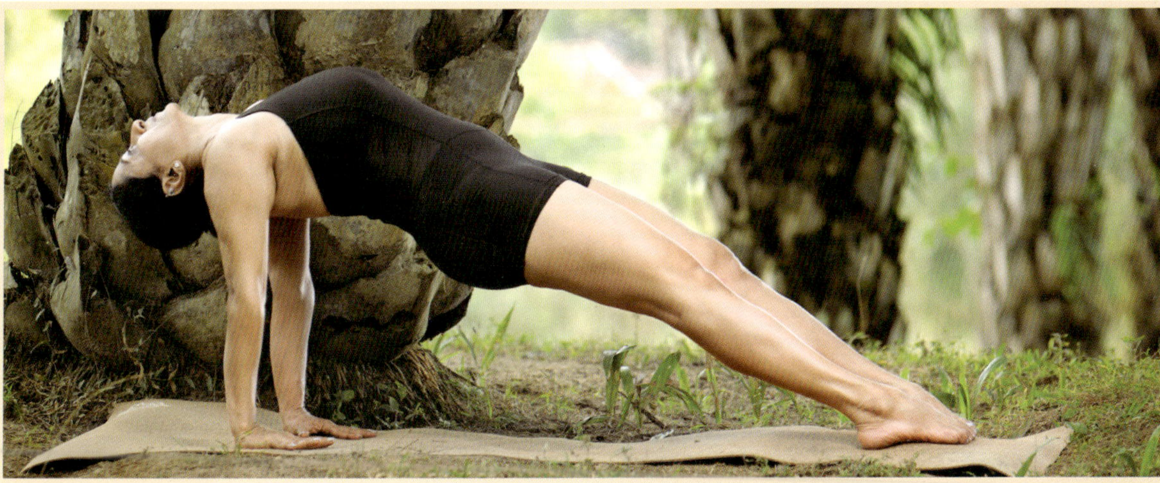

PURVOTTANASANA

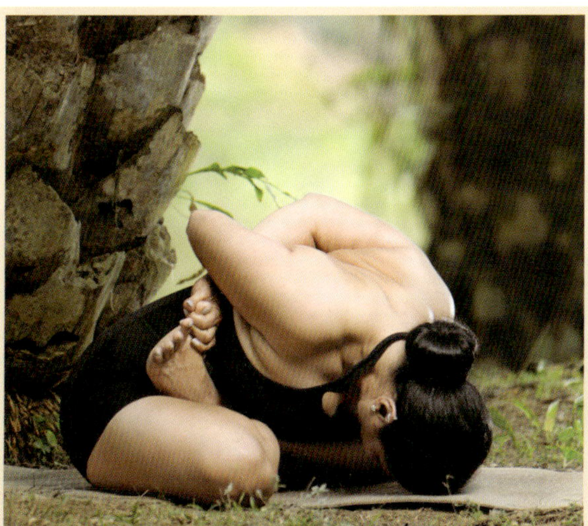

ARDHA BADDHA PASCHIMOTTANASANA

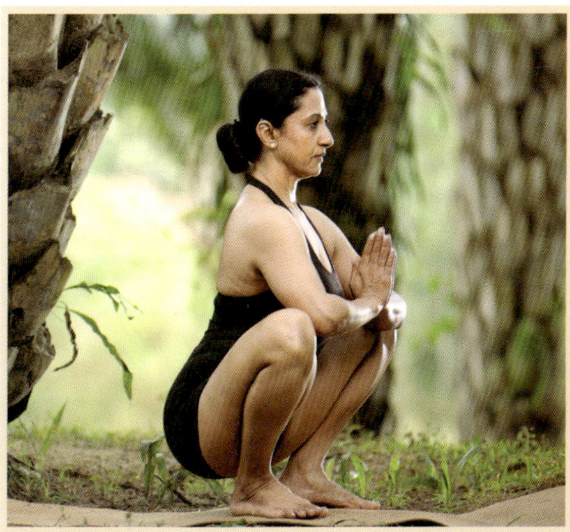

MALASANA

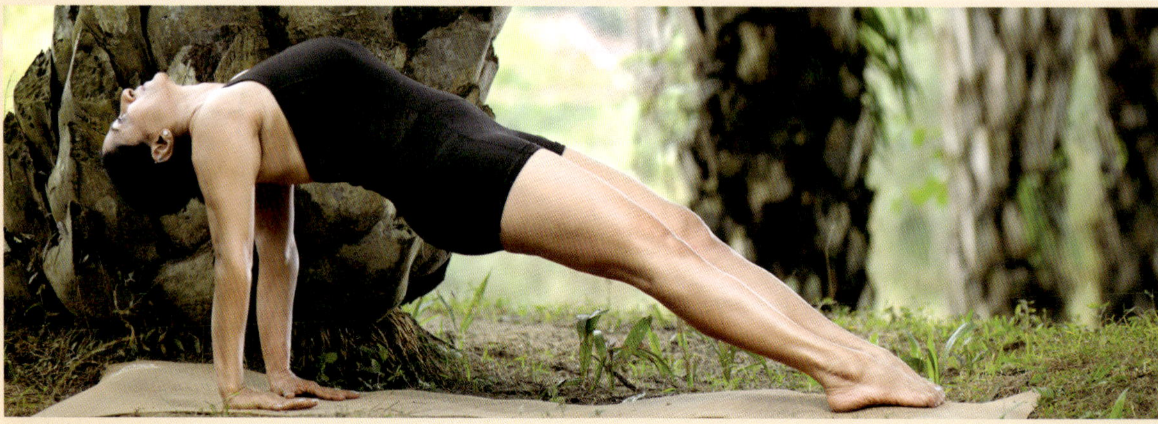

MARICHASANA 1

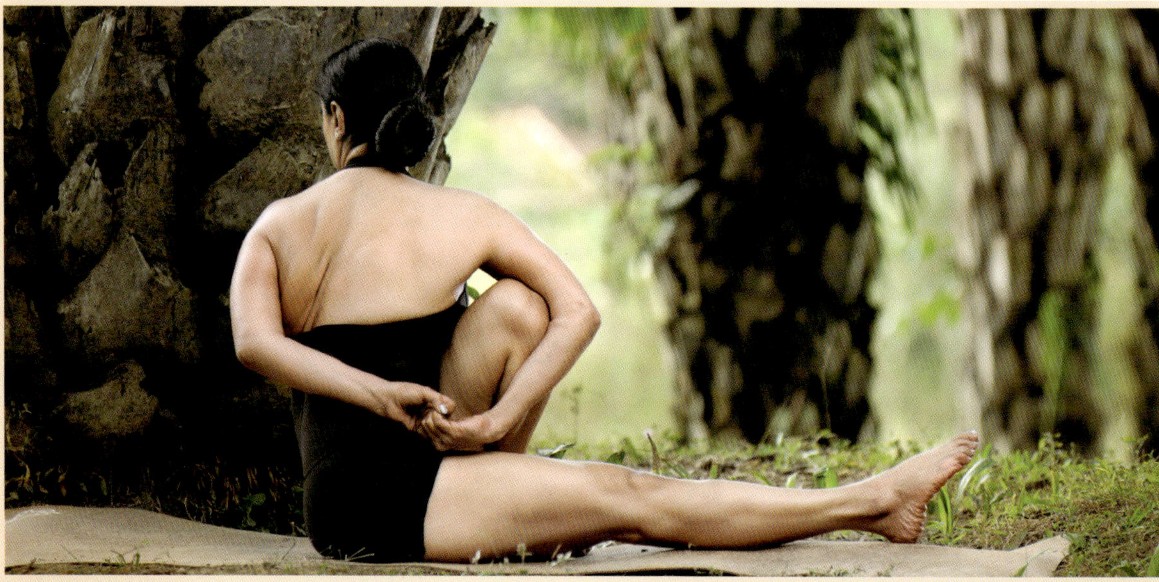

MARICHASANA 2

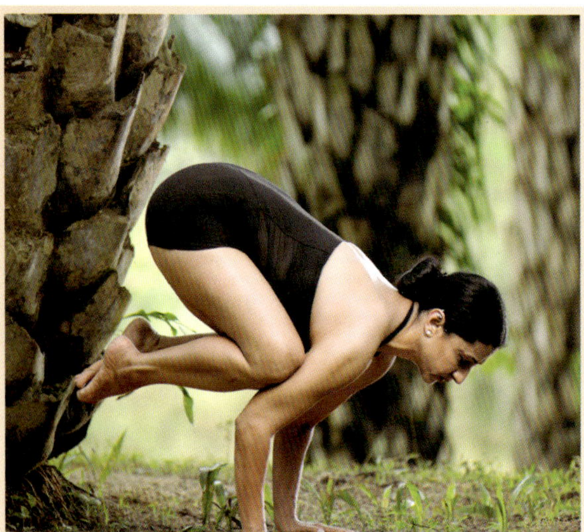

BAKASANA

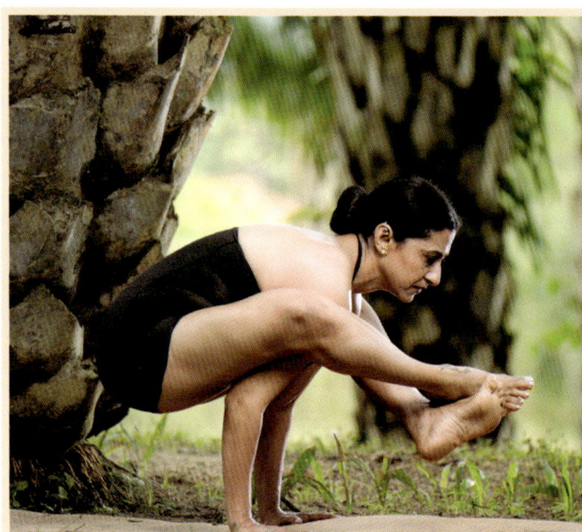

BHUJAPEEDASANA

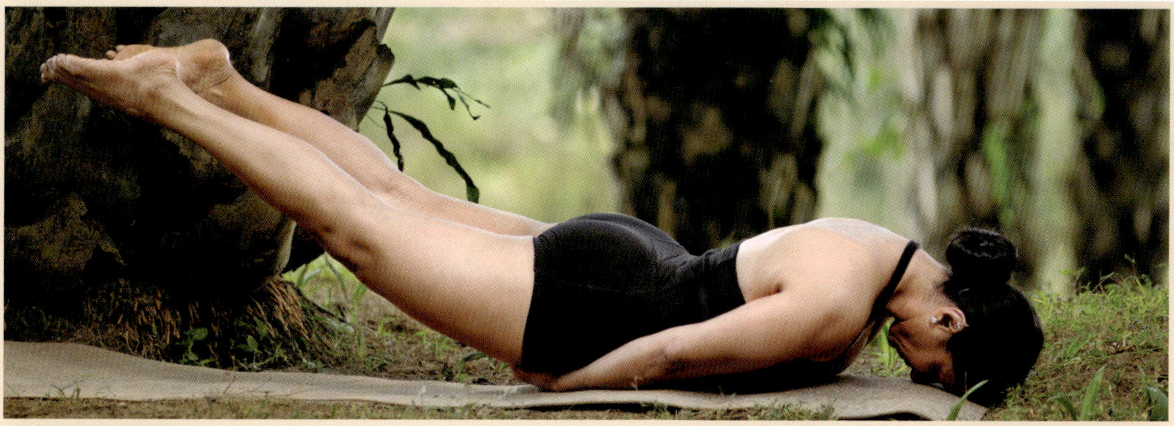

SHALABHASANA

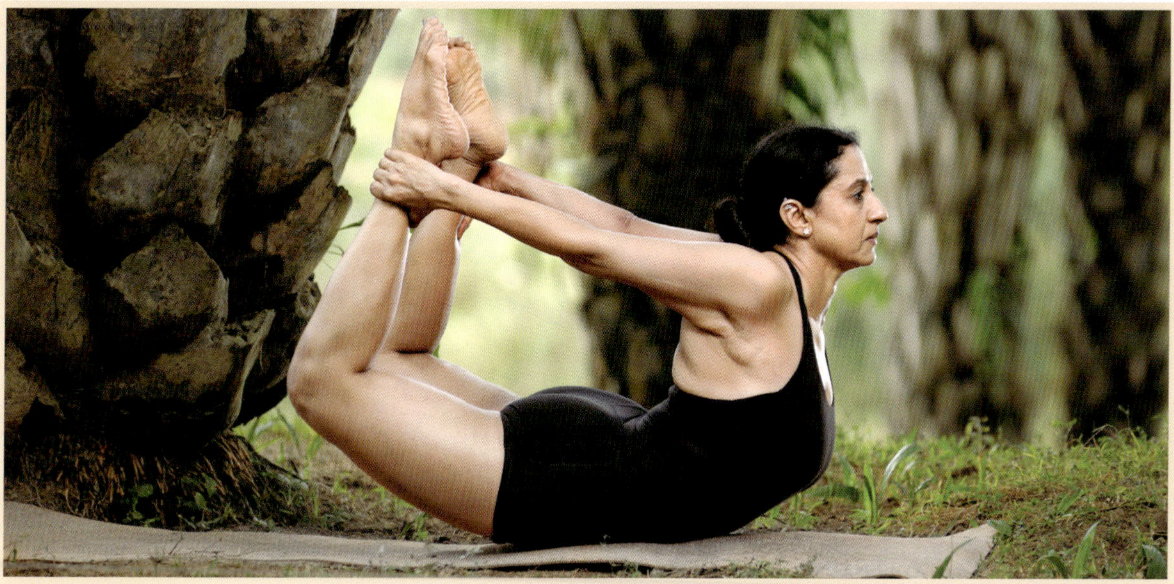

DHANURASANA

Floor Asanas

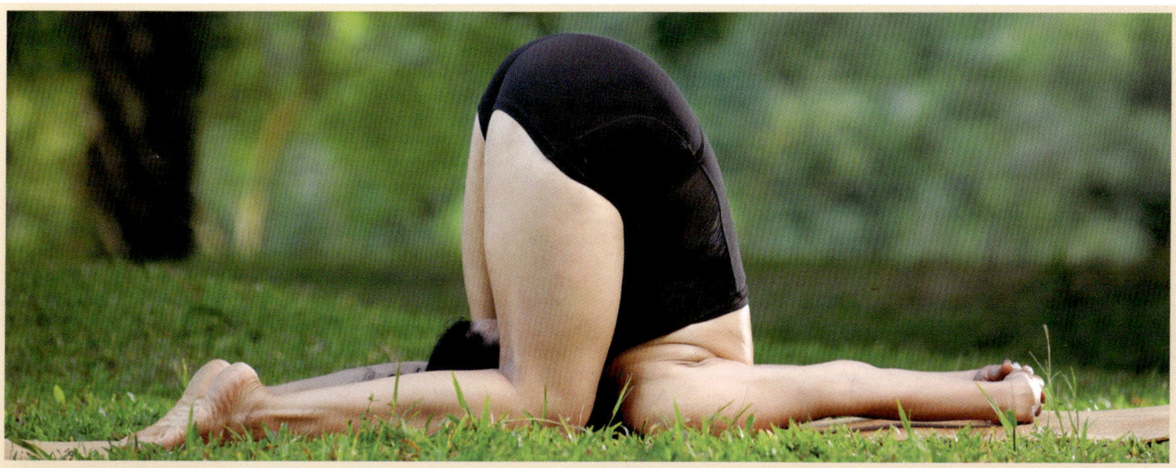

KARNA PEEDASANA

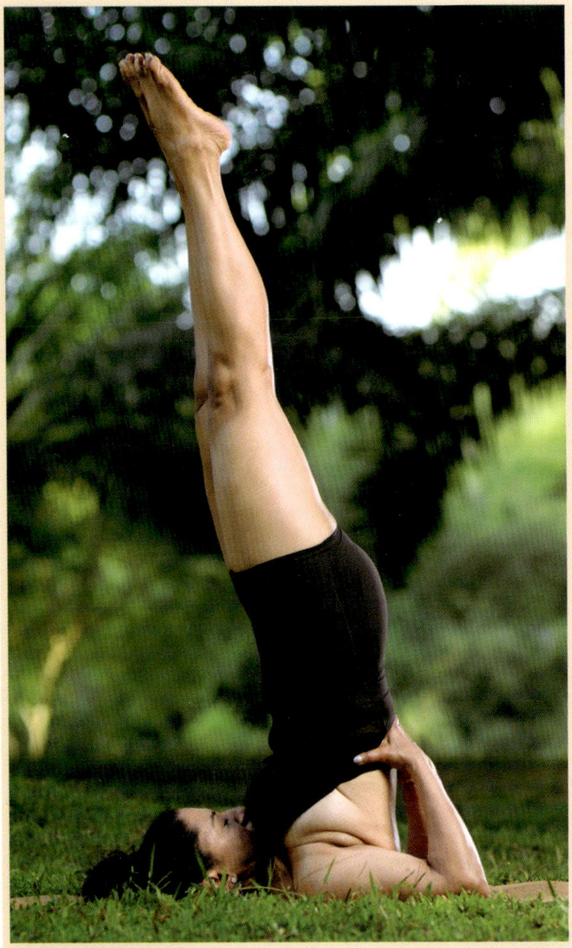

SARVANGASANA

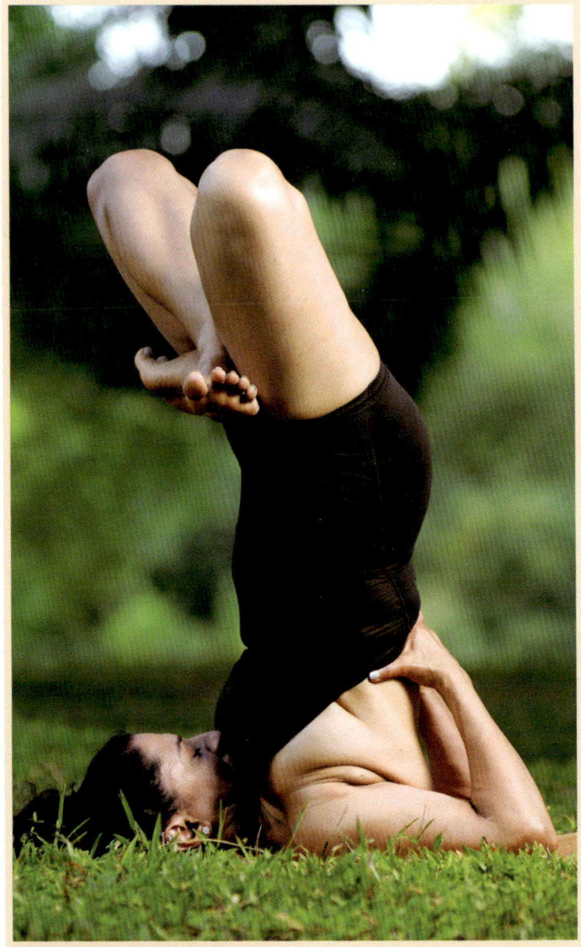

SARVANGA PADMASANA

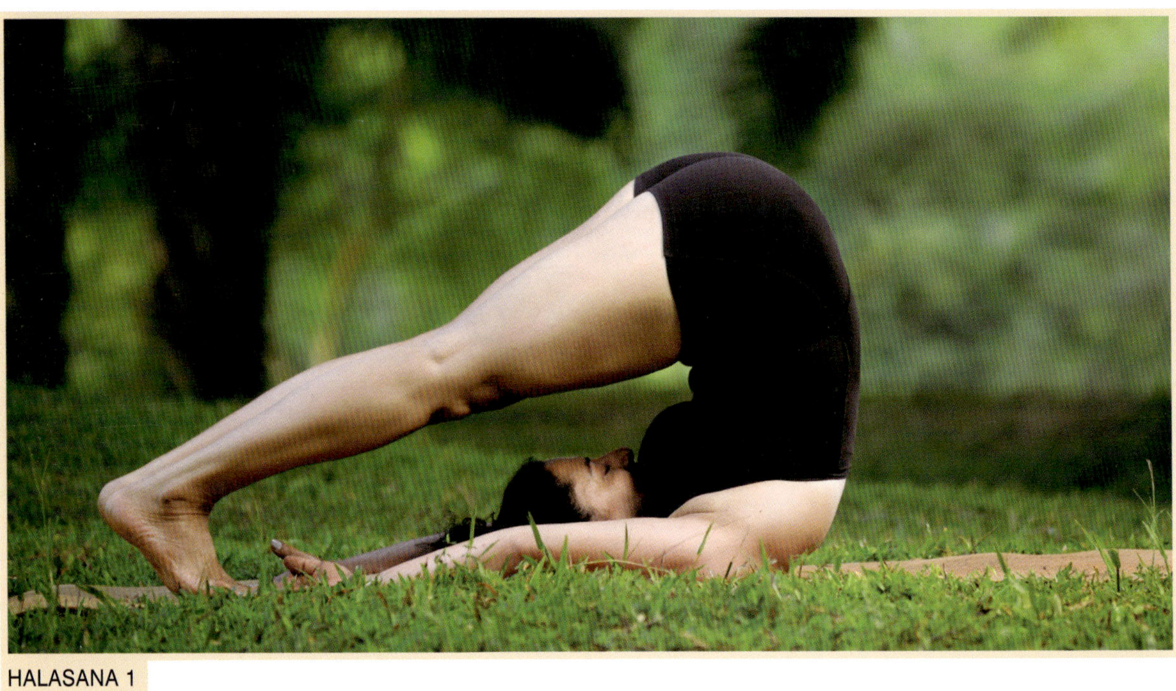

HALASANA 1

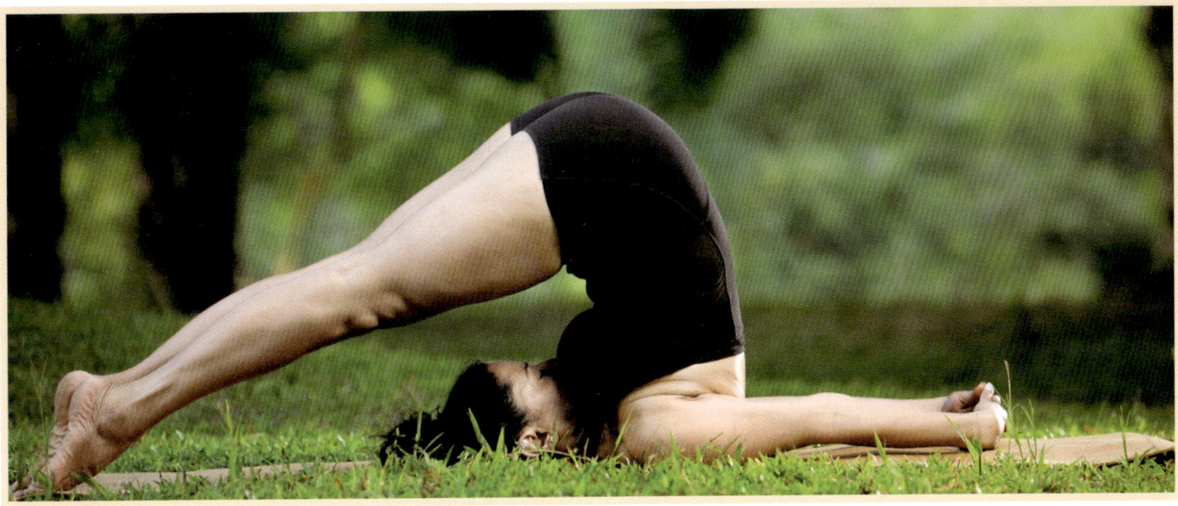

HALASANA 2

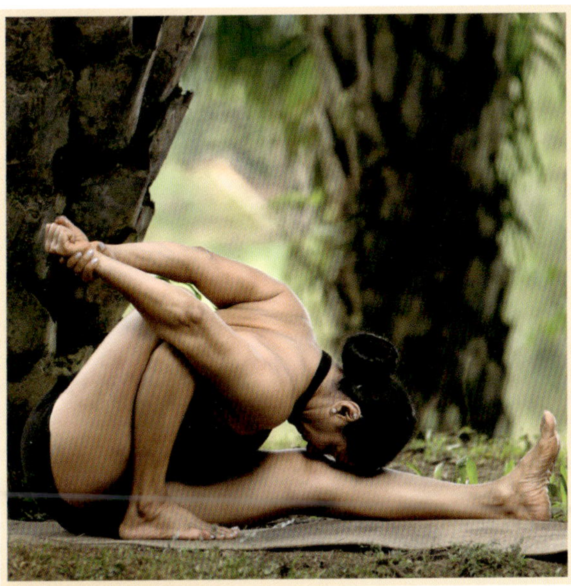

MATSYENDRASANA

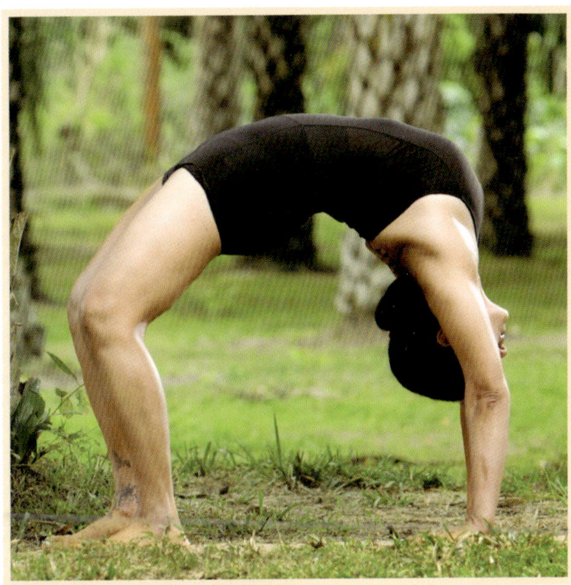

URDDHWA DHANURASANA

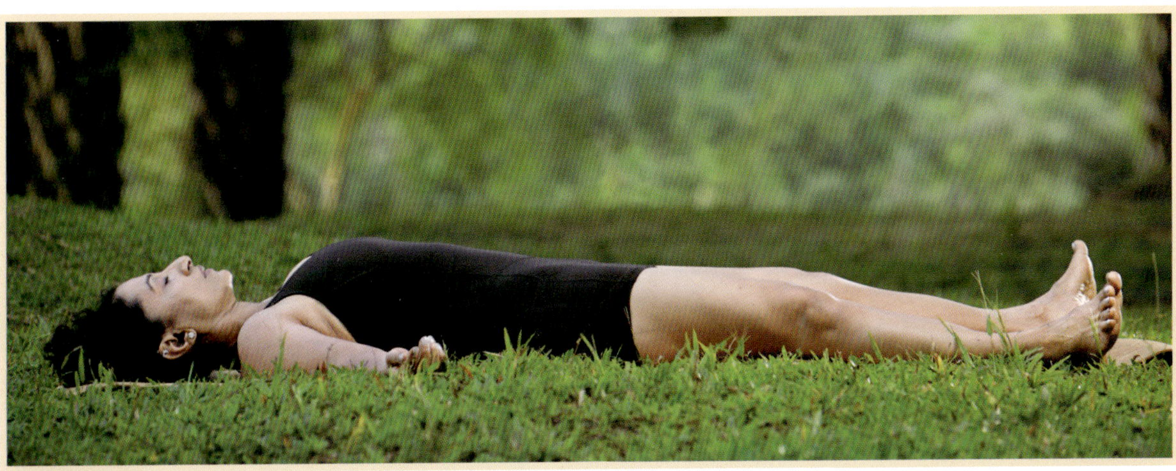

SHAVASANA

Pranayama

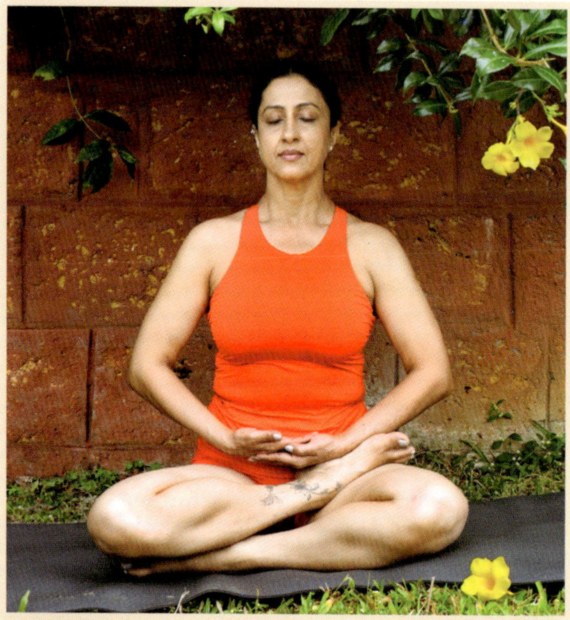

KAPALBATHI

Mudra

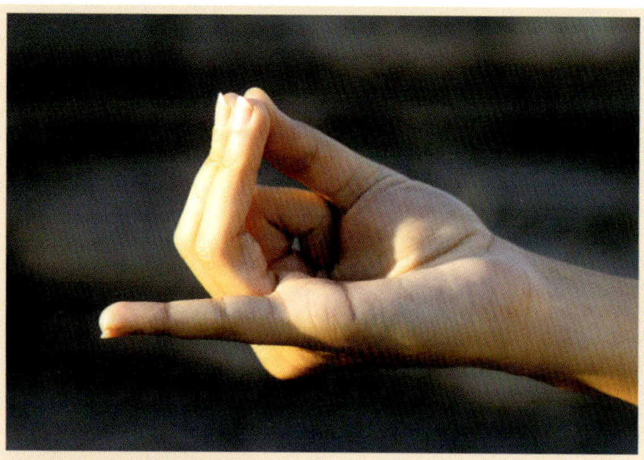

APANA VAYU MUDRA

- This is another variation of holding the apana vayu mudra.
- It involves joining the tips of the middle and the ring finger to the thumb while the index finger rolls in to touch the base of the thumb and the little finger extended.
- Apana vayu mudra promotes downward flow energy.
- A yoga teacher's guidance may introduce mudra variations to cater to diverse needs and abilities.

SAMANA VAYU

Samana vayu, known as the 'middle breath', is active at the navel centre. It exists between prana vayu in the chest and apana vayu in the lower body, harmonizing their energies. Samana vayu governs the absorption and assimilation of nutrients, ensuring that the body receives its vital supplies. Beyond digesting food, it also processes thoughts and experiences, balancing and regulating the information we take in. As a consolidating force, it stabilizes and integrates all forms of energy into our system.

Physical Level

Samana vayu governs digestion and nutrient absorption, converting food into energy. It resides between the diaphragm and navel, moving in a circular pattern to regulate the digestive system. A balanced samana vayu ensures strong digestion and overall well-being.

Subtle Level

Samana vayu is the energy that gives vitality. It processes information and assimilation of knowledge and retains the essence of an experience. This vayu has the power to guide the breath into sushumna nadi. This breath can be harnessed in the asanas by the practice of bandhas and mudras.

Spiritual Level

With an experience, there is always an impression which gets created in our body. Along with this impression, there is usually a learning. Samana vayu, if active, retains such learning and releases unwanted impression.

Imbalanced Samana Vayu

Physically, it affects digestion causing bloating, loose motion, and lack of nutrient absorption. Skin will have less lustre and nails will be brittle.

Mentally, it makes the mind feel weak and disturbed emotionally. Mind gets overhwhelmed with overthinking and it only worsens with disturbed sleep.

Yoga Sequence to Increase the Power of Samana Vayu

- The asana practice for samana vayu in particular is patterned to increase the pranic flow around the navel.
- The selected asanas guide apana vayu upward and prana vayu downward, merging them to awaken the sushumna nadi.
- The integrating of the two vayus will energize and strengthen the body, regulating instinctive urges like hunger and sex.
- The sequence focuses on forward bends, twists and abdomn-strengthening asanas.
- These are most effective when practised during the morning hours.

Standing Asanas

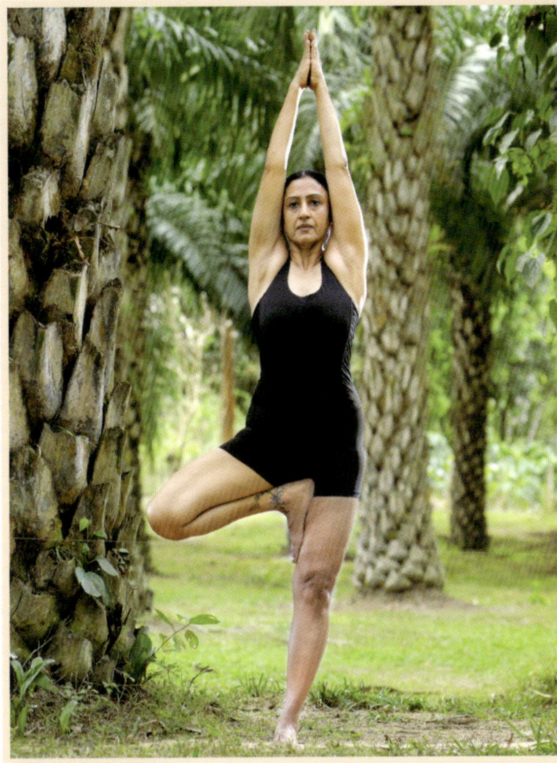

VRIKSHASANA

SURYA NAMASKARA A (FOR REFERENCE, SEE PP. 4–5)

SURYA NAMASKARA B (FOR REFERENCE, SEE PP. 6-8)

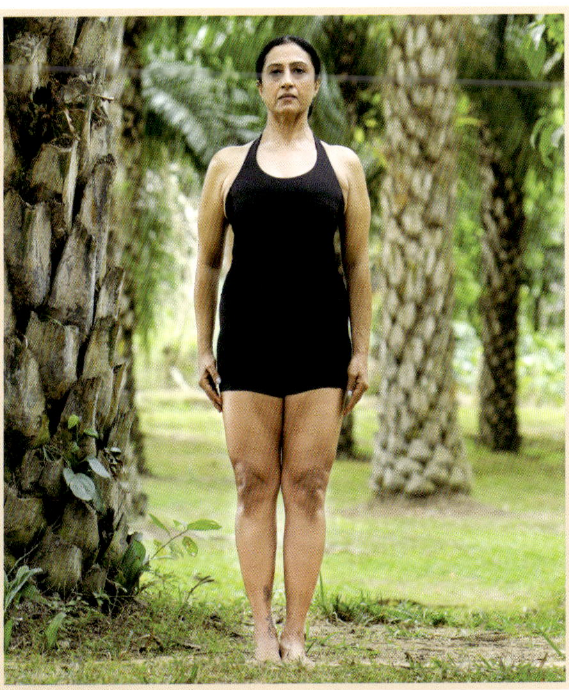

TADASANA

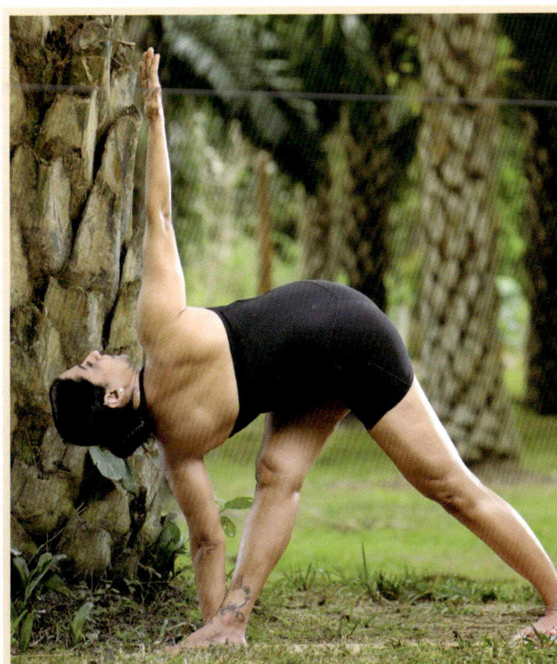

PARIVRTTI TRIKONASNA

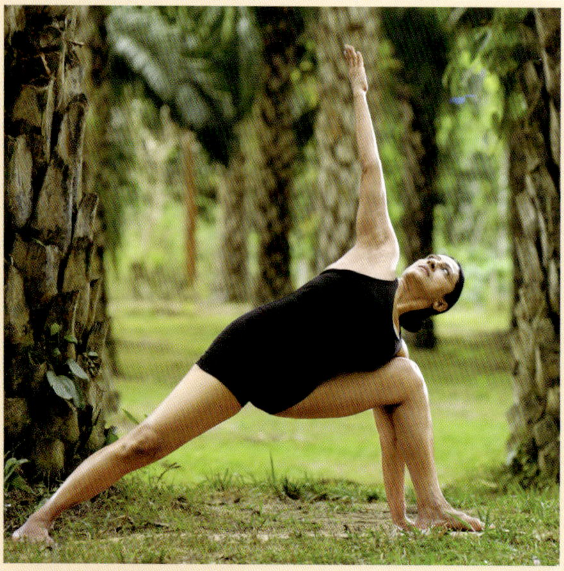

PARSHVAKONASANA 1

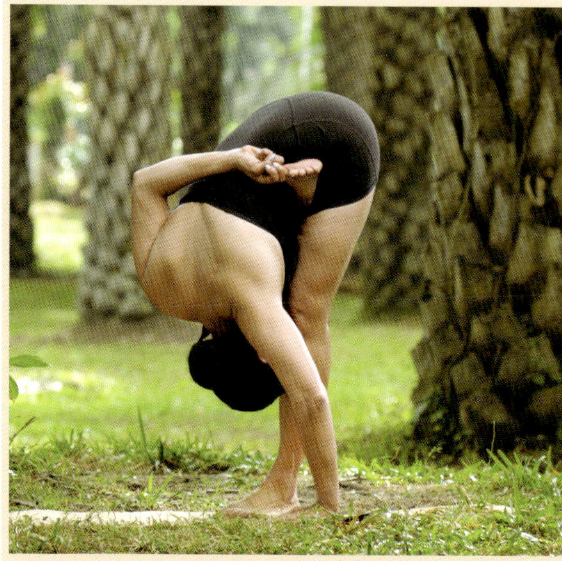

BADDHA PADMA PADANGUSHTHASANA

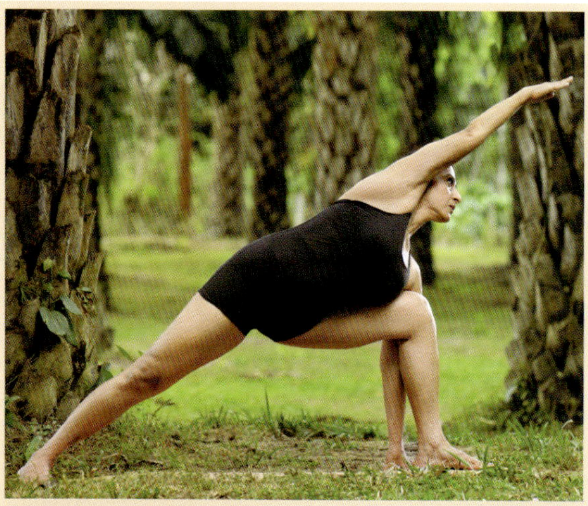

PARSHVAKONASANA 2

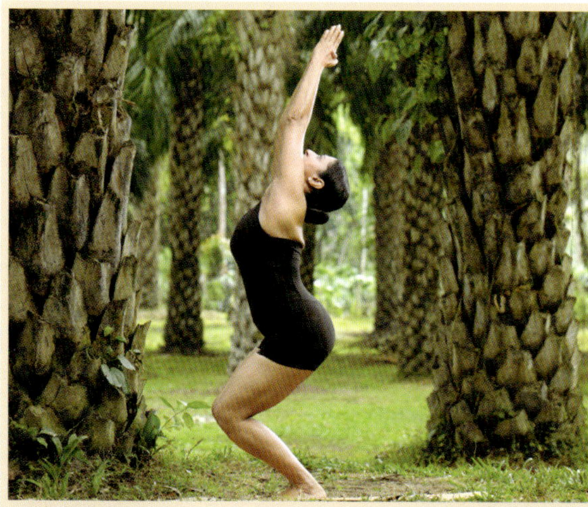

UTKATASANA

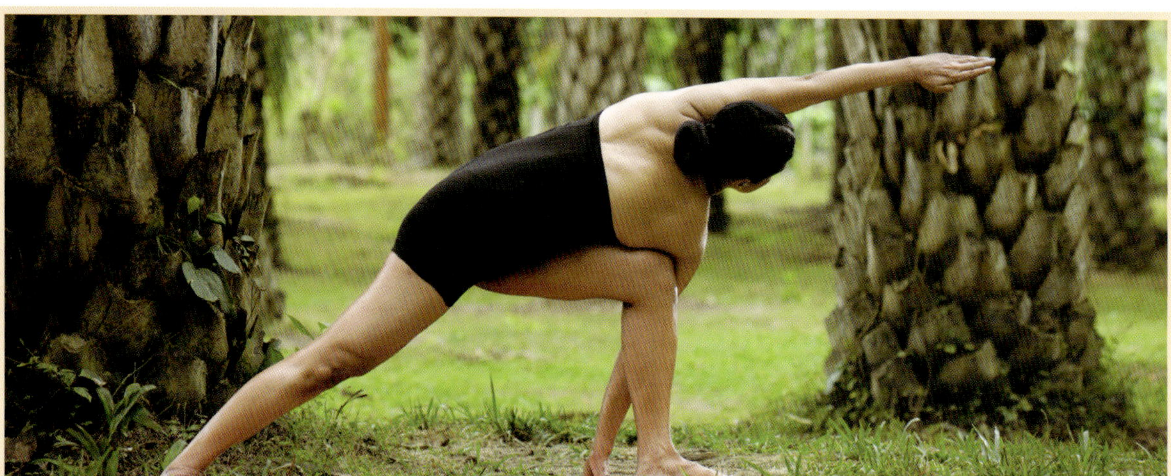

PARIVRITTI PARSHVAKONASANA

Sitting Asanas

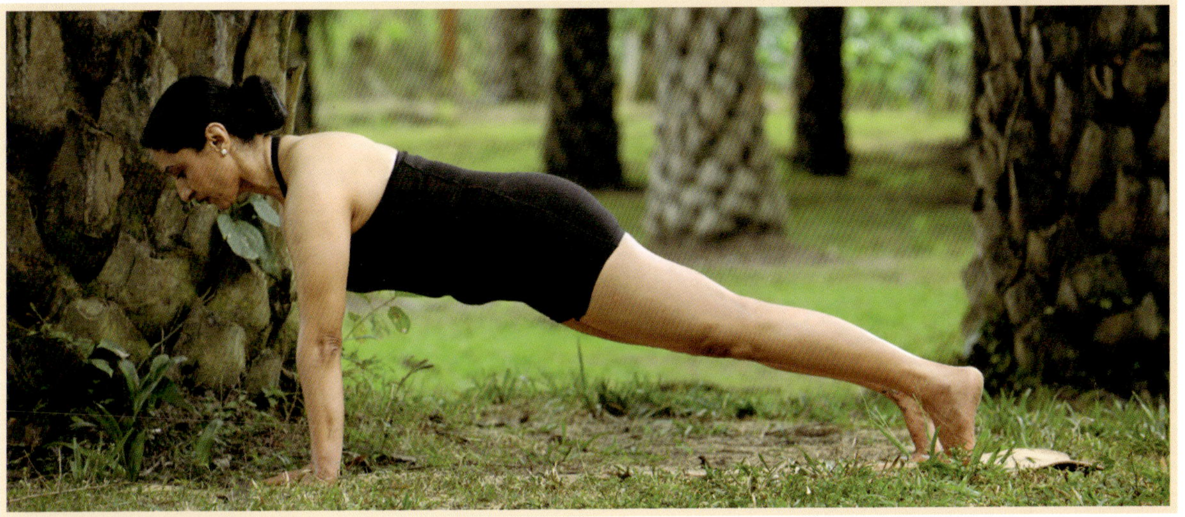

CHATURANGADANDASANA 1

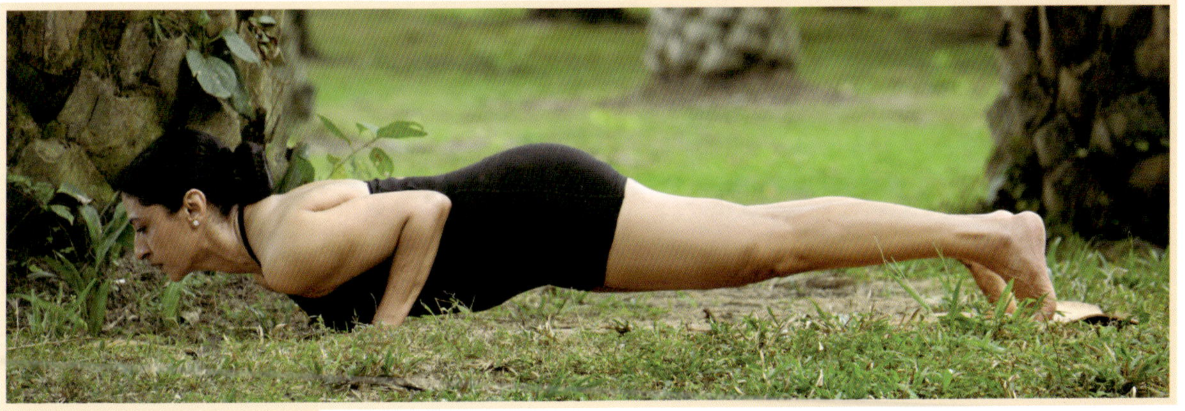

CHATURANGADANDASANA 2

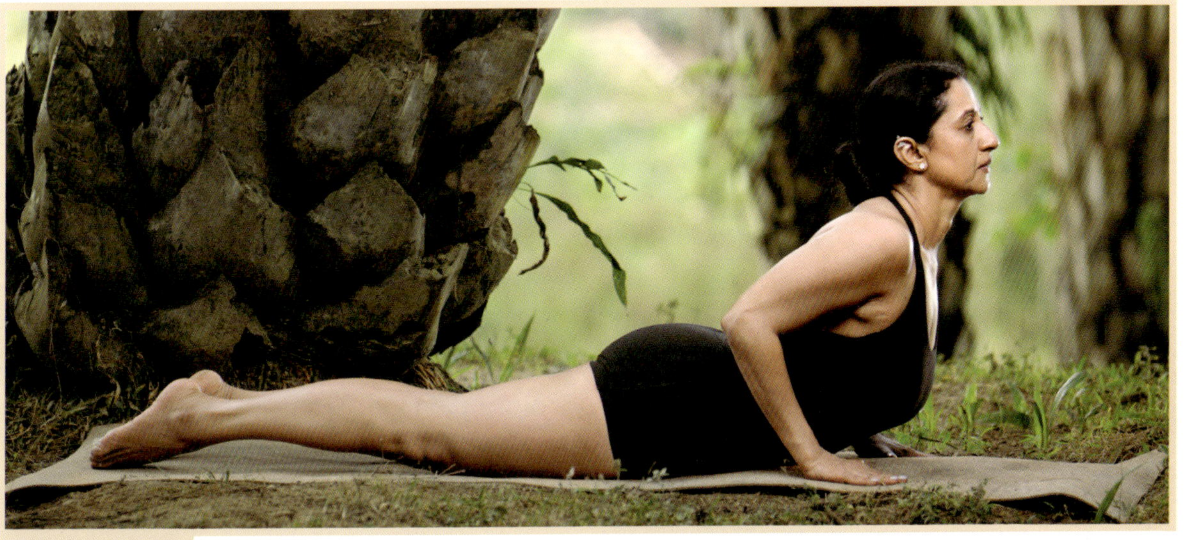

BHUJANGASANA

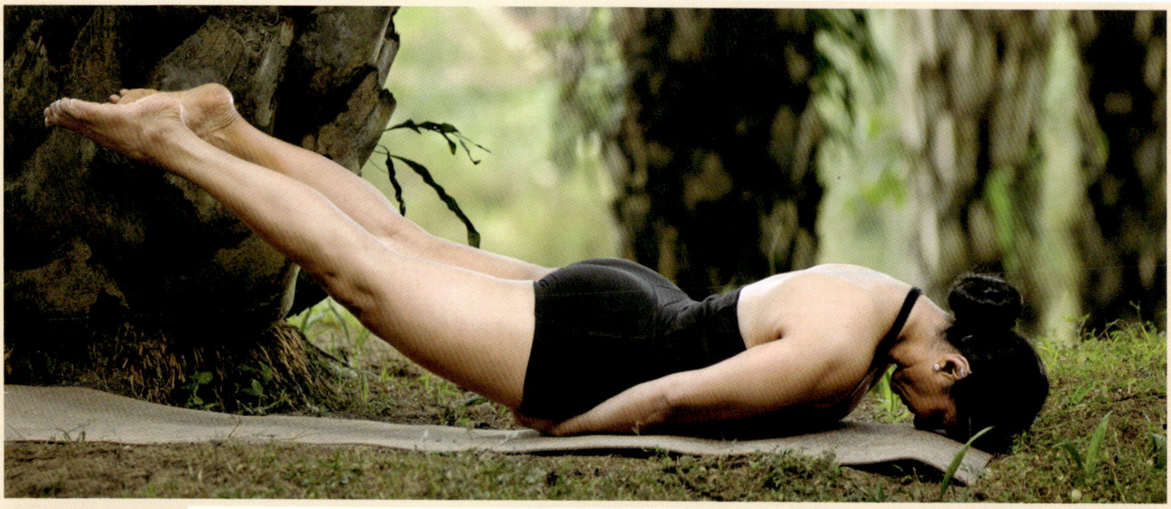

SHALABHASANA

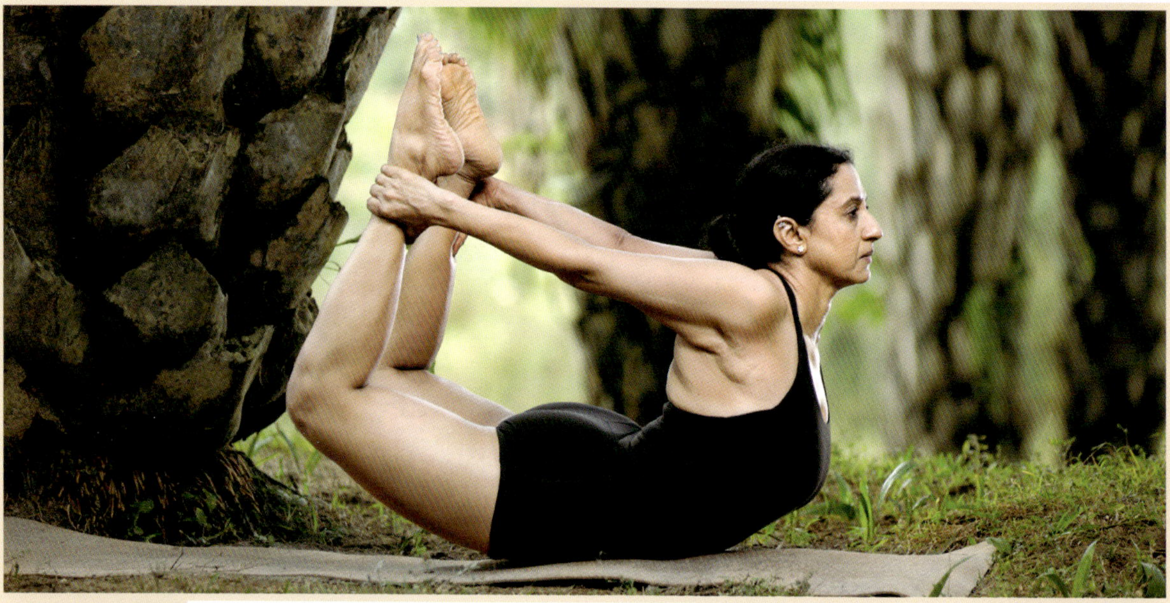

DHANURASANA

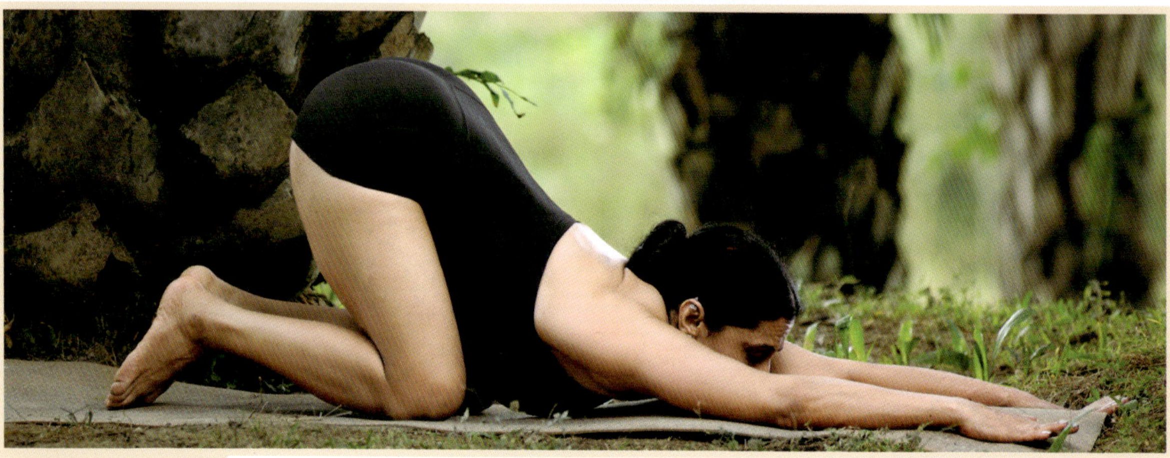

SHASHANKASANA 1

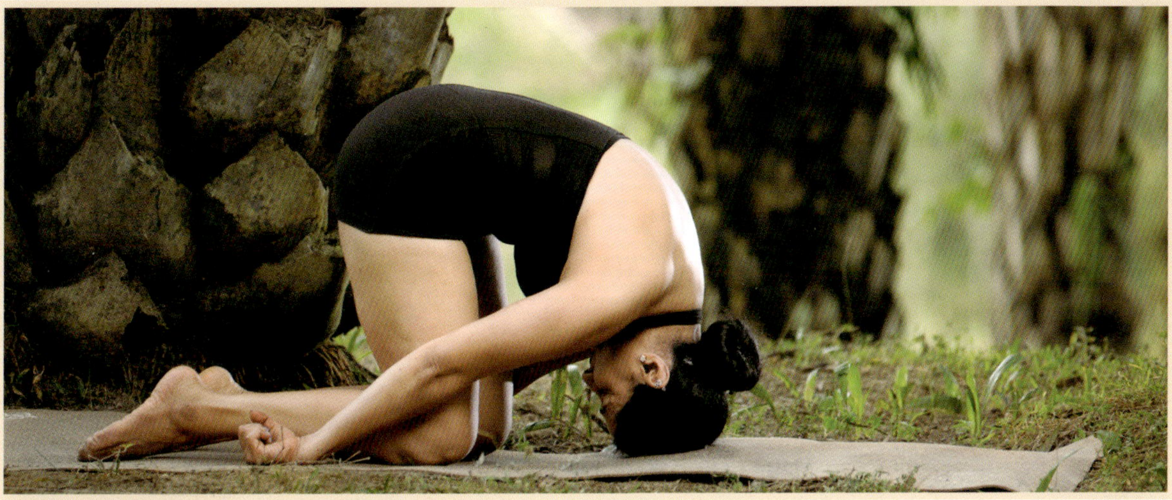

SHASHANKASANA 2

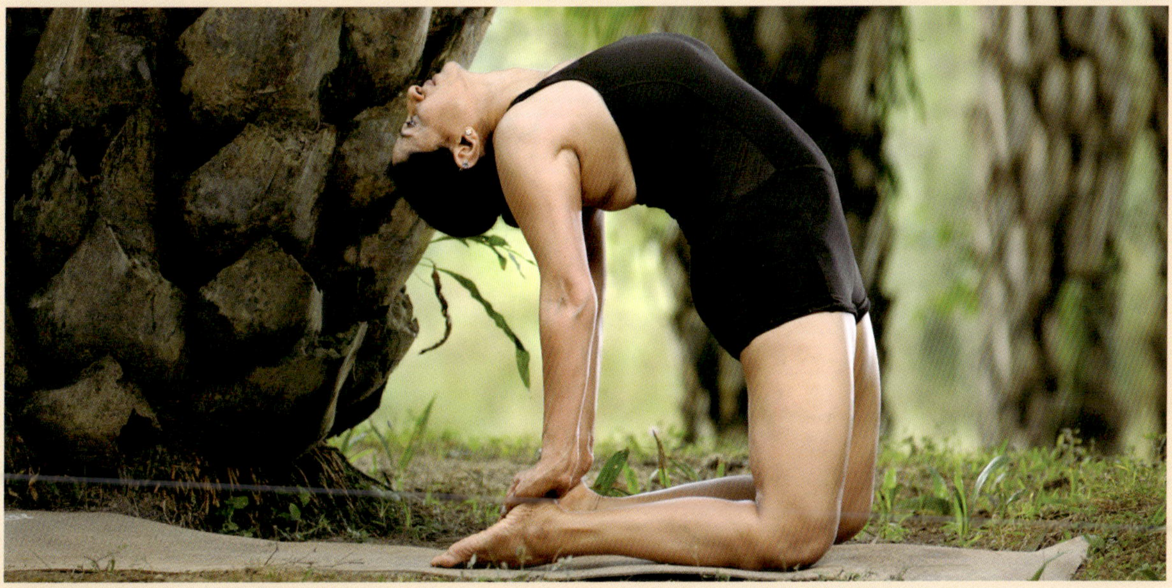

USHTRASANA

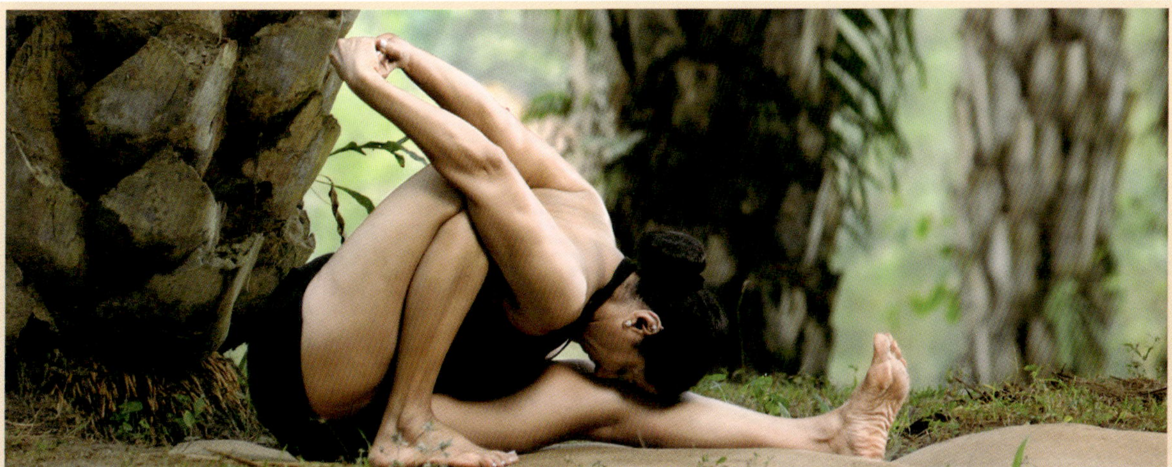

MARICHASANA 1

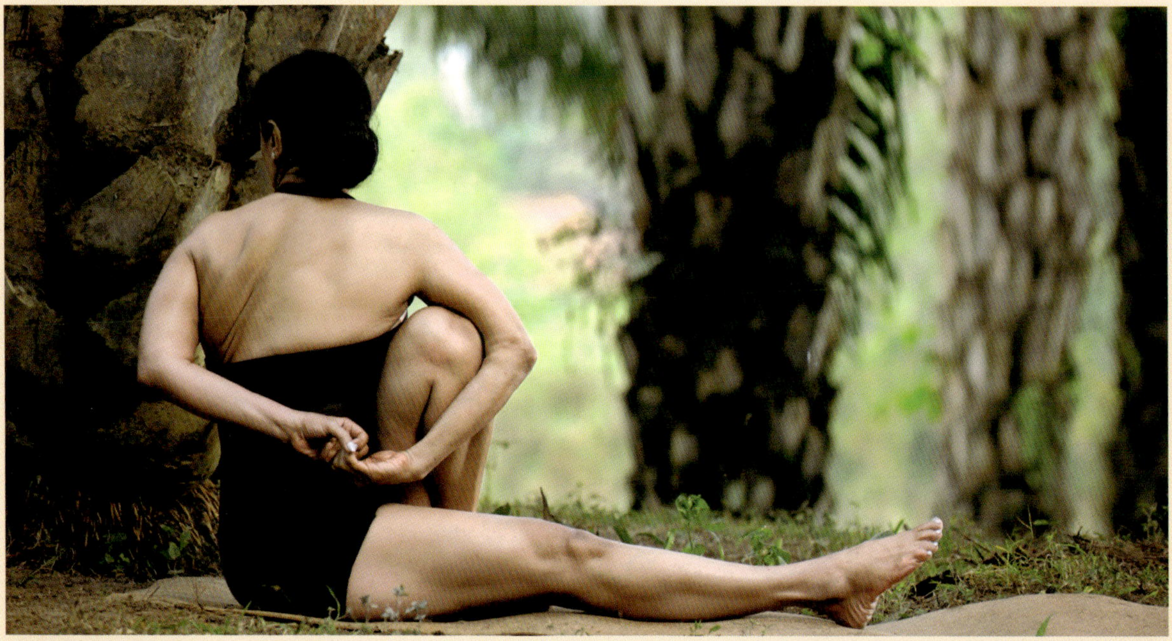

MARICHASANA 2

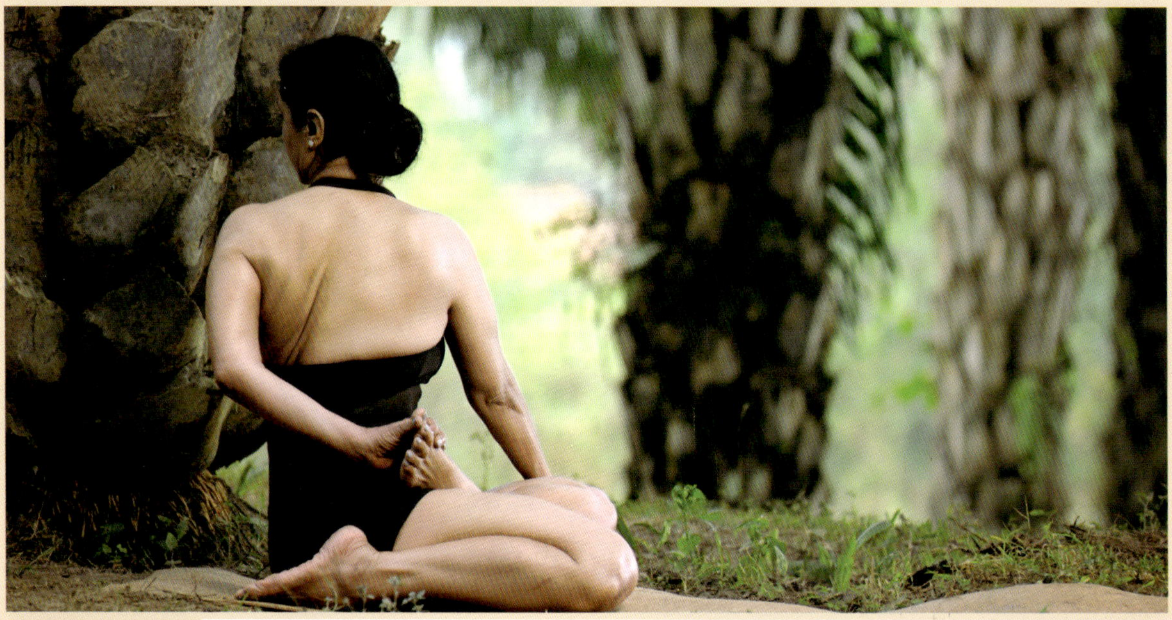

MARICHASANA 3

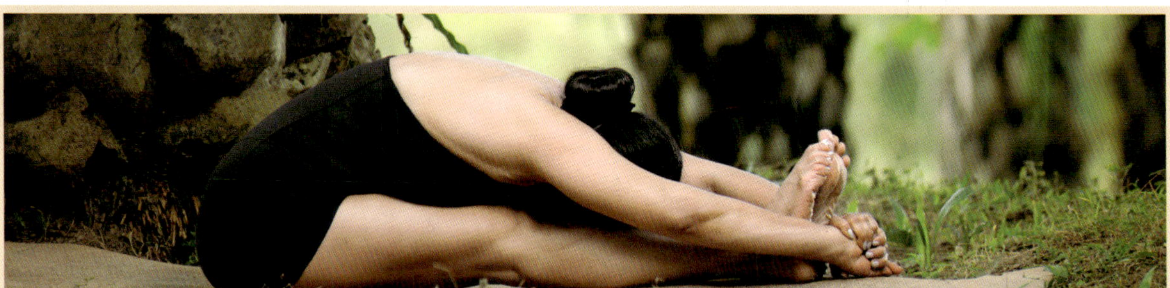

PASCHIMOTTANASANA

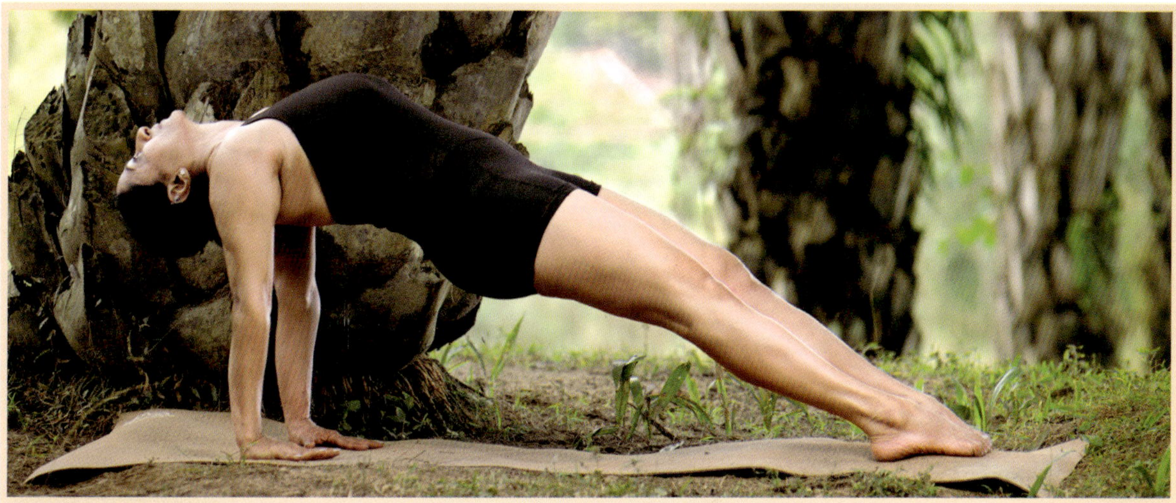

PURVOTTANASANA

Floor Asanas

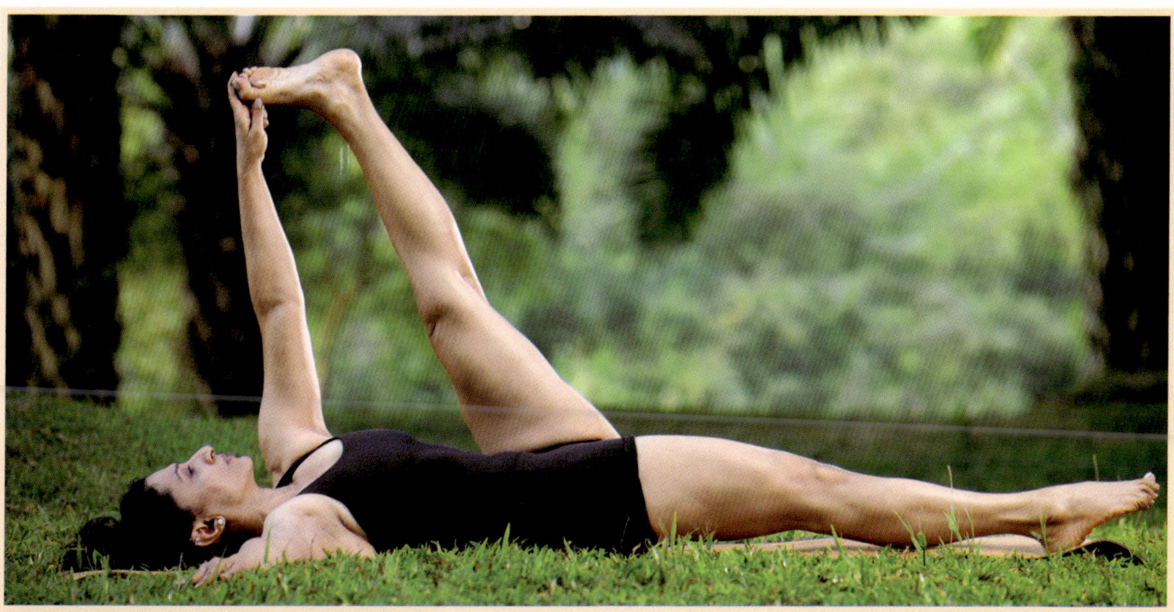

SUPTA HASTA PADANGUSHTHASANA 1

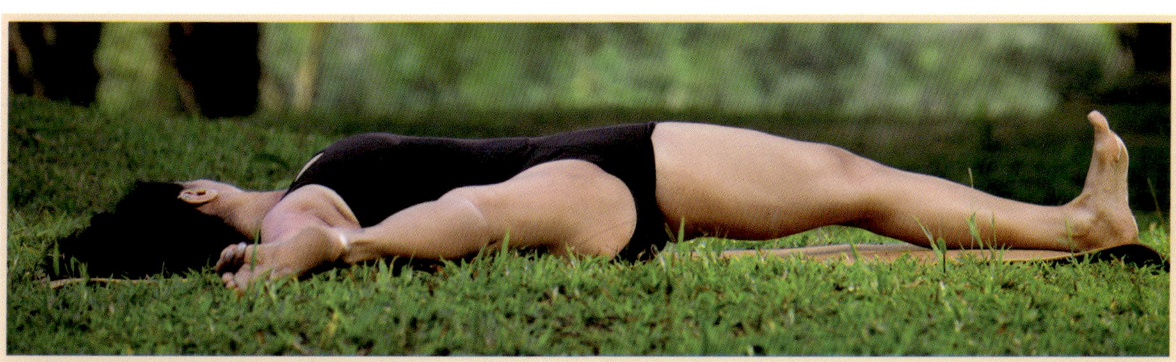

SUPTA HASTA PADANGUSHTHASANA 2

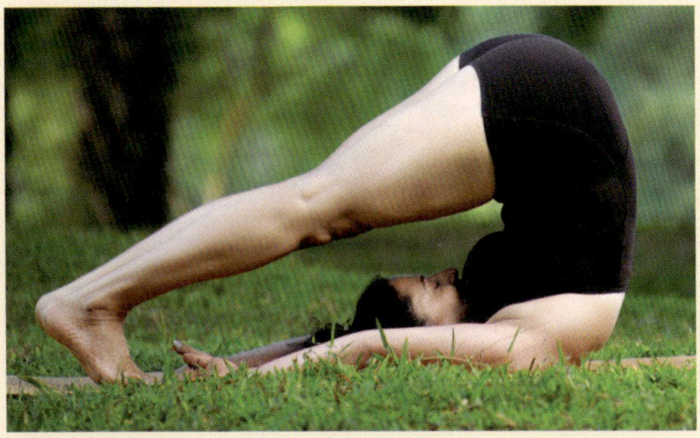

HALASANA

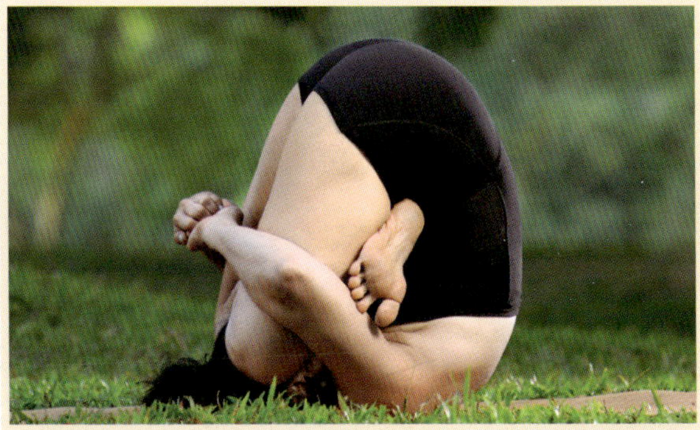

GARBHA PINDASANA (OPTIONAL)

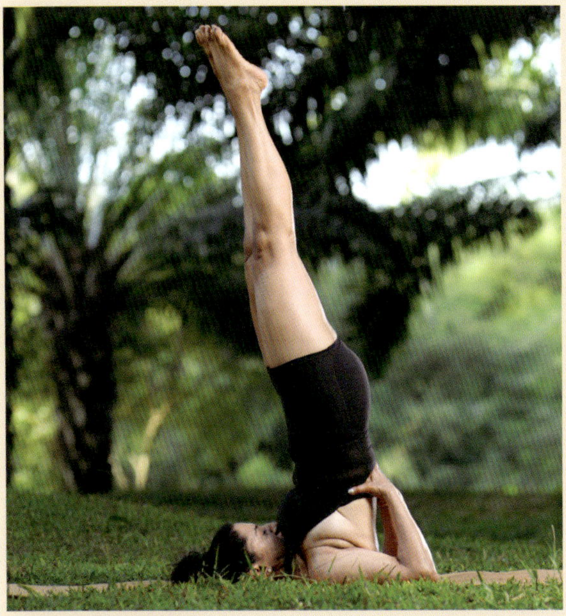

SARVANGASANA

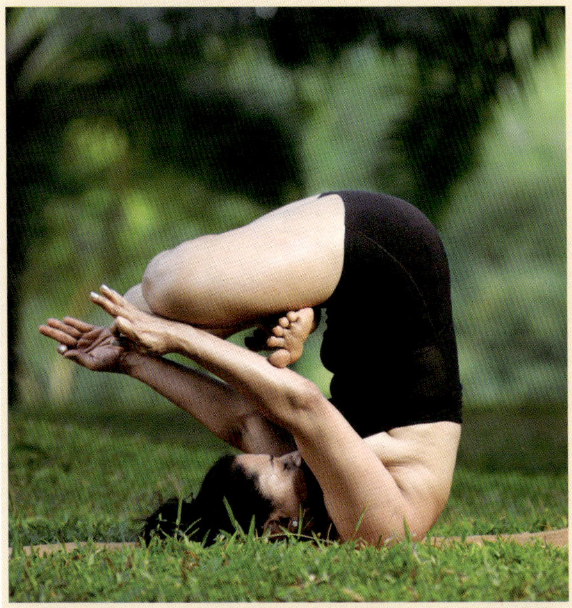

SARVANGA PADMASANA (OPTIONAL)

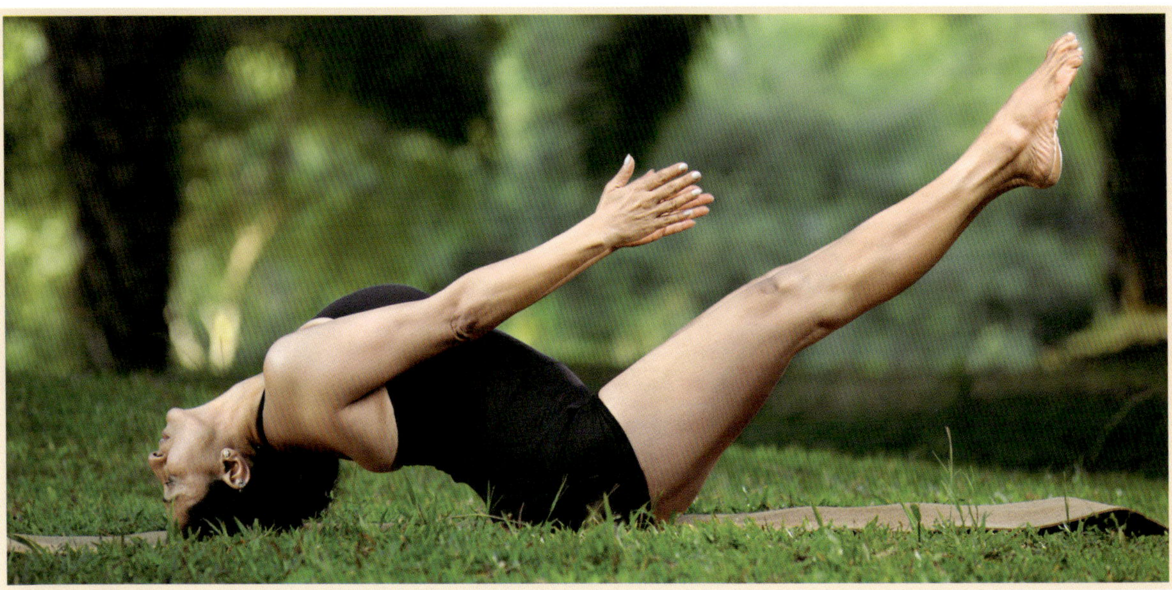

MATSYASANA

Pranayama

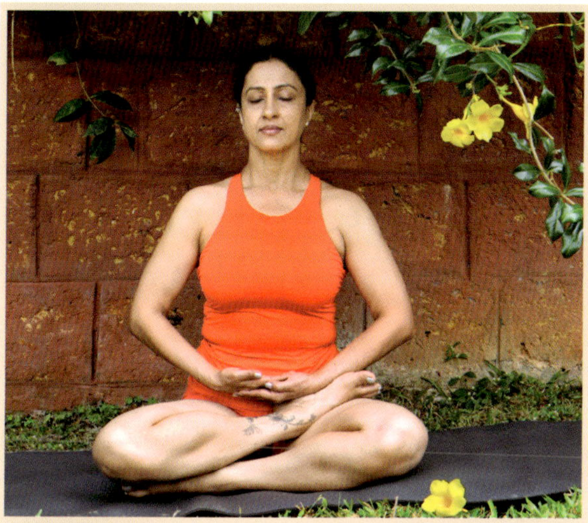

KAPALBATHI

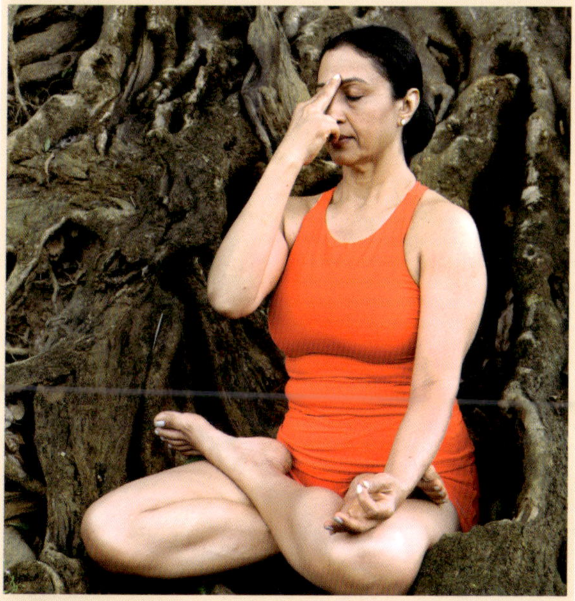

ANULOM VILOM

Mudra

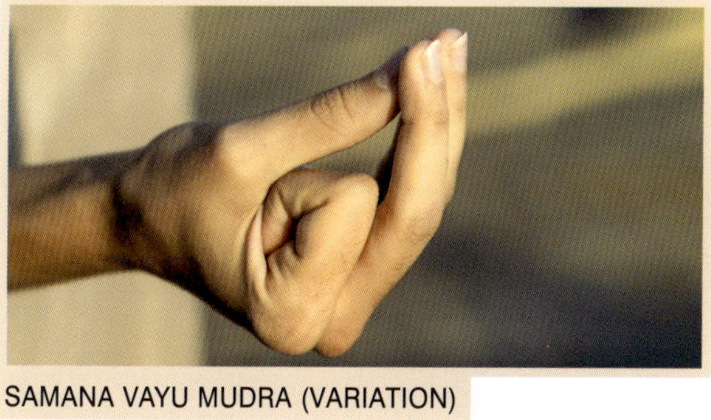

SAMANA VAYU MUDRA (VARIATION)

- Hold Mukula Hasta Mudra and relax your breathing.
- Take a while to visualize forests and valleys, immersing yourself in their tranquillity.
- Focus on deep inhalation and slow, extended exhalations.
- Relax the breathing and stay focused on the visualization.
- Maintain this meditative state for 20 minutes or more.

UDANA VAYU

Udana vayu goes in an upward direction from neck to head. It is located in the area of the diaphragm and thoracic cavity and interacts with downward flowing prana vayu to regulate breath, particularly exhalation. This vayu regulates higher thinking capacities, logical thinking, intuition, and the sense of power and control. This vayu is referred to as the spiritual vayu.

It is responsible for the functions of the nervous system. Its power manifests as speech and expression, growth and metabolism.

Physical Level

This vayu is responsible for the growth of the body. It is crucial to maintain memory, self-expression and speech patterns.

Subtle Level

Udana vayu is the upward-moving vertical breath. This is associated with strength and confidence in the mind. A strong udana vayu keeps agitated thoughts at bay.

Spiritual Level

Udana vayu governs the transition from wakefulness to deep sleep, moving prana from the heart to the head and energizing higher brain centres. When strong, it brings enthusiasm, alertness, willpower and joy.

Imbalanced Udana Vayu

- A weak or dysfunctional udana vayu can manifest as speech difficulties, shortness of breath and diseases of the throat.
- Disturbed udana vayu can lead to lack of expression, uncoordinated movement or loss of balance.
- Negative thoughts, depression, migraine, loss of cognitive skills, excessive talking—all the while feeling anxious—are other ways in which imbalanced udana vayu manifests itself.
- The body appears weak and depleted, while the mind becomes rigid, which is sometimes perceived as arrogance.

Yoga Sequence to Increase the Power of Udana Vayu

- The asanas focus on upward-moving breath.
- Deep and focused breathing is important for the activation of udana vayu.
- Backward-bending asanas are very helpful to establish strength.
- Inversions are very helpful to strengthen udana vayu.

Standing Asanas

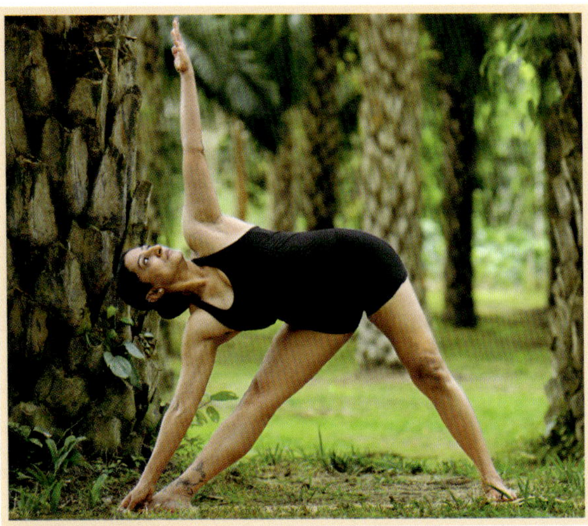

TRIKONASANA 1

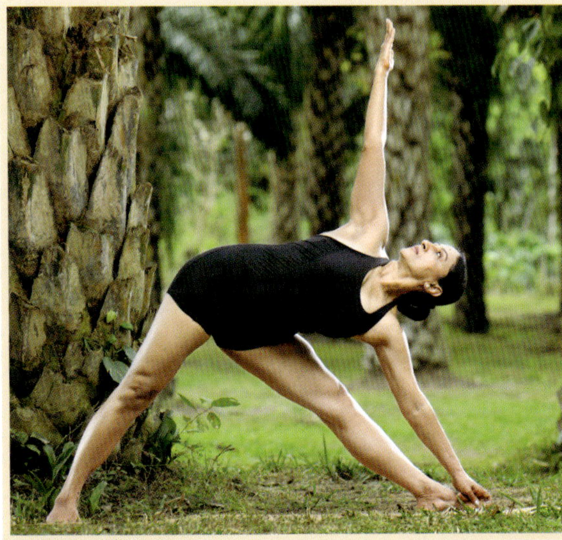

TRIKONASANA 2

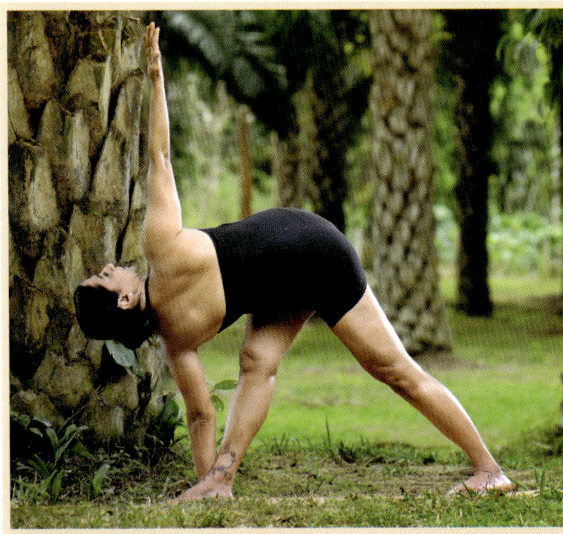

PARIVRITTI TRIKONASANA

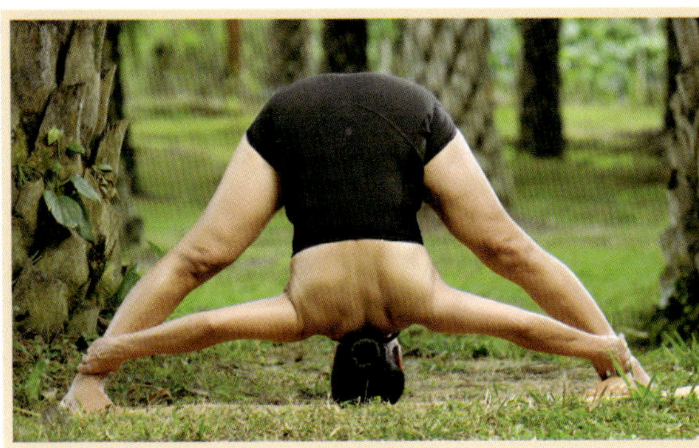

PRASARITA PADOTTHANASANA

SURYA NAMASKARA A (FOR REFERENCE, SEE PP. 4–5)

SURYA NAMASKARA B (FOR REFERENCE, SEE PP. 6–8)

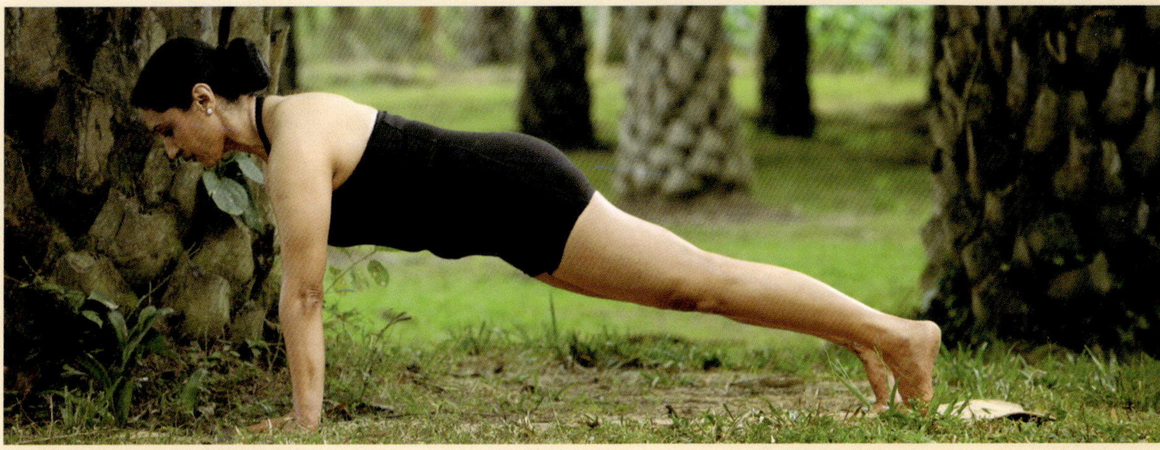

CHATURANGA DANDASANA

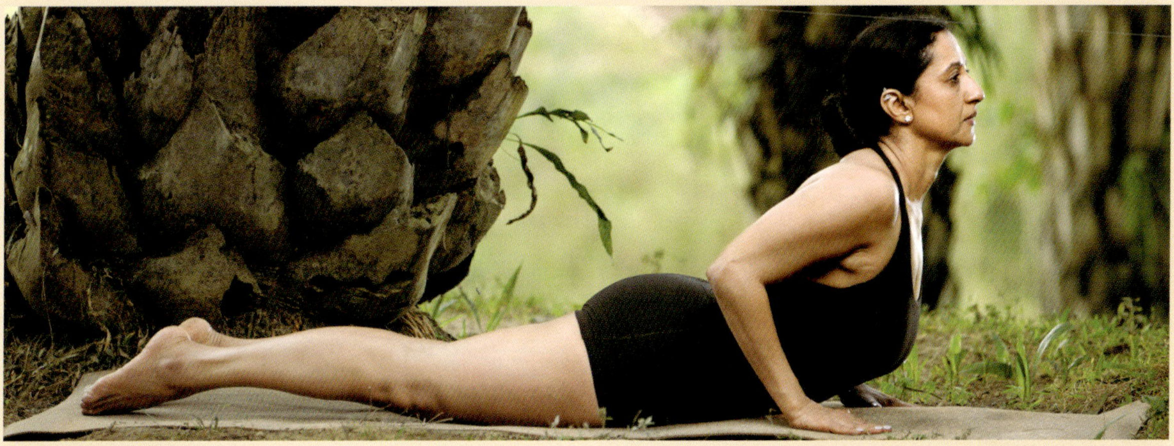

BHUJANGASANA

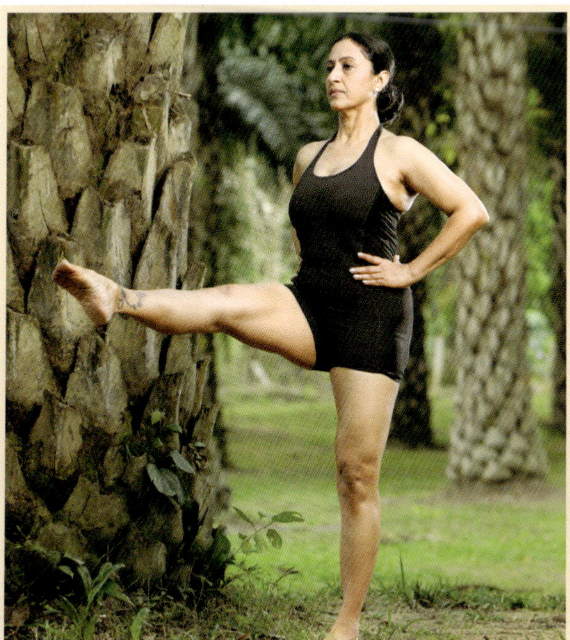

UPADANASANA

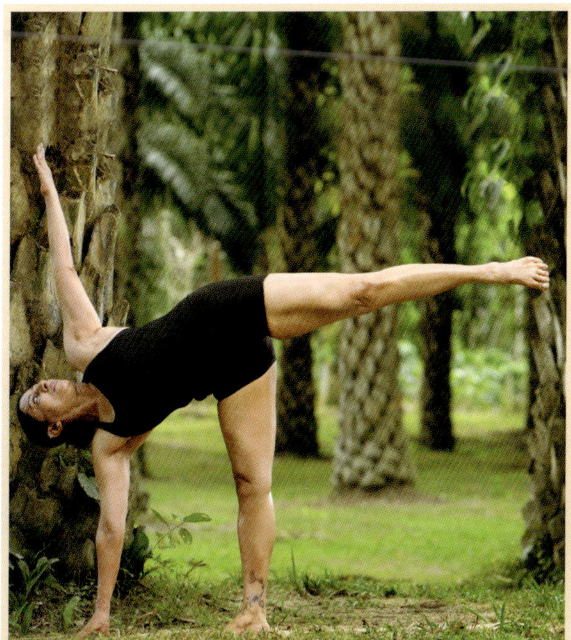

ARDHA CHANDRA CHAPASANA

Sitting Asanas

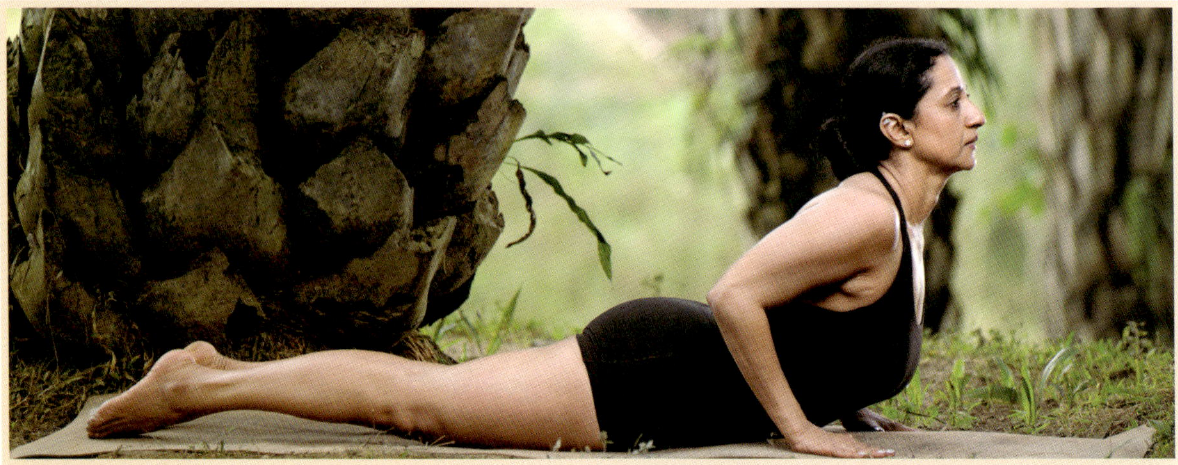

BHUJANGASANA

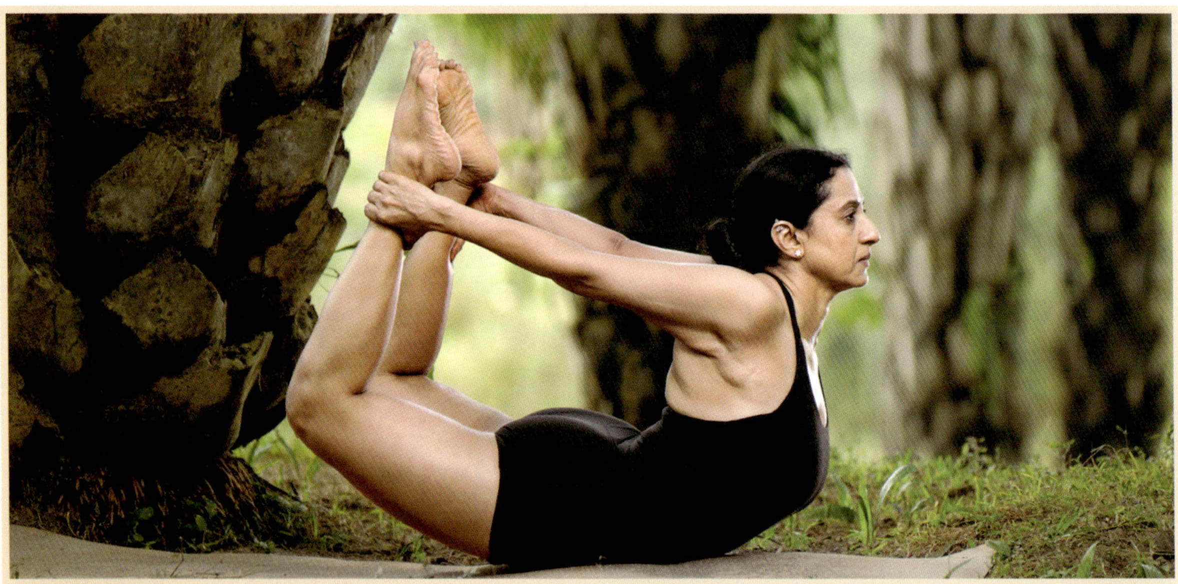

DHANURASANA

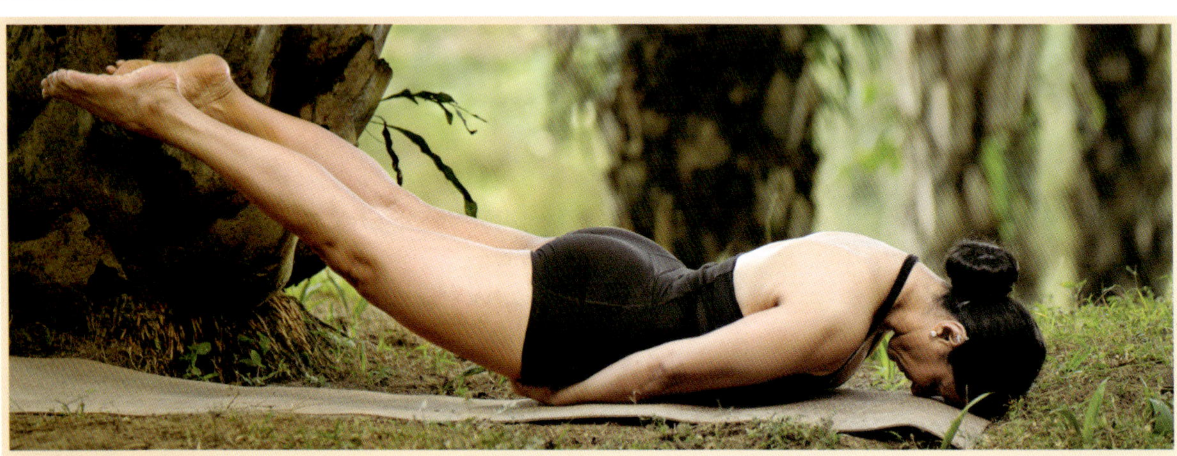

SHESHANKASANA

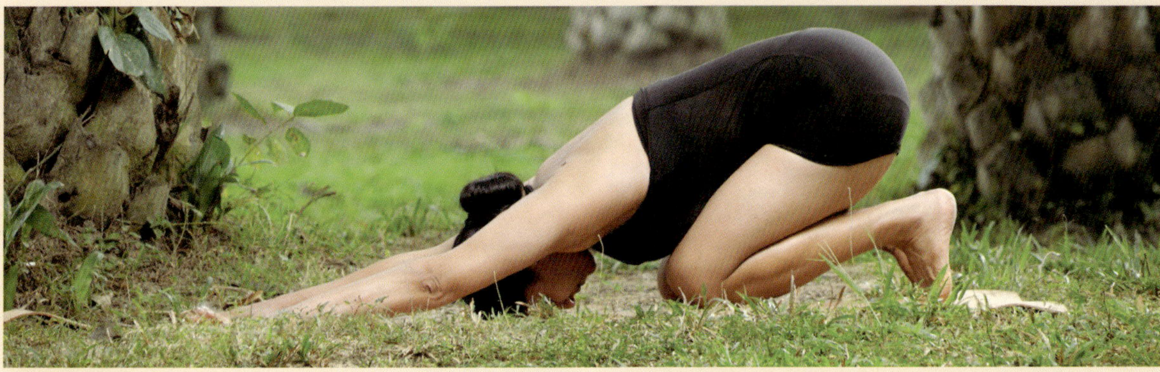

BALASANA

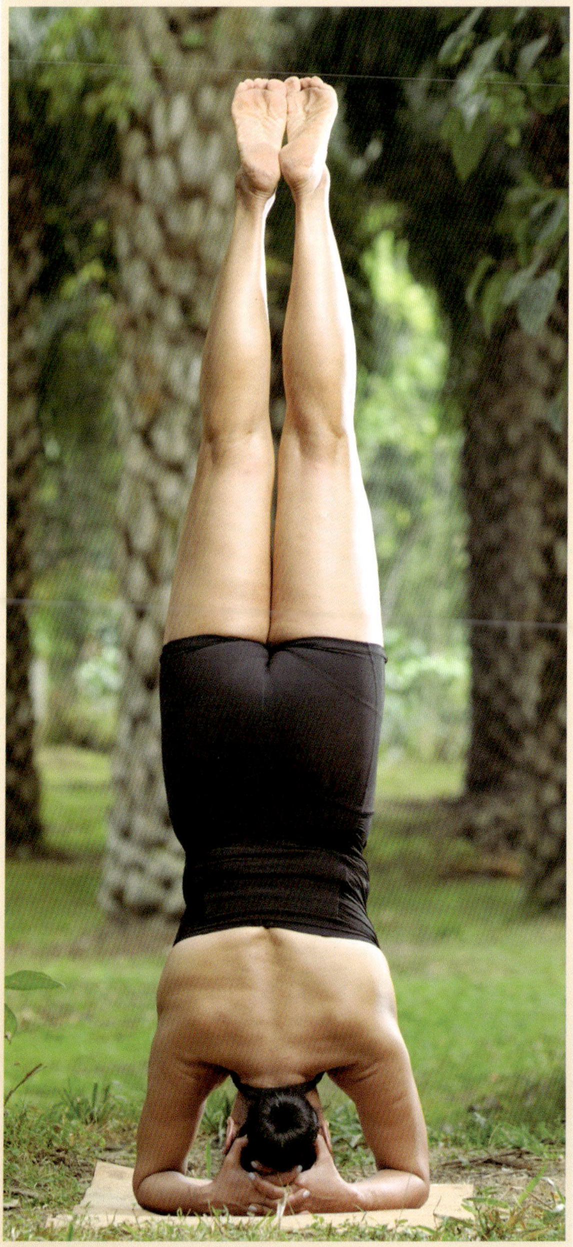

SHIRASANA

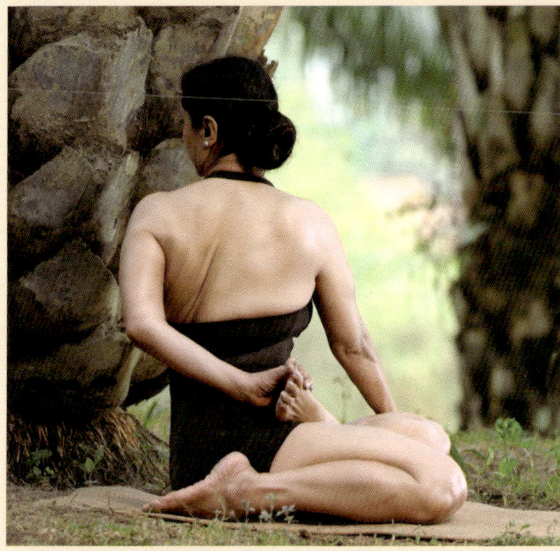

BHARADWAJASANA

Floor Asanas

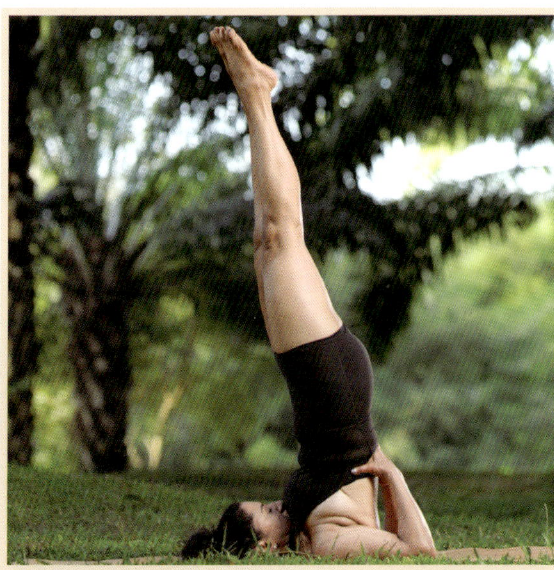

SARVANGASANA

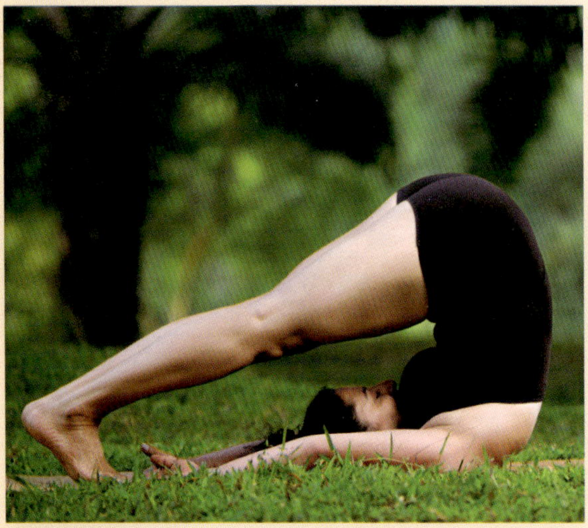

HALASANA

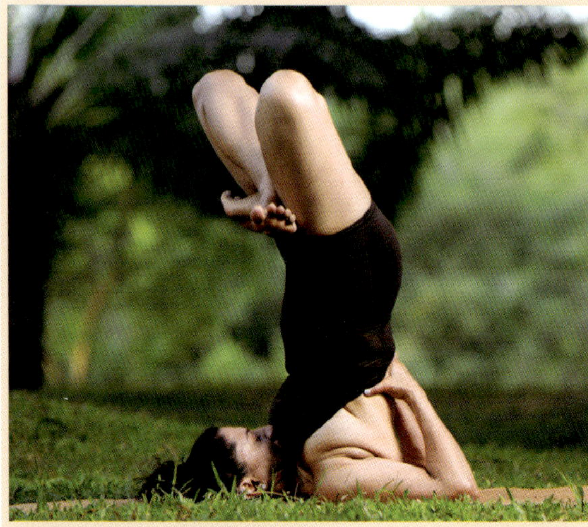

SARVANGA PADMASANA 1

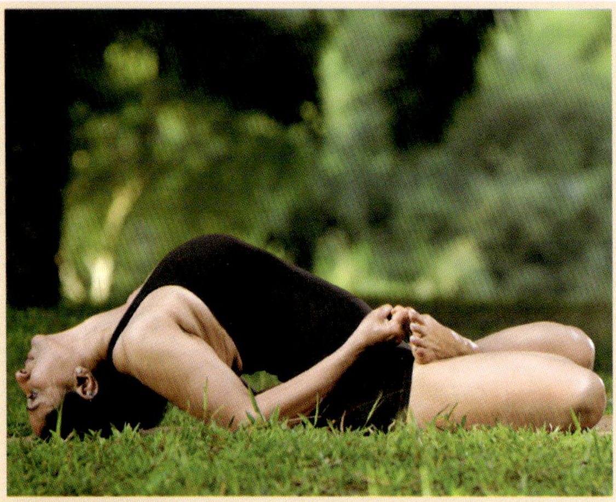

MATSYASANA

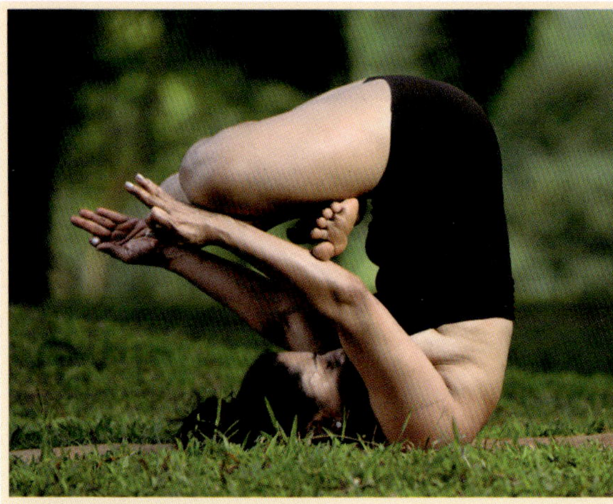

SARVANGA PADMASANA 2

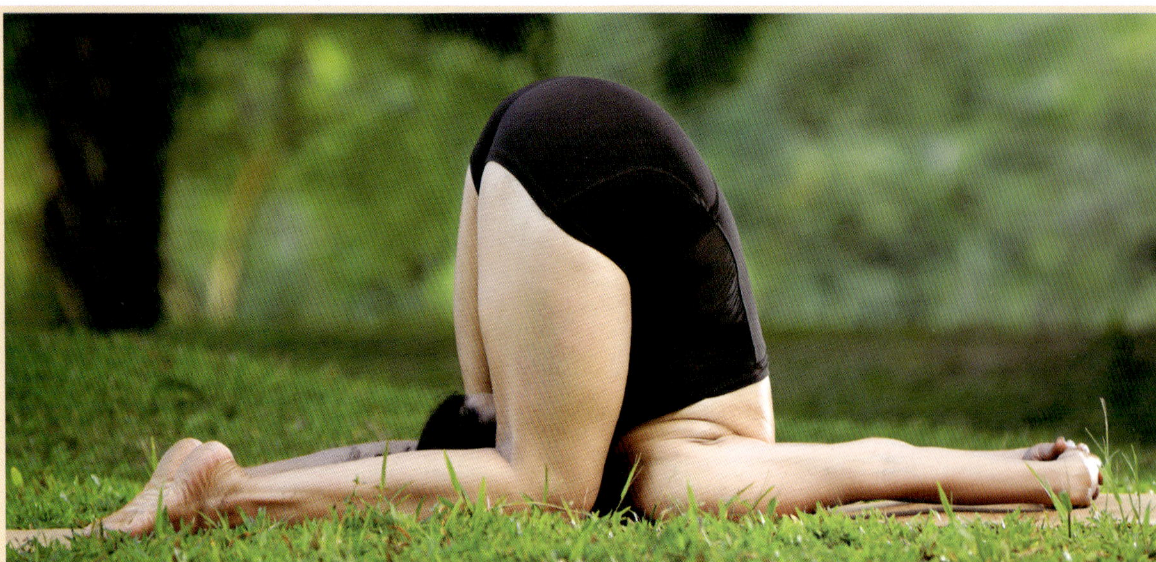

KARNAPEEDASANA

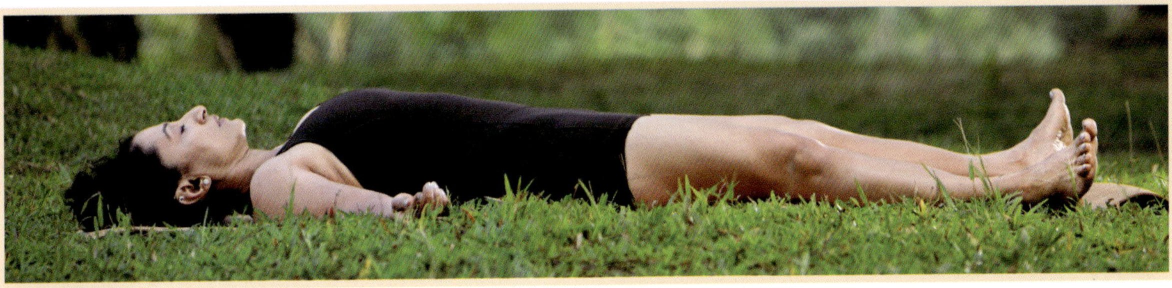

SHAVASNA

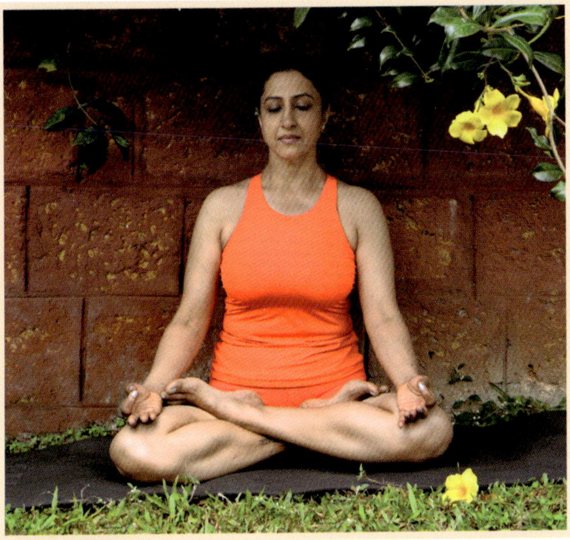

PADMASANA

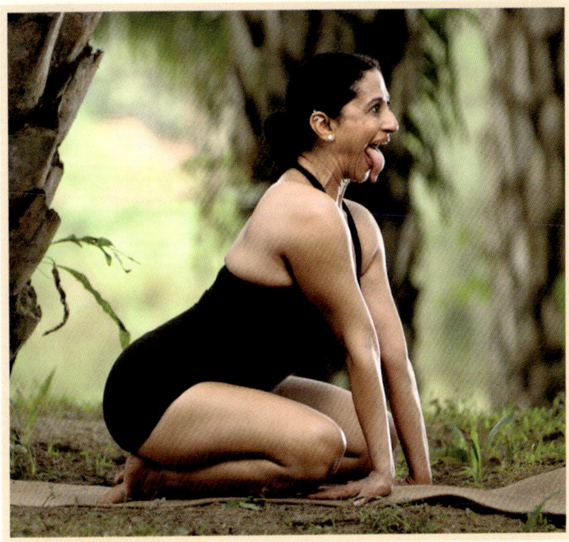

SIMHASANA

Pranayama

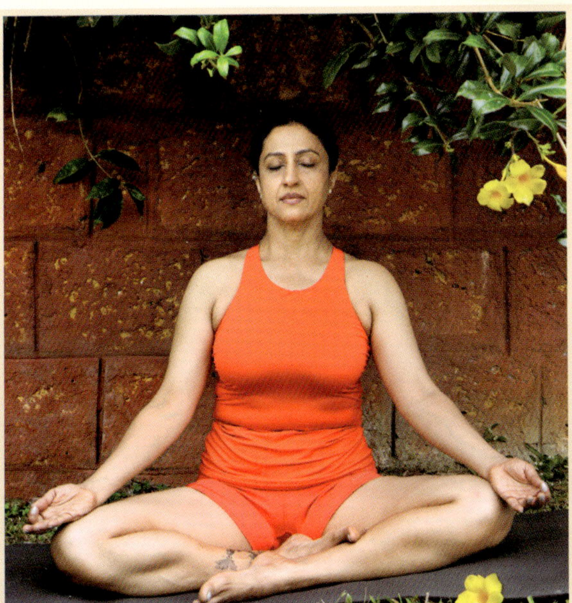

UJJAYI (WITH ANTAR KUMBHAKA)

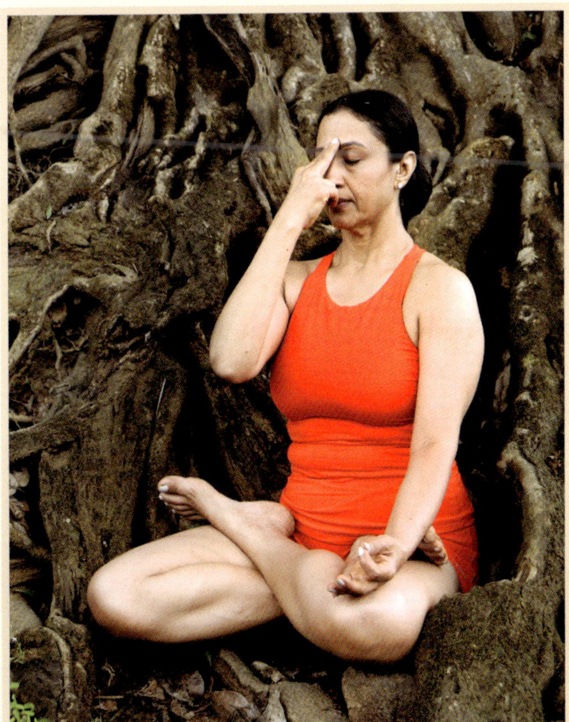

ANULOM VILOM (WITH ANTAR KUMBHAKA)

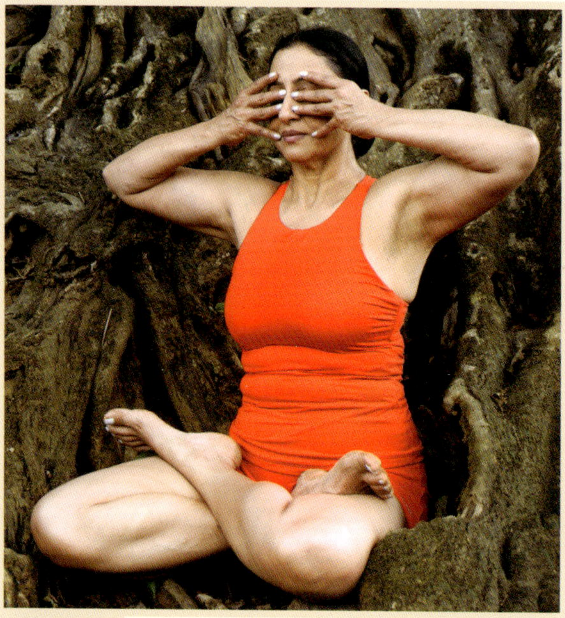

BHRAMARI

Mudra

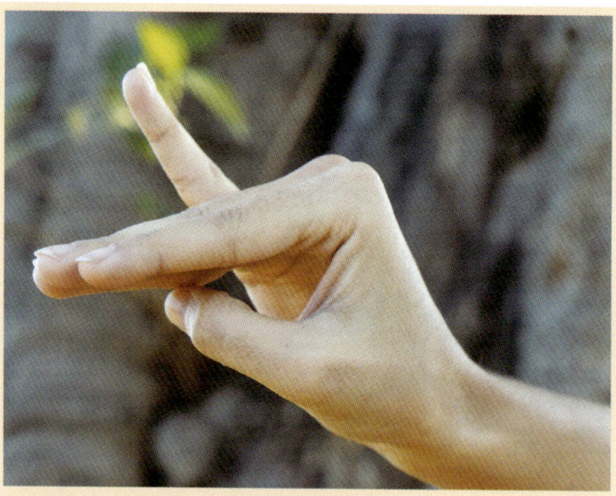

UDANA VAYU MUDRA (VARIATION)

The mind should be completely relaxed for this meditation. Focusing on a spiritual object helps anchor and calm the mind. Holding the mudra while maintaining a steady, relaxed breathing rhythm for five minutes helps balance the udana vayu.

VYANA VAYU

The power of this outward-moving energy is expansive and covers the entire body. The energy that is generated by the prana vayu gets distributed all around the body by vyana vayu. The nadis, nervous system and the circulatory systems get activated by vyana vayu, energizing both voluntary and involuntary muscles. Vyana vayu integrates and coordinates with the other vayus and keeps them balanced.

Physical Level

- It maintains steady blood flow and nutrient distribution.
- It facilitates nerve impulses and coordination
- It supports both voluntary (walking and lifting) and involuntary (heartbeat and digestion) muscle functions.
- It keeps the body flexible and prevents stiffness.

Subtle Level

- Strong vyana vayu dissolves energy blockages and expands awareness.
- It ensures balance across all other vayus.
- It governs movement of thoughts and emotions, enhancing clarity and focus.
- It makes one more receptive to inner and outer energies.

Spiritual Level

- Strong vyana vayu supports deep meditation.
- It facilitates the dissolution of the ego, allowing the mind to move beyond limited identities into a state of vast awareness.
- When vyana vayu is balanced, one feels deeply connected to the divine, experiences effortless intuition, and radiates peace and vitality.

Imbalanced Vyana Vayu

- When vyana vayu is weak, there is a sense of restlessness and anxiety.
- The body feels lethargic and stiff, suffering ailments like joint pain, poor mind–body

coordination, musculoskeletal issues, arthritis, and joint inflammation.

- There is an overhwhelming feeling of alienation and hatred.

Yoga Sequence to Increase the Power of Vyana Vayu

- Standing poses are particularly effective in integrating energy flow.
- Standing poses allow to connect the various movements of the arms and legs.

Standing Asanas

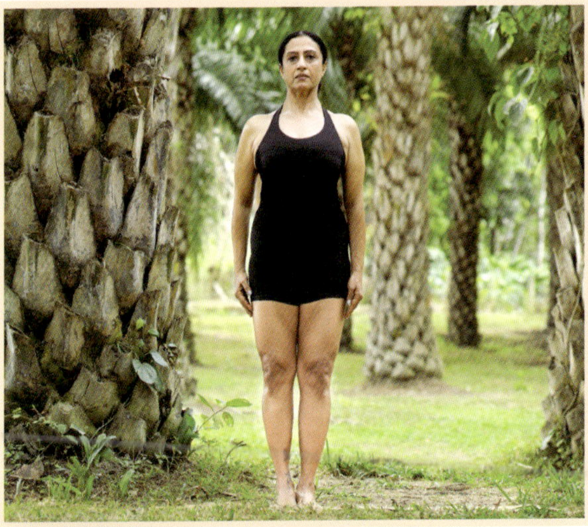

TADASANA

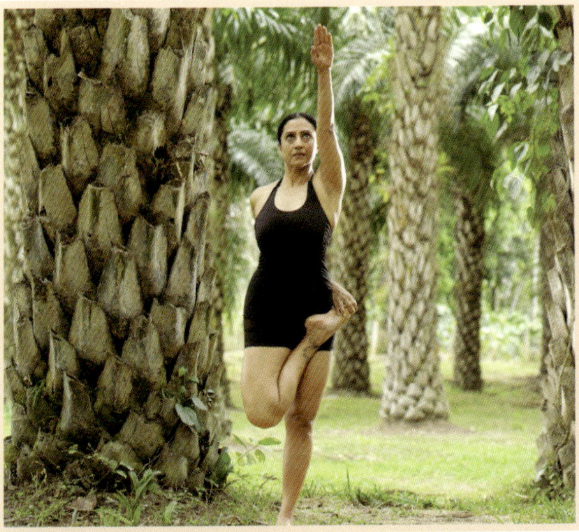

ARDHA PADMA TADASANA

SURYA NAMASKARA A (FOR REFERENCE, SEE PP. 4–5)

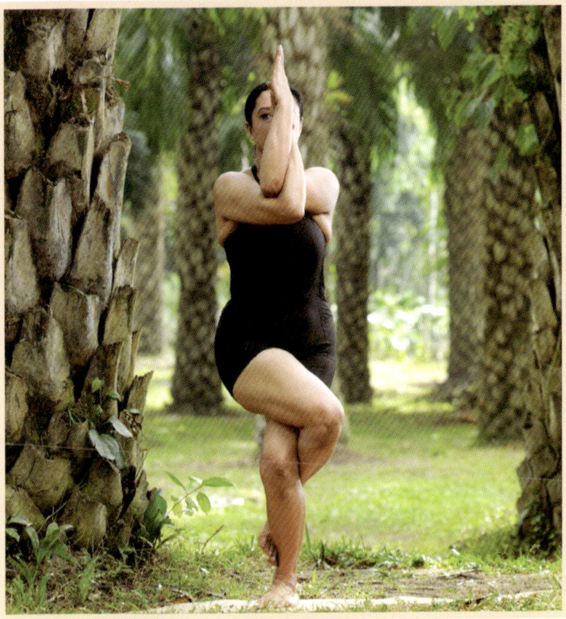

GARUDASANA

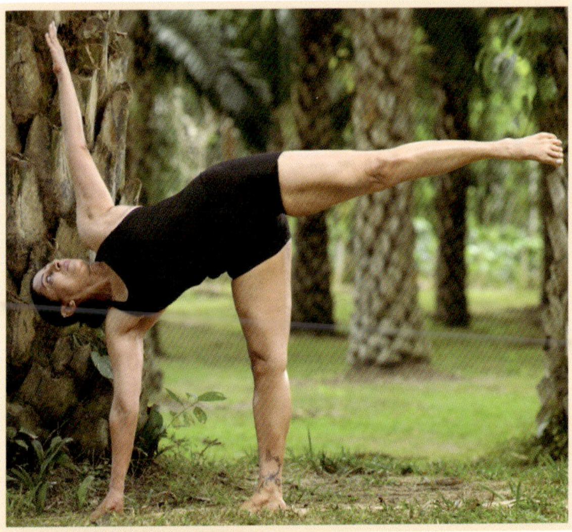

ARDHA CHANDRASANA

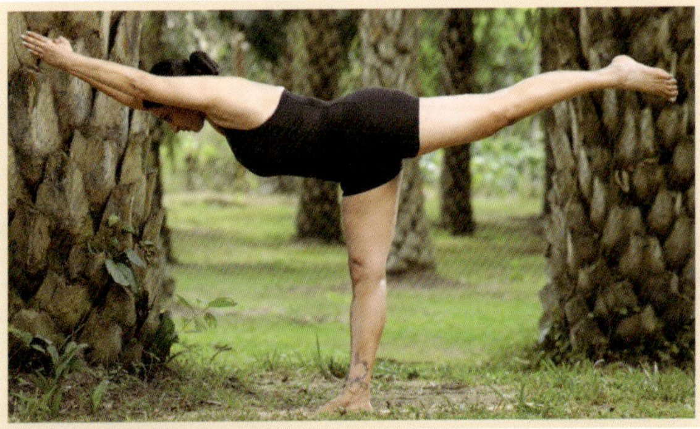

VEERABHADRASANA

Sitting Asanas

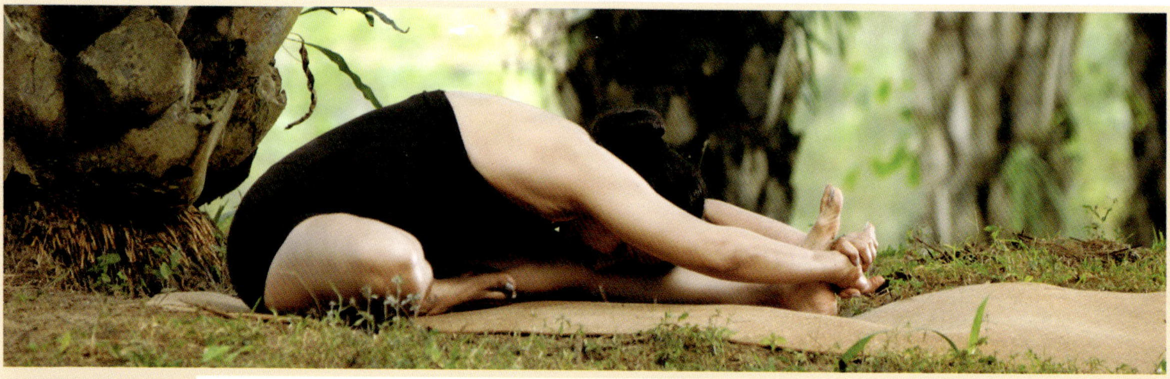

JANU SHIRASANA

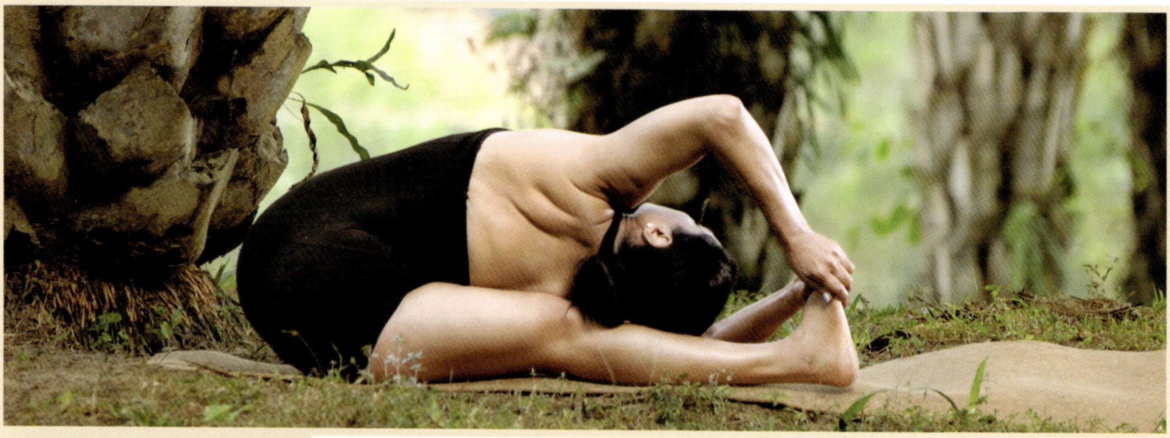

PARIVRITTI JANU SHIRASANA

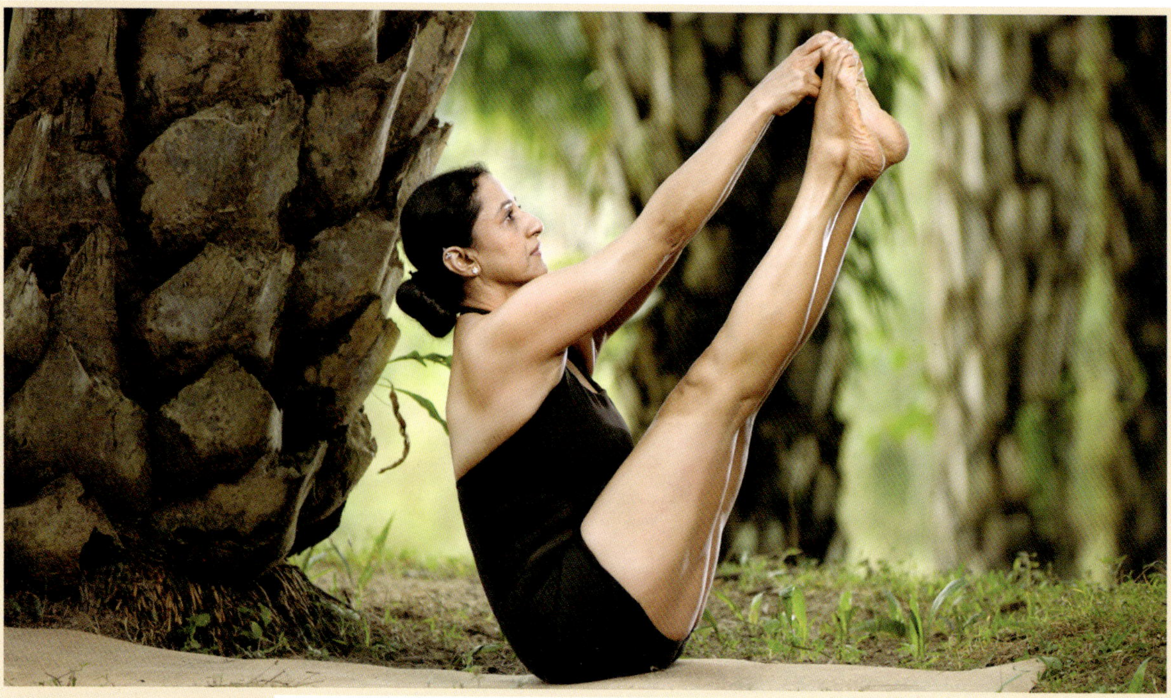

SAMPOORNA NAVASANA

Floor Asanas

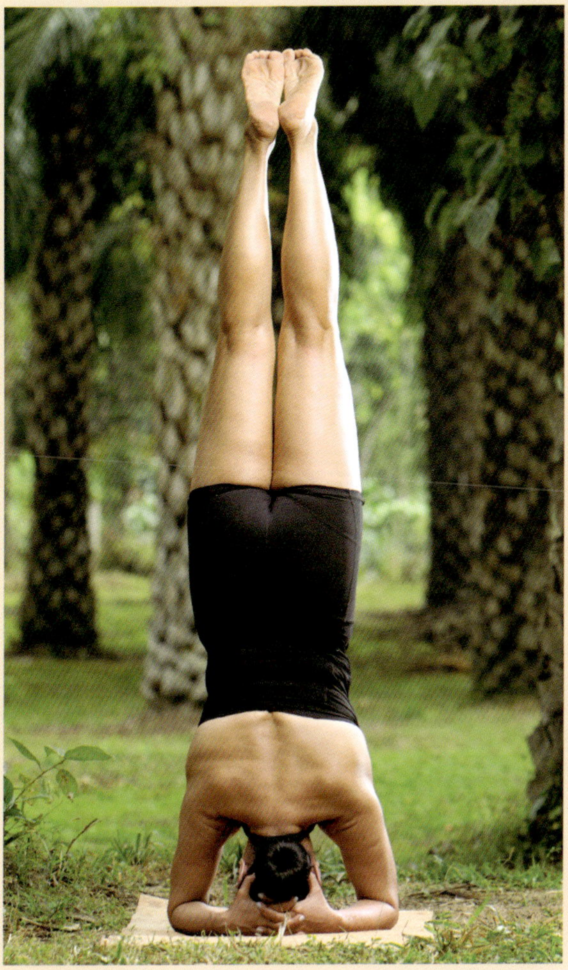

SHIRASANA

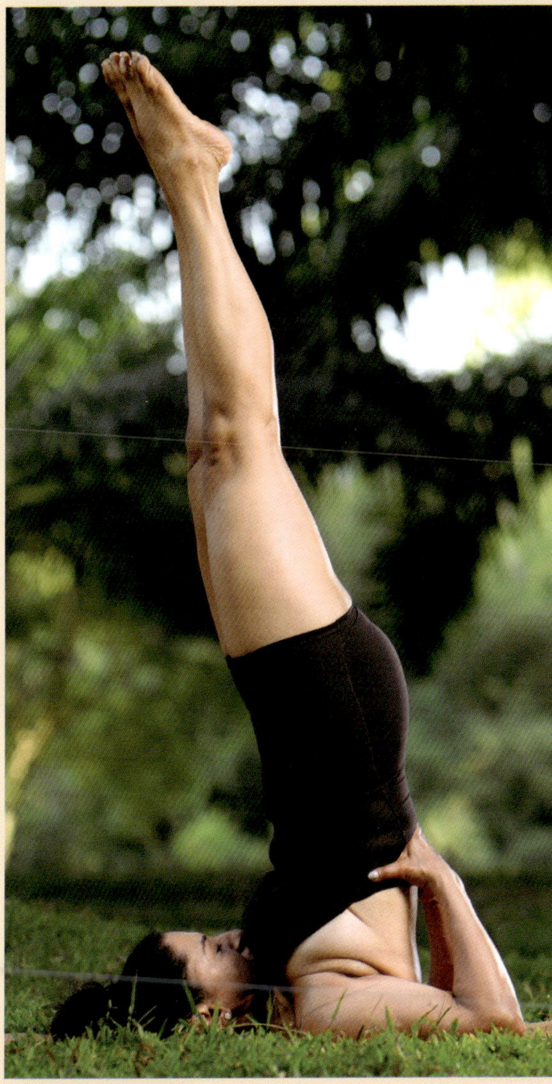

SARVANGASANA

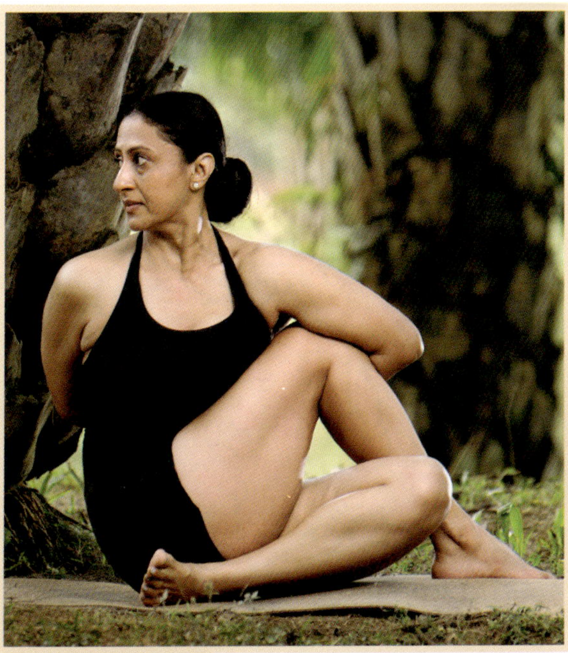

MATSYENDRASANA

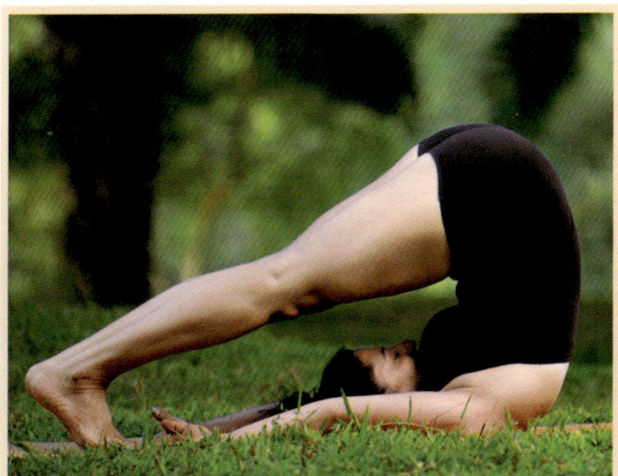

HALASANA 1

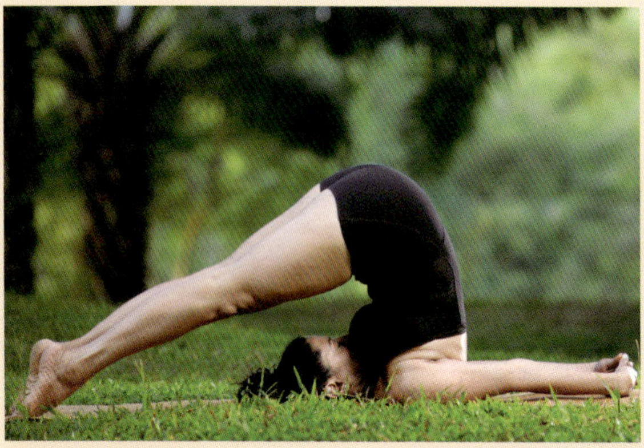

HALASANA 2

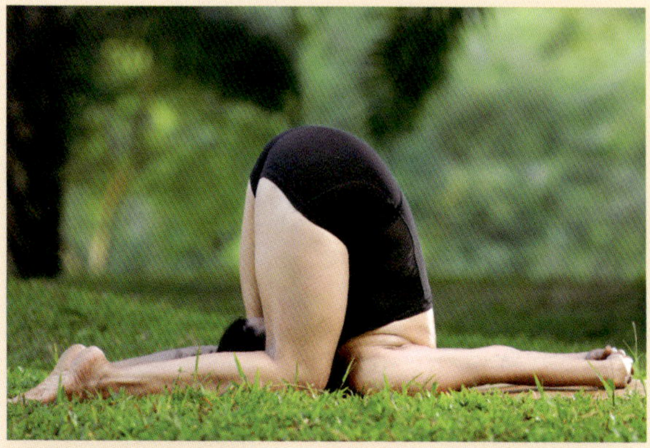

KARNAPEEDASANA

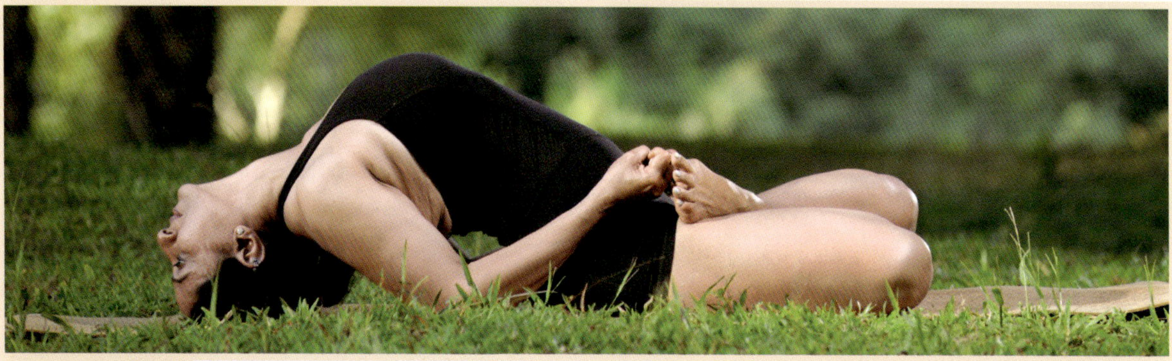

MATSYASANA 1

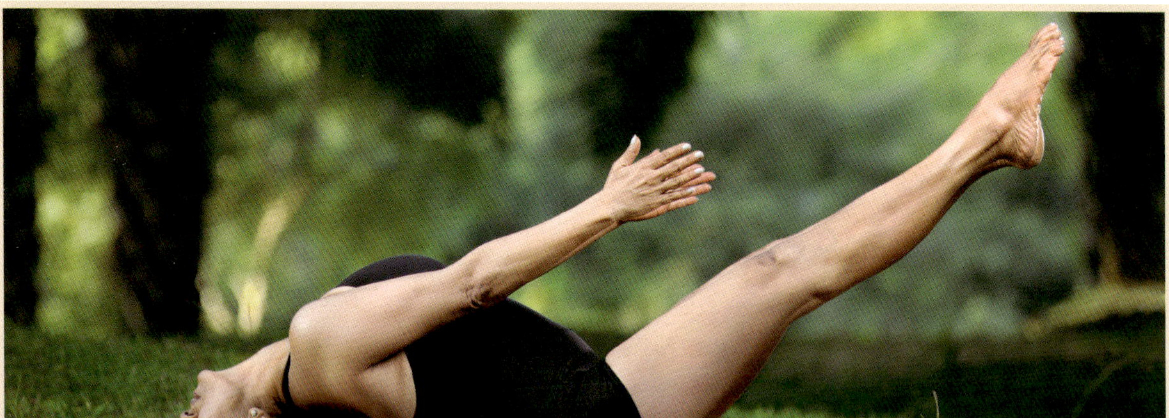

MATSYASANA 2

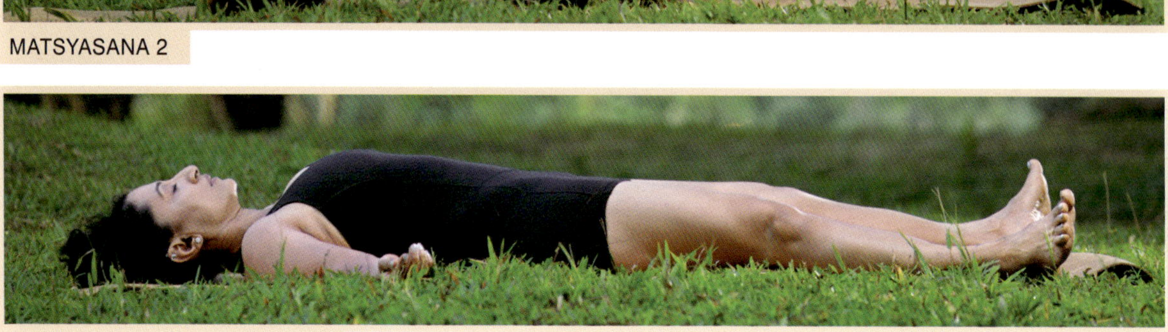

SHAVASANA (FOR 10 MINUTES)

Pranayama

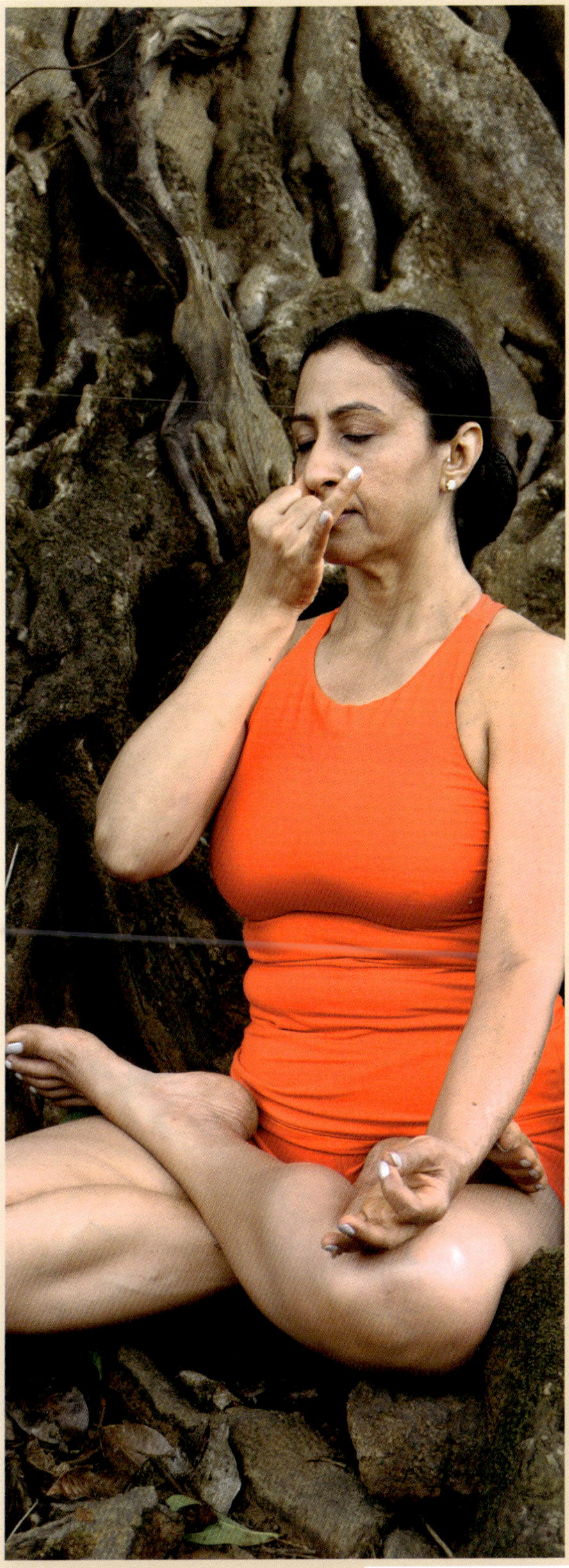

ANULOM VILOM WITH KUMBHAKA (BOTH ANTAR AND BAHYA)

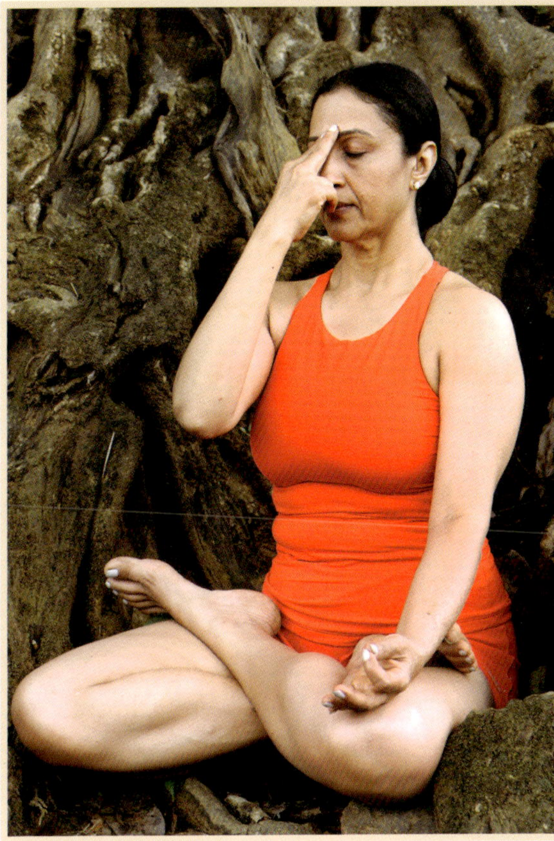

ANULOM VILOM

Mudra

This mudra regulates the vyana vayu. It keeps the energy levels stable and reduces feelings of lethargy and fatigue.

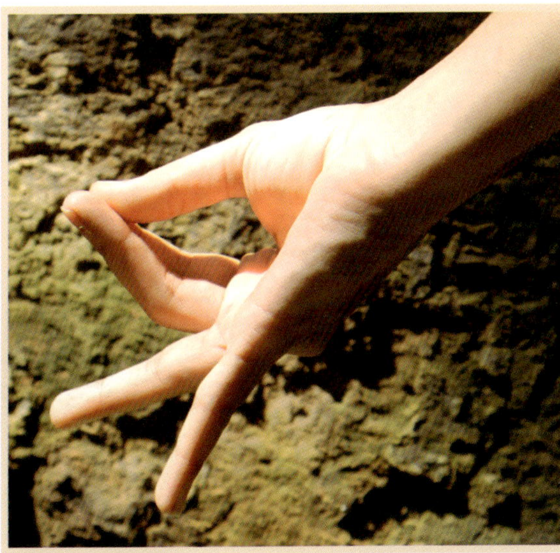

VYANA MUDRA

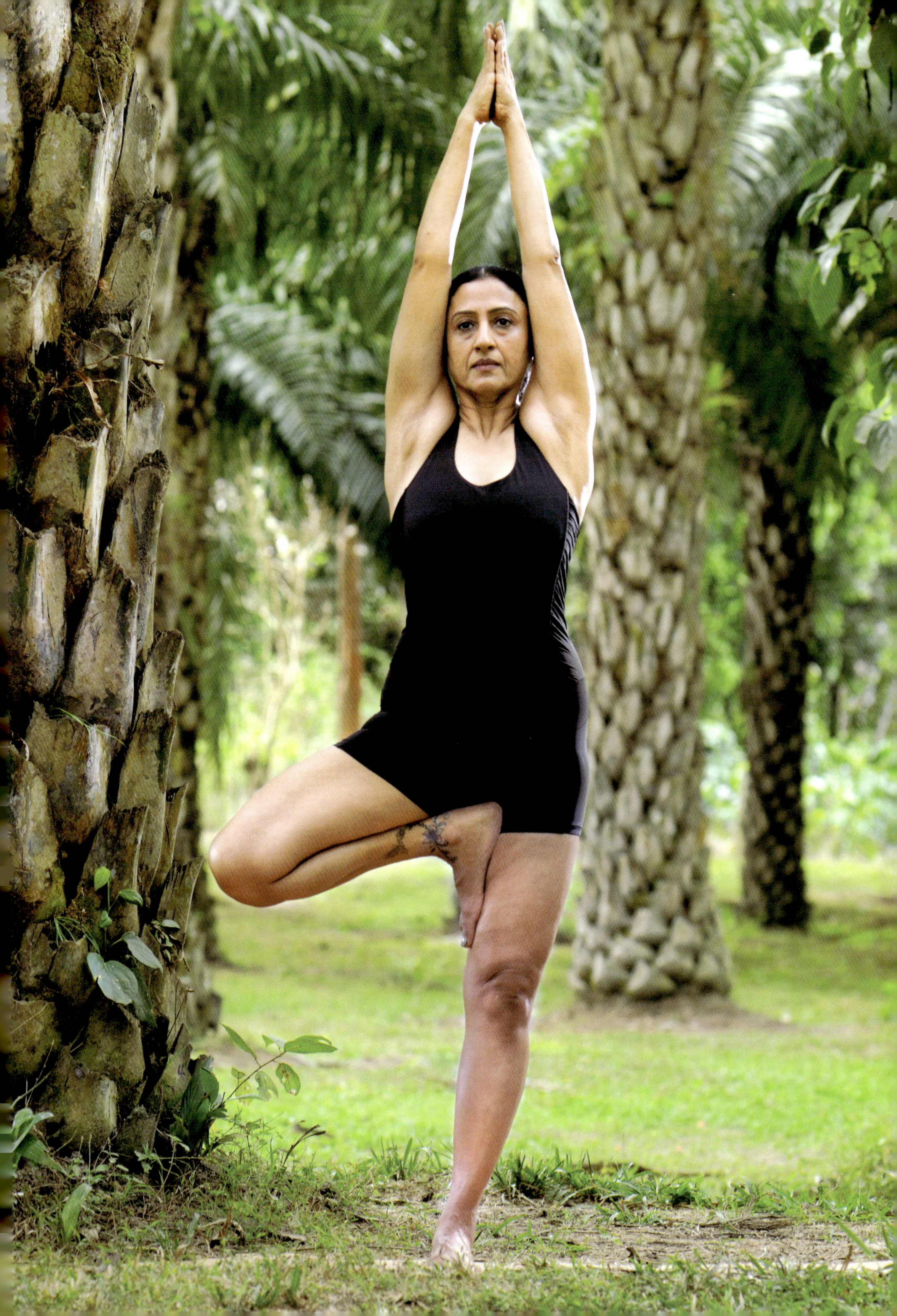

CHAPTER 8

PRANAYAMA

Pranayama, the art of breathing, focuses on expanding life force energy. Unlike asanas, which emphasize muscular and skeletal alignment, pranayama centres on air pressure, energy flow and breath control. *Prana* means 'energy of breath', and *ayama* is 'control'. The process of breathing involves three steps: *rechaka*, *puraka* and *kumbhaka*, or exhalation, inhalation and breath retention.

Pranayama helps a yoga practitioner progress to higher levels of practice. It has various therapeutic benefits. It involves breath control, with focus on timing, duration and frequency of every breath retention. The main purpose of this is to remove toxins from the mind and body, bridging the gap between the two. The benefits of pranayama have been extensively researched. It has been proven that it

- **Increases mindfulness, focus and concentration:** Breathing in and out with total awareness increases mindfulness. Mind wanders from one thought to another, shuffling between the past and future, seldom staying in the present. Pranayama techniques have a very calming effect which supports mindfulness and awareness of the present moment.
- **Decreases the stress levels:** Pranayama decreases stress and anxiety levels, calming the nervous system, as the oxygen intake during pranayama is increased. Regular practice of pranayama improves sleep, increases lung function and regulates blood pressure.

It is easy to add breathing exercises to your daily routine. Mentioned below are some simple tips to consider before you start practising pranayama:

STAGE 1

- It is important to choose the right spot to practise pranayama. It should be ideally in a room where you are getting enough fresh air. However, the immediate environment should not be too breezy, hence avoid open spaces or outdoors.
- A dedicated time and place for practice will help maintain consistency. How much time is put into the practice should not be the primary concern. About five minutes of focused practice is good enough to begin with.
- Pranayama can be practised multiple times in a day but under the guidance of a guru.
- It should be practised on an empty stomach.

STAGE 2

- Sit in a comfortable position. Spine should be straight and not stretched. The body must be relaxed.
- Mind should be calm and focused, refraining from all external and internal disturbances. The focus should remain on breath.
- An understanding of the normal breathing rhythm of a person is essential. Variations in breathing can be practised once normal breathing and rhythm are understood.

SIMPLE BREATHING TECHNIQUES

EXHALATION AND INHALATION (RECHAKA AND PURAKA)

- Ensure the seating arrangement is comfortable.
- Start with normal breathing.
- Inhale and exhale, observing breath.
- Five to ten rounds will help settle the mind.

WHISTLE BREATH (KAKA MUDRA)

- Inhale by flaring the nostril and taking in every breath deeper and stronger.
- Exhale by circling your lips like you are about to blow a whistle with your mouth. Exhale slowly and mindfully.
- Five to ten rounds will help enhance focus.

BELLY OR DIAPHRAGMIC BREATHING

- Sit comfortably, maintaining neutral spine.
- Alternatively, you can practise this while lying down in shavasana.
- Place your left hand on your chest and your right hand just below your navel to enhance breath awareness.
- Inhale deeply through your nose, allowing your abdomen to expand and your right hand to rise slightly.
- Exhale slowly, as if blowing out candles, feeling your abdomen contract as the air leaves your body.
- Observing this breathing pattern helps calm the mind and deepen relaxation.

Do this five times. This breathing technique is very helpful for quality sleep when practised right before bedtime.

TRADITIONAL PRANAYAMA TECHNIQUES

UJJAYI

Ujjayi, often translated as 'victorious breath', is also known as 'ocean breath' due to the soothing, wave-like sound it produces during practice. This is a very important breathing technique for a yoga practitioner. In asana practices, breath is sometimes more important than the posture itself. Ujjayi technique of breathing has the potential to override disturbing and floating thoughts and help bring back focus and concentration. It helps synchronize movements of the body with breath. This also has the potential to oxygenate the body and heal it.

Practice

- Sit in a calm spot.
- Gently constrict the throat to regulate airflow, creating a soft, rushing sound that resembles ocean waves.
- Keep inhalations and exhalations equal to begin with.
- Gradually extend your exhalations to twice the length of your inhalations while maintaining the same sound and throat constriction.
- The sound produced should resemble gentle ocean waves or the rhythmic breath of deep, peaceful sleep.

Benefits

- Improves concentration.
- Calms the mind.
- Releases trapped tension in the body.
- Warms up the diaphragm and the body.
- Regulates temperature during asana practice.

Caution

- When the body is high on pitta dosha, ujjayi should be practised with a slight variation.
- Inhale using the ujjayi technique of constricting air, and exhale through the mouth, making a sound like 'hhaa' or 'ufff'.

NADI SHODHANA—ANULOM VILOM

This breathing technique involves gently closing one nostril while breathing in through the other, then switching sides for the exhale. (As shown

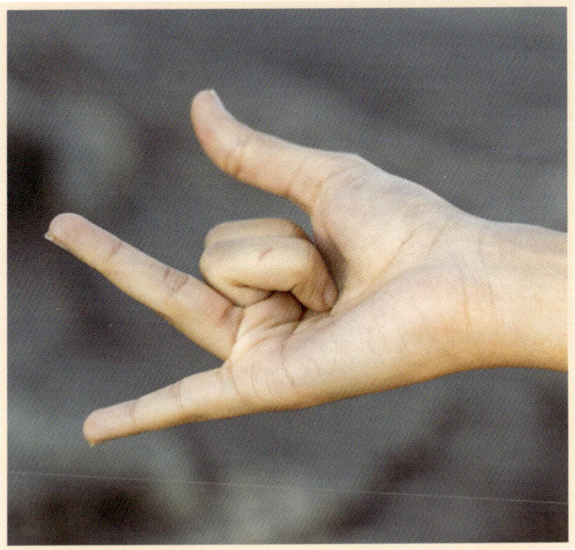

VISHNU MUDRA

in Vishnu Mudra) You can place your index and middle fingers on your forehead between your eyebrows, using your thumb and ring finger to alternately open and close each nostril.

Method

- Seating should be comfortable.
- Close the right nostril with the right thumb.
- Breath out from the left nostril.
- Steadily breath in through the left nostril.
- Close the left and breath out of the right nostril, removing the thumb.
- Breath in from the right nostril, with ring finger on the left.
- Breathe out from the left, removing the finger and the right nostril closed with the thumb.
- This makes it one round.
- Repeat for at least five rounds, and then take a short break before repeating another five rounds.
- Breathing should be mild and calm, producing a gentle sound.
- The practice should be done for at least 10 minutes and not exceed 15 minutes for beginners.

Antar Kumbhaka

- This involves holding of breath after every inhalation.
- Inhale through left nostril and close both the nostrils and hold it for a count of five seconds (for beginners), and then release thorough the right nostril.
- Inhale through the right nostril and close both the nostrils and hold it for a count five seconds (for beginners), and then release through the left nostril.
- Maintain a comfortable ratio. For example, start with a two-second inhalation, four-second hold, four-second exhalation. If comfortable, gradually progress to two-second inhalation, six-second hold, four-second exhalation.

Benefits

- The most important benefit of anulom vilom is the balance it brings about in the body's constitution. Most of the diseases in the body are due to the imbalance in the doshas.
- It helps regulate the body's temperature which may fluctuate due to environmental changes.
- It helps calm the mind.
- It facilitates better focus, concentration and memory.
- It enhances the digestive power.
- Cardiovascular health immensely benefits from this.

Caution

- Kumbhaka should be practised only when one has significant experience in practising anulom vilom for atleast a year.
- Any prolonged discomfort should be taken up with the doctor or with a yoga teacher, to ascertain possible diagnosis.

BHRAMARI

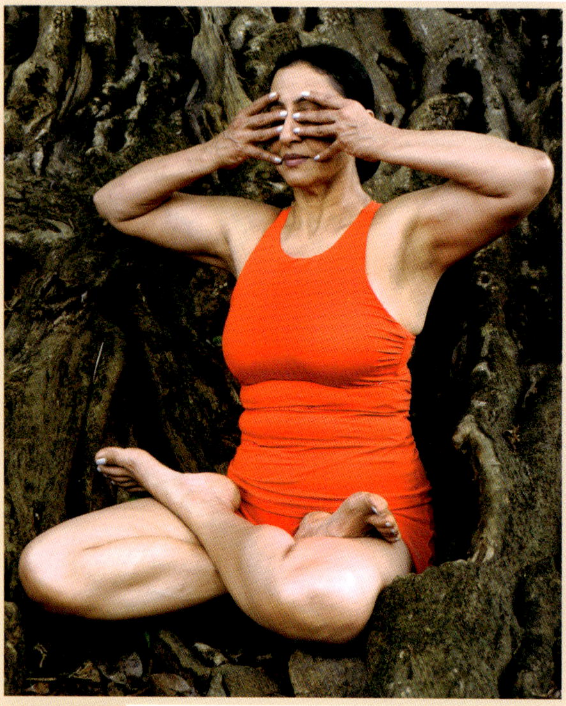

BHRAMARI

Bhramari involves imitating the humming sound of a bee. This simple yet calming breathing technique not only has a soothing effect but also influences the flow of prana.

Method

- A quiet place in the open air will be ideal.
- Relax your facial muscles and expressions.
- Place your thumb on the cartilage (tragus) of your ears, your index finger on the eyebrows, middle finger on the eye lids, ring finger below the bridge of the nose, and the little finger on the sides of the lips.
- Inhale as you gently press the cartilage with your thumb.
- Exhale with a humming sound with your lips closed.
- Let the hum last as long as the breath does.
- Take a deep breath and repeat again.
- Do it for three times initially and do not exceed more than six times in a single sitting.
- Bhramari can be prasticed lying down as well.

Benefits

- This breathing technique is highly beneficial for those suffering from thyroid issues.
- It reduces blood pressure.
- It reduces anxiety, anger and frustration.
- Quality of sleep improves.
- People battling hypertension should practise bhramari.

Caution

- Do not continue the buzzing bee sound if there is an irritation in the throat or if there is an infection, like ulcers, in the mouth.
- It is not ideal to practise bhramari in the afternoon.

SITALI

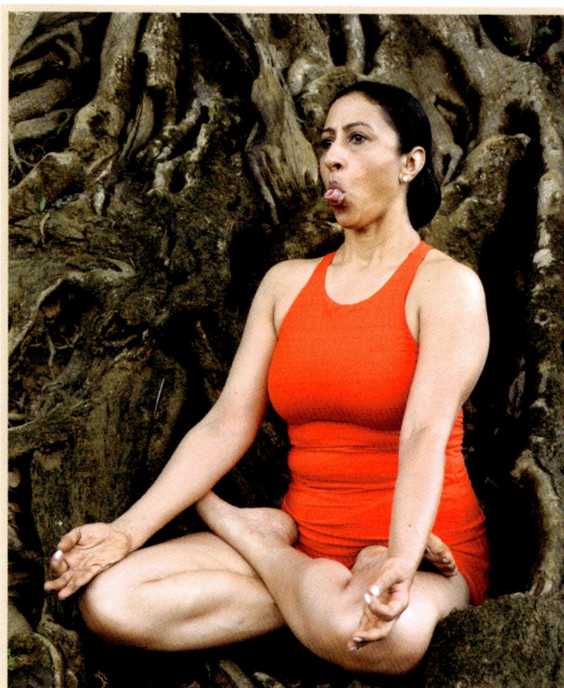

SITALI

Sitali is a cooling breathing technique in yoga that helps regulate body temperature, calms the nervous system and reduces stress. It is especially useful in hot weather, during times of emotional stress, or to balance excess heat (pitta dosha).

Method

- A comfortable seating position is important.
- Calm the existing breathing (especially if this is being performed after an asana practice).
- Work on rolling the tongue to resemble like a tube. If this is difficult, then clench your teeth and keep lips slightly parted.
- Press the tongue to the back of the teeth.
- Inhale slowly through the tongue or between the teeth, as if drawing air through a pipe.
- Pull the tongue in and press the tip of the tongue to the palate and exhale gently through the nostrils, making the sounds of ujjayi.
- After each try, rest for 20 seconds before the second round.
- Do not exceed more than five rounds in a single sitting.

Benefits

- It cools the body.
- It helps relax muscles and nerves.
- It is beneficial for people suffering from blood pressure.
- It aids in digestion.

Caution

- Do not practise this breathing technique during winters. It might result in a bad cold.
- Avoid practising this technique after the body has cooled down.

KAPALBHATI

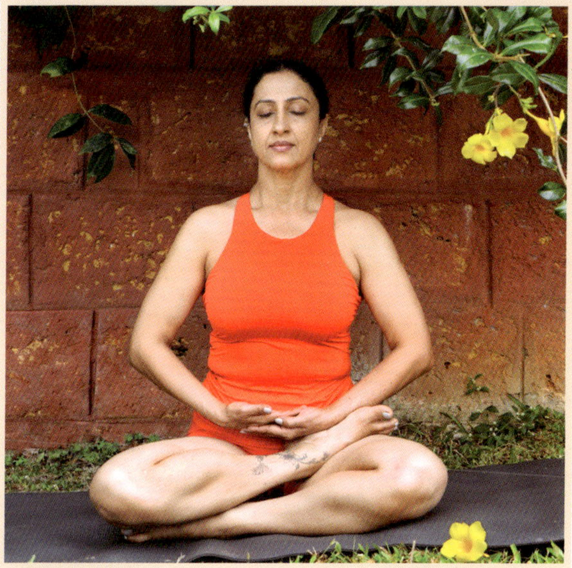

KAPALBATHI

Kapalbhati is also called the 'breath of fire'. The literal translation of the term *kapala* means 'skull' and *bhati* means Illuminating. This breathing technique generates heat in the body and dissolves waste and toxins from both body and mind.

Method

- Comfortable seating on a hard surface is a requirement.
- Place your palms on top of one another, holding them over your lap.
- Focus on the belly region and observe the breathing, studying the movement of the belly.
- Inhale steadily and fill both lungs with air.
- Pull stomach in and back as if taking it close to the spine, contracting the abdominal muscles.
- As you relax your muscles, exhale forcefully through your nostrils in short, sharp bursts, producing a strong hissing sound.
- Go as far as possible and stop.
- Repeat after giving enough rest to the body.
- Do this for about two minutes without losing focus.

Benefits

- This practice dissolves waste and toxins from the body and mind.
- Blood circulation increases significantly.
- Weight loss becomes more achievable.
- The digestive fire strengthens.
- The mind feels uplifted.
- Warmth spreads throughout the body.
- The texture of the skin and hair improves.

Caution

- Stop if you feel dizzy or experience a mild headache, especially if you have high blood pressure.
- Stop when there is a pain in the abdomen.
- Heart patients should slow down the kapalbhati and do it for shorter counts.
- It should be practised on an empty stomach
- It is important to learn this technique from a certified teacher.
- Do not practise this technique if there is ulcers in the body.
- Asthma patients should first seek guidance from a yoga teacher.

BHASTRIKA

This method of breathing involves rapid forceful breathing in and out. The sound of the breathing during inhalation and exhalation is audible and strong.

Method

- A comfortable seating position with a steady, neutral spine is essential.
- Inhale deeply and forcefully for at least five seconds. Engage the facial muscles to enhance the strength of your breath through the nostrils.
- Exhale with the same force and for the same length of time, mimicking panting for breath.
- Do not exceed more than five breaths per sitting.
- Take enough break and rest between each sittings.

Benefits

- This technique oxygenates the body and increases blood supply to the lungs.
- Excess phlegm gets drained from the lungs.
- It calms the mind and cools the body.
- The lungs grow stronger.
- Abdominal organs become toned and strengthened, improving their function.

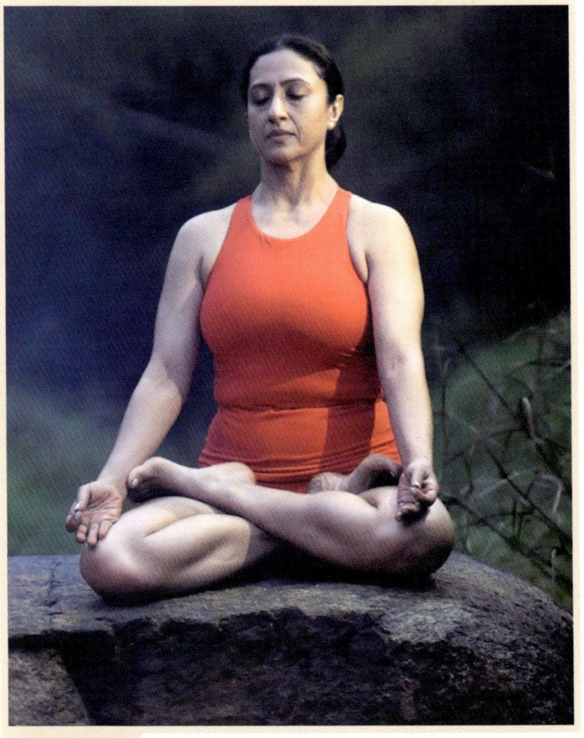

BHASTRIKA

Caution

Do not practise this pranayama if you suffer from hypertension, heart ailments, intestinal disorders, spinal abnormalities, eye problems, vertigo, cardiovascular problems and asthma.

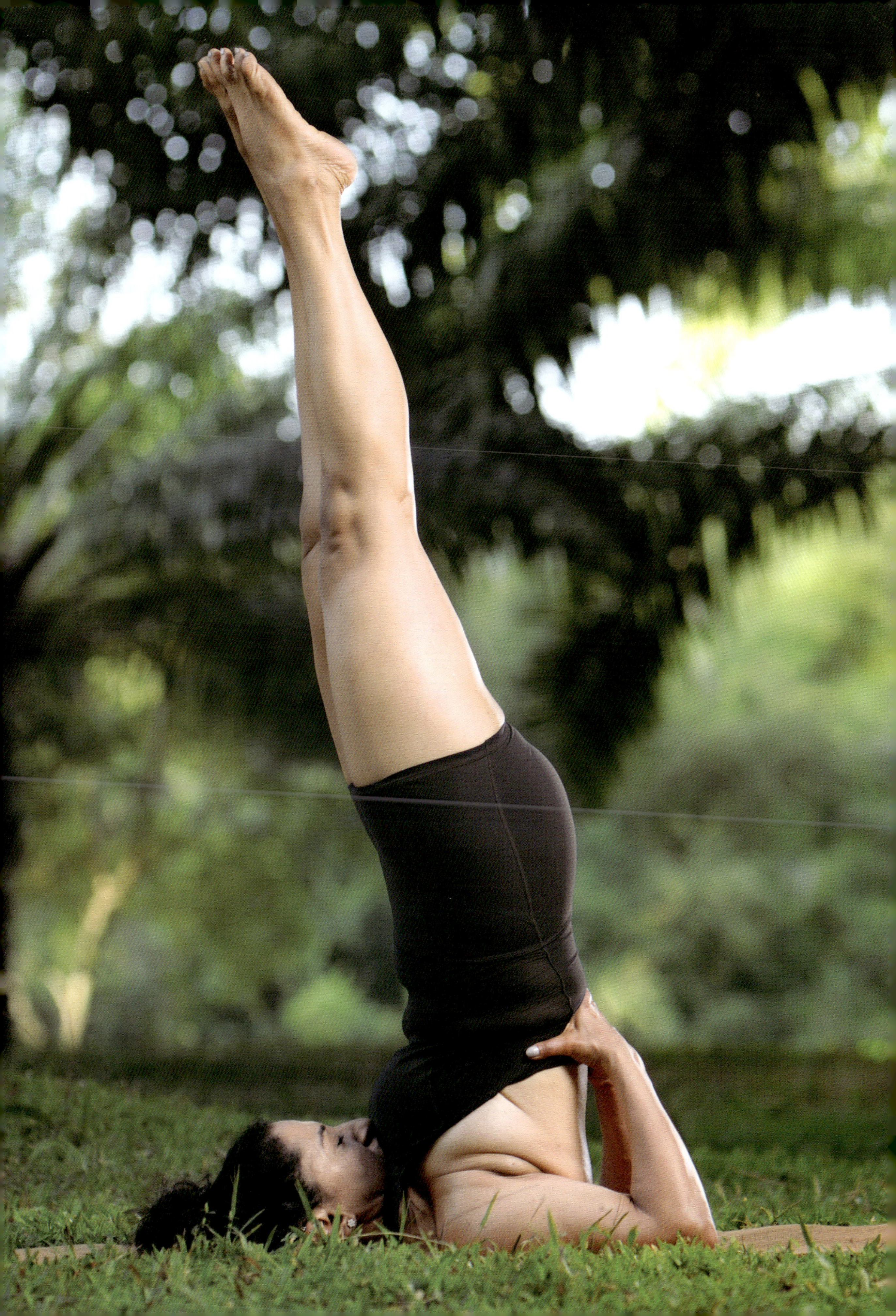

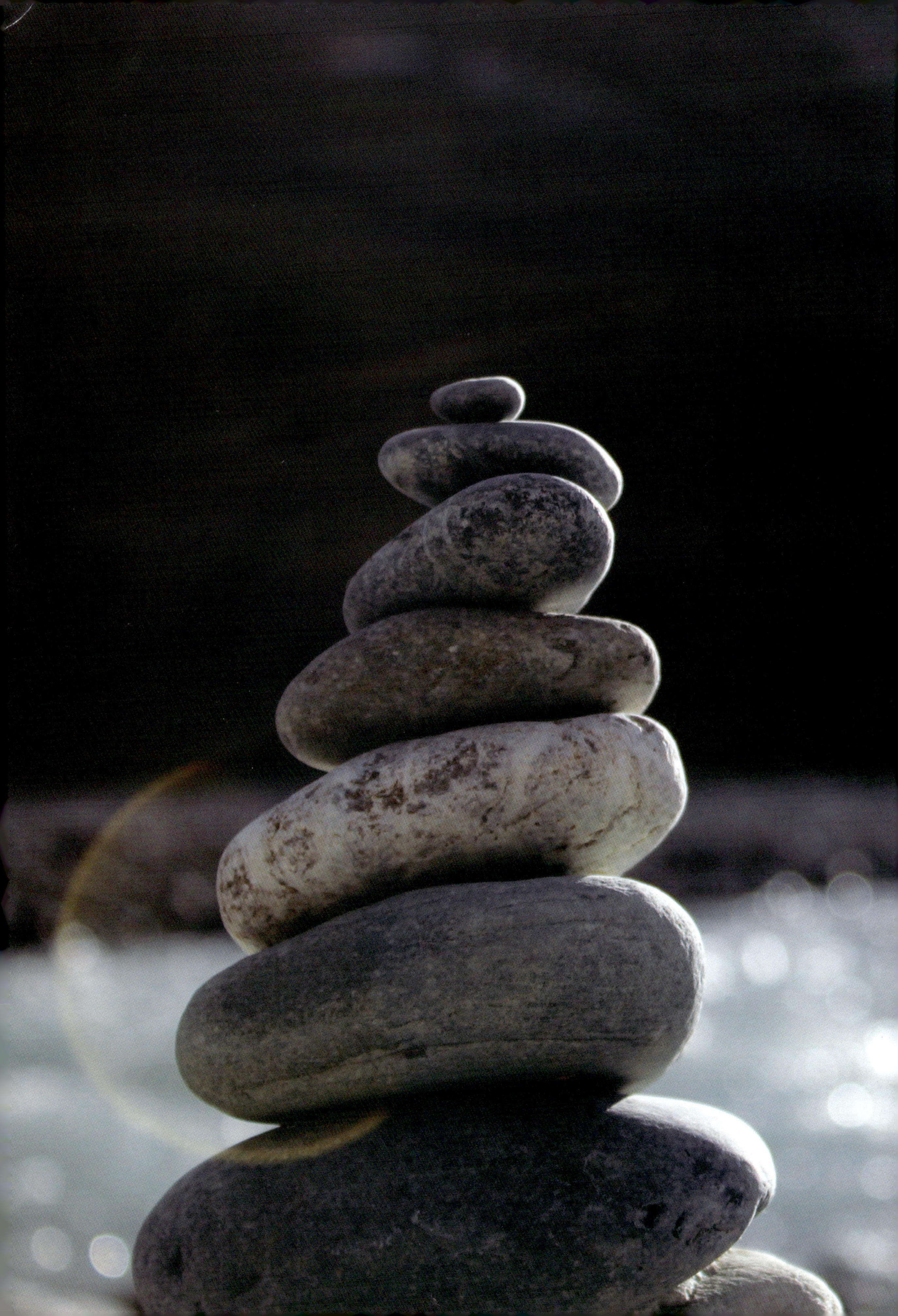

SECTION C

KARMIC LANDSCAPE OF THE BODY

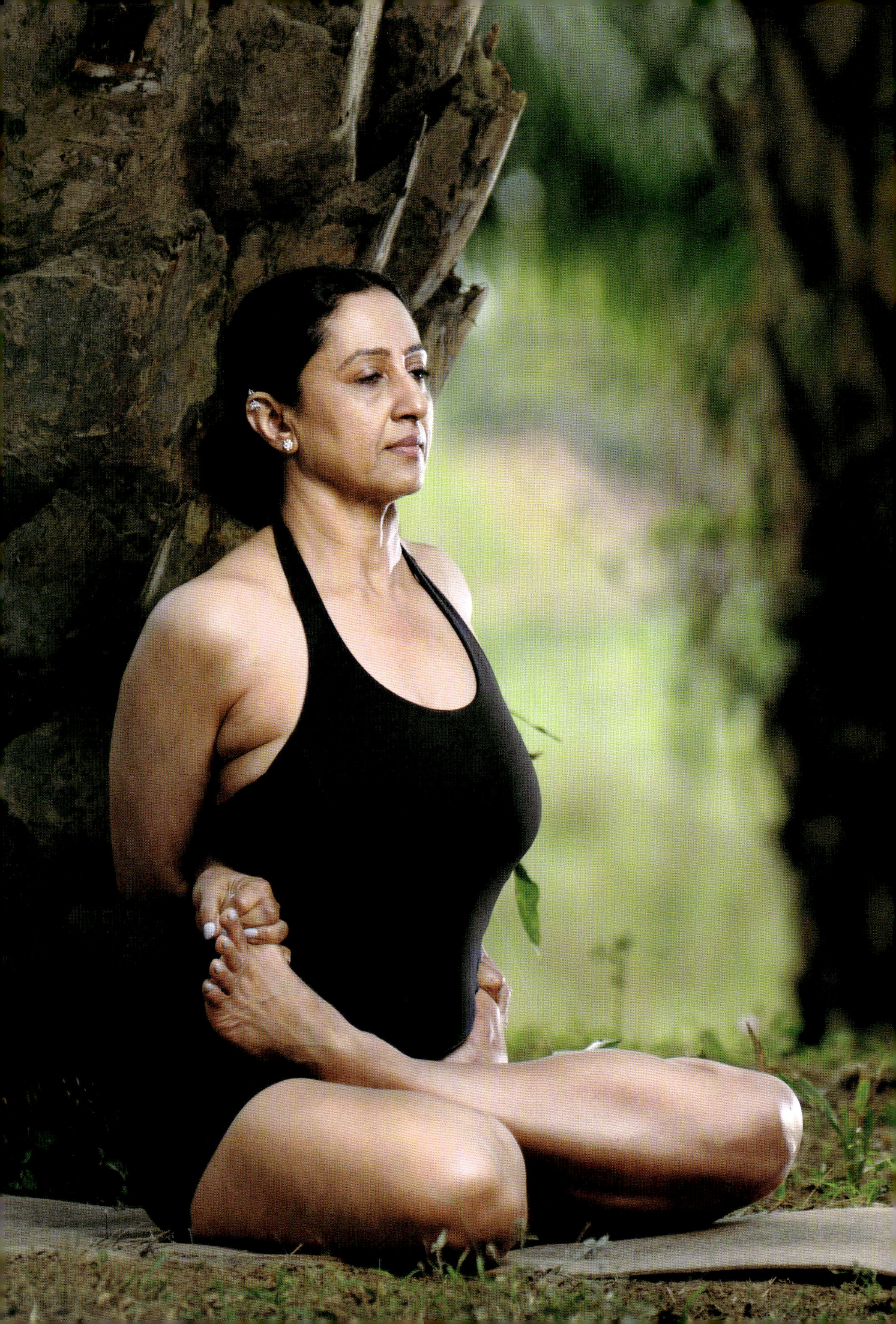

CHAPTER 9

KARMASHAYA

The study of the principles of karma is an ongoing and complex pursuit, yet it is essential for understanding the key questions that often arise among yoga practitioners. No single text fully encapsulates the principles of karma, as various ancient scriptures explore it from different perspectives. Much of the information in this book is drawn from personal study of classical texts, scholarly discourses, and insights from epics and mythology.

The most important and constant explanation of the doctrine of karma is that it is based on cause and effect: 'For every karma, there is a corresponding *phala*'. The word 'phala' literally means the 'fruit' or 'the result of an action'. It may seem like a simple principle, but when all its causes come together, the results become complex. Every karma can lead to multiple outcomes—some aligning with expectations, some exceeding them, some falling short, and others deviating entirely. The unpredictability of these results arises from unseen factors influencing them. What we often call luck or random events may, in fact, be effects of karma.

Studying the texts on karma gives the impression that sages deeply contemplated the events unfolding around them. Their reflections led to reasoned insights, which were then documented. These texts offer numerous interpretations and explanations, highlighting the circumstantial nature of karma's causes. However phala can be understood in two ways:

- *Drishta:* It can be seen or experienced in immediate surroundings. The consequences manifest in the present life, often occurring soon after the action is performed.
- *Adrishta:* It cannot be seen or experienced immediately. It is what one experiences in later stages of life, or in the next life.

AUTHOR'S NOTE

The scope and doctrine of karma cannot be definitively proven or disproven, making it a matter of faith. This understanding should be approached with respect, as there is no absolute right or wrong.

According to karmic principles, everyone born will undergo some undeserved joy and undeserved sorrow. Everybody is subjected to the law of karma. Understanding the principles of karma helps us make sense of the unexpected and undeserving events of our lives. When there are instances where our carefully planned actions do not yield the results or when we are beset by some kind of tragedy, these teachings help us to be more patient, more composed and more resistant, and could help us navigate towards a higher understanding of one's purpose in life.

PRINCIPLES OF KARMA

According to the laws of karma, thoughts are the core energy that give rise to actions, while emotions represent this energy in motion.

There is no single, universally agreed-upon number of principles of karma, but in modern spiritual teachings, 12 principles of karma are commonly referenced.

1. **Law of cause and effect:** *As you sow, so shall you reap.* Good thoughts will produce good energy and bad thoughts will produce bad energy.
2. **Law of creation:** *Life doesn't just happen.* Things don't magically happen on their own—effort is the key. You, as an individual, are the creator of your destiny.

3. **Law of humility:** *Accepting existing circumstances is vital.* Being humble enough to accept that the current life circumstances are the result of past actions is necessary.
4. **Law of growth:** *One has control over how to deal with life but none over the final results.* Here, the ultimate focus is not on the circumstances or the results but how one needs to navigate through the circumstances and deal with it.
5. **Law of responsibility**: *Take responsibility of whatever happens in life and never depend on others.* The choices one makes to deal with life is the focus in this law.
6. **Law of connection:** *Life is always connected to the past, present and future.* Whatever one does in the past will bear results in the future.
7. **Law of focus:** *Do one thing at a time.* Maintain goal-oriented focus on what should be done in life.
8. **Law of giving:** *Happiness is when people around us are happy.* Everything in the world is shared—we share the land, we share the air we breathe, food, etc.
9. **Law of here and now**: *Embrace the present.* Dwelling in the past and worrying about the future are not healthy for life to move on smooth.
10. **Law of change:** *Change should not be feared.* Change is an important step to progress in any aspect of life.
11. **Law of patience:** *Calmly accept the fact that everything takes time.* Nothing happens with immediate effect.
12. **Law of purpose:** *Contribute to the higher purpose of life.* Everyone is born with some special skill and talent that have to be recognized and used to fulfill themselves.

Life can push anyone into unimaginable situations. Understanding the possible reasons behind these challenges and learning to steady the mind, rather than reacting impulsively, can be invaluable. Gaining insight into the laws of karma provides the spiritual strength to face adversity with patience, resilience and wisdom.

AUTHOR'S NOTE

The principles of karma are not studied as precise mathematical equations. It can be understood in various ways, depending on how it is studied. Self-studying the scriptures is interesting to begin with. However, being open to scholarly interpretations of the scriptures by gurus and teachers is what makes a huge difference.

TYPES OF KARMA

Karma is a widely discussed topic among those who practise yoga and and embrace spiritual or holistic approaches to enhance their lifestyle. Understanding this can provide clarity on seemingly inexplicable life events. This awareness helps cultivate calmness, focus and a deeper sense of duty while navigating life's challenges.

The Vedic concept of karma offers a perspective on the various events unfolding in the world around us. Understanding karma can offer deeper insights into yoga philosophy. The points below are drawn from the author's personal study, though multiple interpretations exist in the scriptures, reflecting diverse schools of thought.

- **Sanchita Karma:** This is the aggregate sum total of karmas collected from many past lives. Every conscious choice made by a human being gets registered as karma, like in a container or a file, and this is called *karmashraya*. These are stored as good impressions and bad impressions. It is explained in the scriptures that this container is carried for lifetimes, like a baggage.
- **Prarabdha Karma:** Each time life takes a new form, it offers an opportunity to repay a portion of the accumulated karma within a single lifetime. However, it is important to note that

only a fraction can be resolved, as new karmas may also be created in the present life.

- **Kriyamana Karma:** The choices one makes in a lifetime lead to destiny. This is kriyamana karma, where one is able to initiate a new course of actions that have the potential to modify and even nullify the effects of karmic baggage.
- **Adhyatmika Karma:** It refers to the karma that unfolds immediately or in the near future as a direct result of one's actions. For example, if you help someone in need, you will be certainly helped when you are in need. If you rob someone, you will see losses in your own life too.
- **Adhibhautika Karma:** It pertains to the sufferings and challenges arising from interactions with other living entities and the material world. These miseries are inflicted by external sources, such as other people, animals or environmental factors. Adhibhautika karma can also refer to the collective karma created by groups of people, such as families, communities or nations, affecting individuals within these groups.
- **Adhidaivika Karma:** This refers to 'acts of nature'. It is believed that even our planet has its own karma that manifests in different forms. It could be in the form of volcanic eruptions, tsunami, earthquakes, etc.

AUTHOR'S NOTE

Karma is not a simple, linear equation but a complex web of interwoven causes and effects, shaped by countless permutations and combinations. While this may give the impression that life is entirely predetermined, that is not the case. Kriyamana karma—the actions performed in the present—are fully within one's control and actively shape future outcomes. Therefore, living with responsibility, dispassion and commitment is essential in navigating life with awareness and purpose.

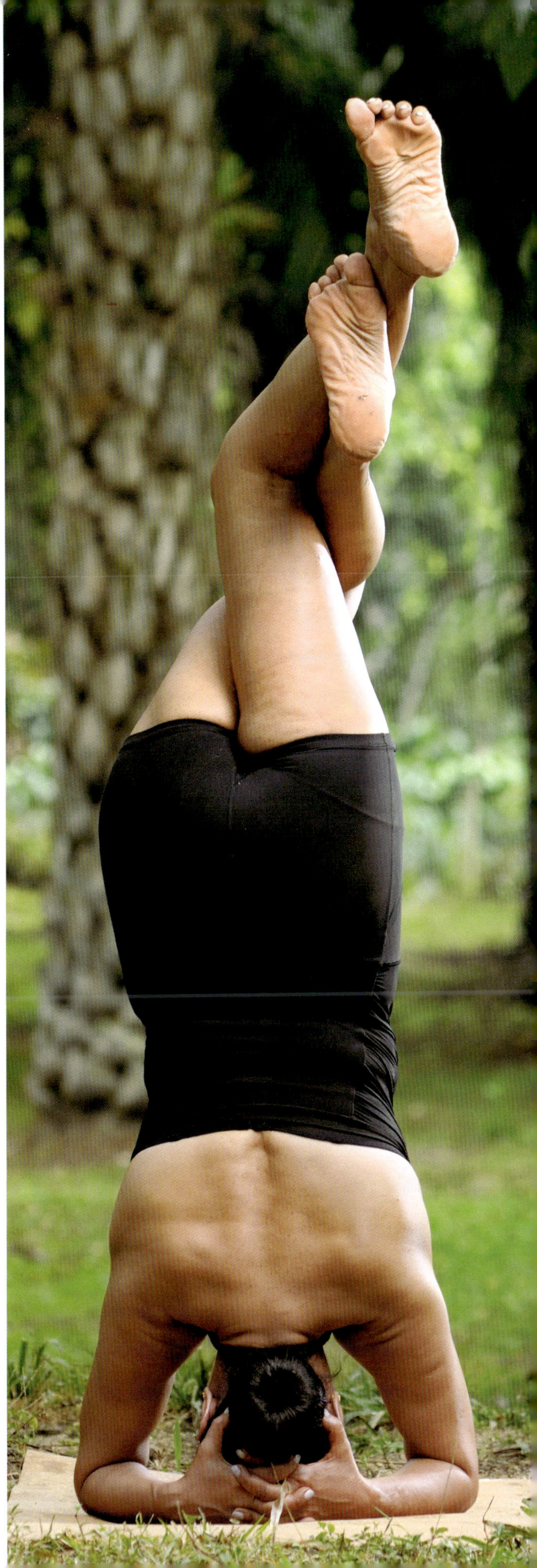

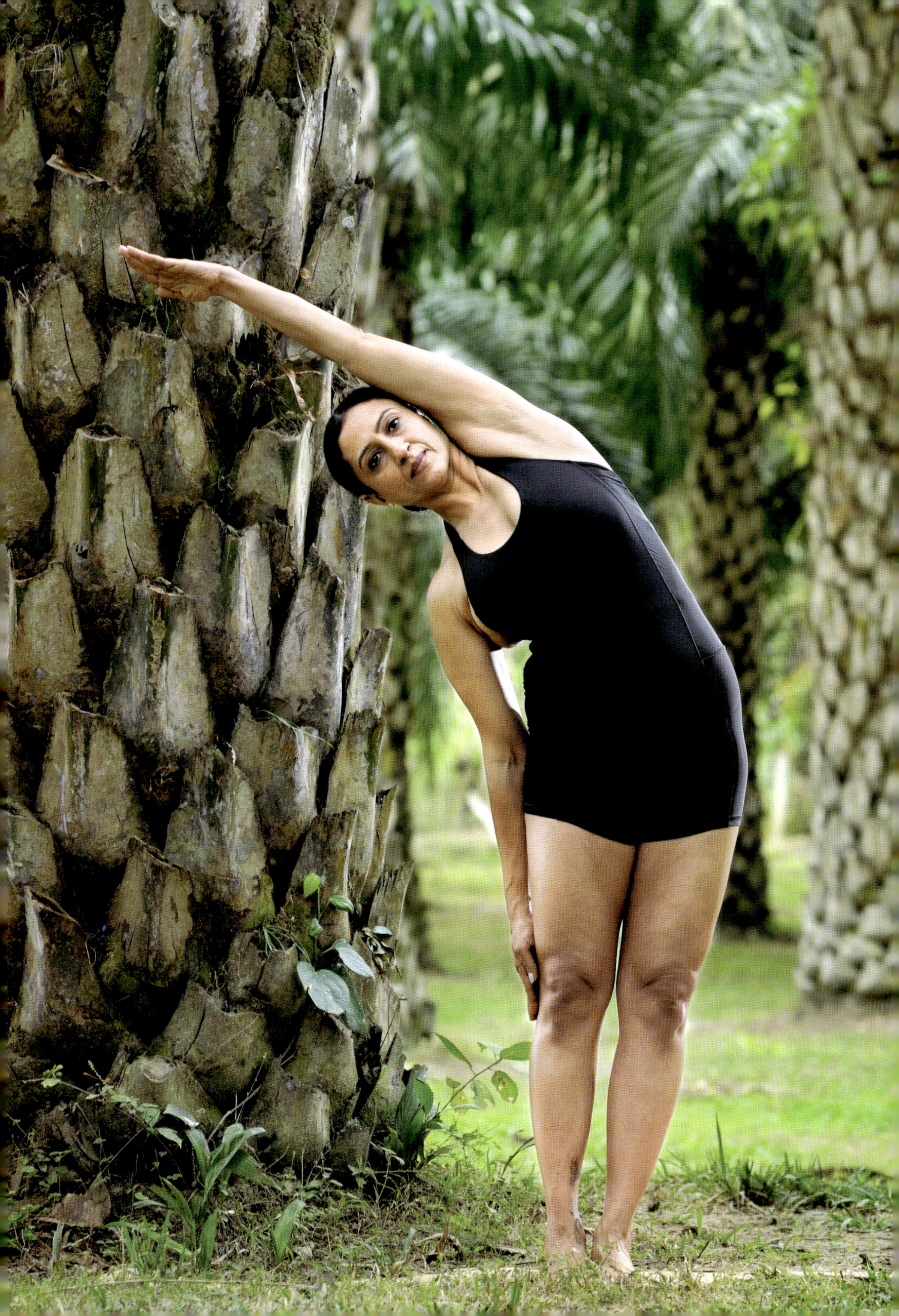

CHAPTER 10
PHILOSOPHY OF YOGA

The philosophy of yoga is not derived from a single text but is a vast body of wisdom compiled by ancient scholars. It serves as a guide to understanding the body, mind and spirit. Nearly every ancient text contributes to the knowledge of yoga in some form. Whether through asanas, pranayama, mantra or dhyana, these practices are designed to deepen perception and reveal the inherent unity between life and nature.

There are several texts that discuss the philosophy of yoga. The following are some of the most important ones:

1. The Vedas, Upanishads, *Agama Shastra*, Tantra, *Natyashastra*, the great epics—Ramayana and Mahabharata, along with the Bhagavad Gita, Ayurveda and Siddha traditions are regarded as the most valuable and sacred sources of foundational wisdom for the practice of yoga.
2. The *Yoga Sutras* compiled by Patanjali, who codified 195 sutras or threads of knowledge, is another significant text. These are divided in four sections:
   - Samadhi Pada: The 51 sutras explain the various states of samadhi and the types of sadhana that leads one to such states.
   - Sadhana Pada: The 55 sutras explain the practices and approaches required to study, understand and attain oneness with the universe. This sections also explains the various obstacles one may experience in the practice and how to overcome it.
   - Vibhuti Pada: The 55 sutras explain the attainments and powers one may unlock in the practice of yoga. This section lists out the powers and clearly mentions that such attainments can become obstacles on the path to higher spiritual realization. It also provides guidance on how to navigate them.
   - Kaivalya Pada: The 34 sutras explain the final state of attainment. This is the state where one can understand what it means to feel the complete union with the true nature of existence.
3. *Hatha Yoga Pradipika*, authored by Swami Svatmarama, is a more practice-oriented book that contains the details pointing to yoga sadhana. It carries 383 shlokas, called *upadeshas*, meaning 'guidance'. It explains about some very effective asanas, pranayama and the six methods of purification called the Shat Karmas. The various mudras and their benefits are also talked about. The book is complete with explanation on the process of dhyana, *dharana* and understanding the state of samadhi.
4. The 355 shlokas of *Gheranda Samhita*, by Sage Gheranda, explains the progressive steps to attain the state of yogic consciousness or bliss.
5. The 3,2000 shlokas in Yoga Vashishtha, by Sage Valmiki, have complete explanation as to what yoga is and what its philosophy encapsulates.
6. Samkhya Philosophy, attributed to Sage Kapila, is one of the oldest and most influential philosophical systems, profoundly shaping the beliefs, values and foundational concepts of yoga.

STUDYING THE SCRIPTURES

The decision to study and practise yoga is a transformative journey—one that leads to knowledge and freedom from ignorance. The scriptures reveal that ancient sages were on a quest for this very understanding. Through deep study and contemplation, they uncovered profound insights into the purpose of life. Their wisdom offers guidance for life's most challenging situations—those beyond ordinary intelligence.

The scriptures encapsulate the collective wisdom of thousands of saints and sages across millennia. They outline a structured approach to studying them, comprising four key steps:

- *Adhyayana:* Learning or studying with the help of a guru
- *Manana:* Reflecting upon the meaning by self-study
- *Pravachana:* Listening to the teachings of various scholars
- *Vyavahara:* Applying the learnt ideas in daily life.

There are numerous encyclopedic scriptures from various sources across our land. However, encompassing that vast expanse of knowledge within this book is impossible. Therefore, this chapter presents carefully selected insights from the Vedic scriptures.

Every word and aphorism holds immense value. Here, we explore four major forces at play—key to understanding the significance and purpose of life.

LIFE'S PURPOSE

Vedic wisdom is essential for understanding yoga philosophy. In human life, the Vedas serve as a guiding manual, offering knowledge and purpose. They are broadly classified into four categories:

- Rig Veda: This is the oldest Veda, involving philosophical questions and answers about virtues—all of which help in leading a happy and content life.
- Sama Veda: This Veda is considered to be the storehouse of melodious chants. The Indian classical music has its roots in this Veda.
- Yajur Veda: This Veda encompasses the knowledge of worship and rituals performed for various life events, such as marriage, agriculture and victory.
- Atharva Veda: This Veda has the magical formulas for medicines. It also has sections on charms and spells.

Understanding the purpose of life is the key concept in all four texts.

Purushartha

Purushartha originated from Vedic wisdom but became explicitly structured only in later Hindu philosophical texts. It serves as a guiding principle for leading a balanced, meaningful life, integrating duty, material success, desires and spiritual liberation.

Purushartha literally means 'the purpose of life' or 'life's goals'. It encompasses the four objectives of human life, which are classified into four categories:

- Dharma
- Artha
- Kama
- Moksha

Every human being on earth is born to attain the above four goals. These goals make for valuable guidelines to transform life to a more structured and purposeful one.

Dharma

Walking the path of dharma empowers an individual to lead a purposeful life. The scriptures define dharma as the duties and responsibilities that uphold societal harmony and cosmic order. It is an expansive and profound area of knowledge that requires thoughtful application.

According to the scriptures, the moment a being takes birth, they are placed in a specific environment, with a particular physical form and circumstances—all aligned with their inherent dharma. However, one's purpose is not always immediately evident; it must be realized through wisdom, self-inquiry and conscious effort.

AUTHOR'S NOTE

Dharma is difficult to translate into English, as its meaning varies across different scriptures. Some texts define it as an individual's duty in life, others as justice, faith, the law of creation, or obligations. Each interpretation offers a unique perspective on its depth and significance.

However, true understanding of dharma comes through the study of scriptures, self-reflection, and the practice of righteous living. As one applies dharma in daily life, its meaning becomes clearer over time.

Artha

If dharma states purpose, *artha* is 'the means to fulfil purpose'. It encompasses both material wealth and intellectual pursuits, including knowledge. The scriptures clarify that seeking wealth is not contrary to the spiritual path. Poverty can hinder progress when basic needs like food, shelter and clothing remain unmet. Enough wealth is required to take care of the basic necessities in life. The important thing is to stay unattached and not too obsessed with generating more than what is required. Most of the texts explain artha as a study of social welfare.

Kama

'Kama' means desire, the driving force behind all actions—whether mundane ambitions or spiritual aspirations. According to the scriptures, desire itself is not wrong, but it must be aligned with dharma to be constructive and meaningful. When approached wisely, kama supports artha, helping to fulfil one's purpose without leading to excess or imbalance.

Suppressing desires entirely can cause disharmony, so the scriptures suggest two ways to manage kama:

- Fulfilling desires in a balanced and ethical manner, and
- Transcending desires through self-awareness and spiritual growth.

Fulfilling kama may seem straightforward, as its results are tangible and satisfaction is easily recognized. However, transcending desires is a far more challenging path, requiring discipline and self-awareness.

Moksha

The scriptures say the ultimate goal of a human life is to attain liberation from the cycle of birth and death. Liberation is not death but the realization of the potential of life and the knowledge which is essential for freedom from life's suffering. Moksha is also referred to as *mukti* in some texts and in Samkhya Philosophy.

This is the stage where dharma, artha and kama are in total alignment with the 'self', fulfilling a divine purpose.

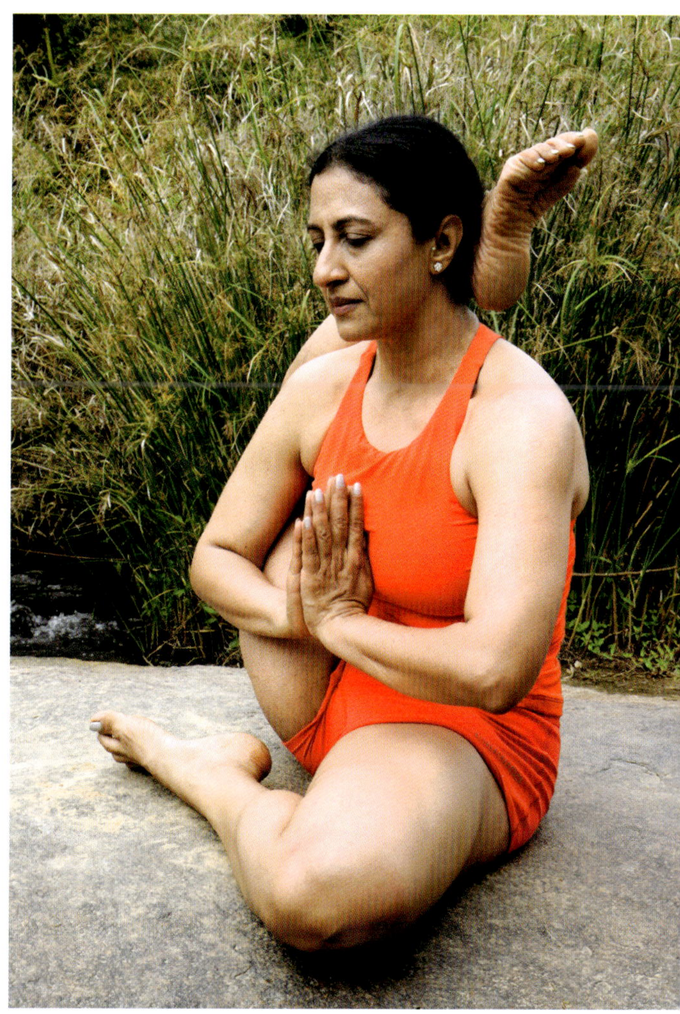

SAMSKARA AND VASANA

The concepts of *samskara* and *vasana* are very significant in understanding yoga philosophy. These explain that every action or decision in life has an impact in some way or the other to create a personality or a thought pattern in an individual. What one sees, what one hears, touches or smells assimilate into the chitta or the subconscious mind.

The main concept of yoga philosophy is in *Yoga Sutra* no. 1.2:

Chitta Vritti Nirodha

Yoga is the cessation of the fluctuations of the mind.

Understanding the concepts of samskara and vasana is key to training the chitta with greater clarity. They help identify the sources of mental distractions, making it easier to recognize and manage the patterns that shape the mind.

Samskara

Samskaras are the deep-seated mental impressions—left by past actions or experiences—that contribute to a personality. Repeated samskaras get further reinforced and create a groove in the mind field, which further become a habit or a pattern. Every action or life decision can be traced to that groove that exists as samskara.

Samskara is a universal concept. Human beings are creatures of habit. The physical, mental and emotional attitudes depend on the positive and negative samskaras we have gathered. As long as we live, we are continuously performing some action or the other—some with awareness and some without. Most of these actions and decisions have the potential to leave behind such strong samskaras that they could even be carried to the next life as karmic imprints.

Every experience in life is associated with circumstances that produce either positive, negative or neutral results. Regardless of the nature of the outcomes, it leaves an impression in the mind. Neutral expressions are short-lived and they slip out the memory field. But the actions that create a stronger impression and that which has taken place with full awareness are the ones that form strong samskaras. As time passes, memory activates the dormant samskara which produces a desire to either repeat or avoid the experience.

Each time an action is repeated, a strong impression is created. The stronger the habit gets, the mind seals them into the memory, which eventually starts influencing life in various ways via emotions, speech and actions. They become determining factors of how the world is perceived.

AUTHOR'S NOTE

We do see people who are caught up in destructive habits and some even struggle to create positive and healthier behavioural patterns. Understanding samskara helps identify repetitive patterns and transform them for the better. Yoga principles and asana practice serve as powerful tools in overcoming negative samskaras, allowing for growth and inner transformation.

Stages of Samskara Formation

- The **action** caused by a situation—*kriya*
- The **experience** caused—*anubhava*
- The **impression** created by the situation when it gets into the subconscious mind—*samskara*
- The situation and the experience repeat themselves leading to an **outcome** (could be positive or negative)—*vasana*
- The desire component which takes form of **character**—*ichchha*

Vasanas

A group of samskaras become a vasana, or a behavioural pattern. Samaskars are formed by external impulses, the end product of which is vasana. Samskara and vasana together form human experience, thereby having a great influence on the spiritual life of the person.

The contents of the minds are referred to as colours of perception (vasanas) in the texts. Even the discriminating faculty of the brain or the intellect is coloured. The spontaneity or effortlessness sometimes observed in thoughts, speeches and actions are all in accordance with those coloured impressions.

A Few Methods to Transform Samskaras and Its Vasanas

Sankalpa (Strong Declaration/ Intention)

Sankalpa literally means an 'intention with a strong declaration'. Changing samskaras is not easy. Therefore, a strong and a deep-rooted intention, deep from the heart, has to be set. Every action from that point needs to be aligned to this intention. Sankalpa is set under strong planning, strict monitoring and is to be carried out with precision until the purpose and goal are attained. The intention set with sankalpa has the capacity to unite the mind with those deeper parts of the self that are harder to access. Consciously taken sankalpa is a compelling way to communicate and emotionally guide the intention.

Tapas/Vrata (Intense or Austere Practice)

Tapas is an intense discipline to ignite a psychological process to sustain the discipline required to change a samskara. As soon as a decision is made to refrain from repeating a particular samskara, a concentrated energy from within is required to refrain from engaging in the habit. This energy fans the flame of awareness, bringing the inner wisdom to light.

It is important that tapas is practised with knowledge and awareness to be able to observe the change in the energy pattern. Tapas is the practice of wholehearted commitment to self-transformation. It involves discipline, self-restraint, and conscious effort to break old patterns and cultivate positive change. Practical approaches include abstaining from negative thoughts, emotions and behaviours, staying vigilant of samskaras that need transformation, and resisting distractions that hinder growth.

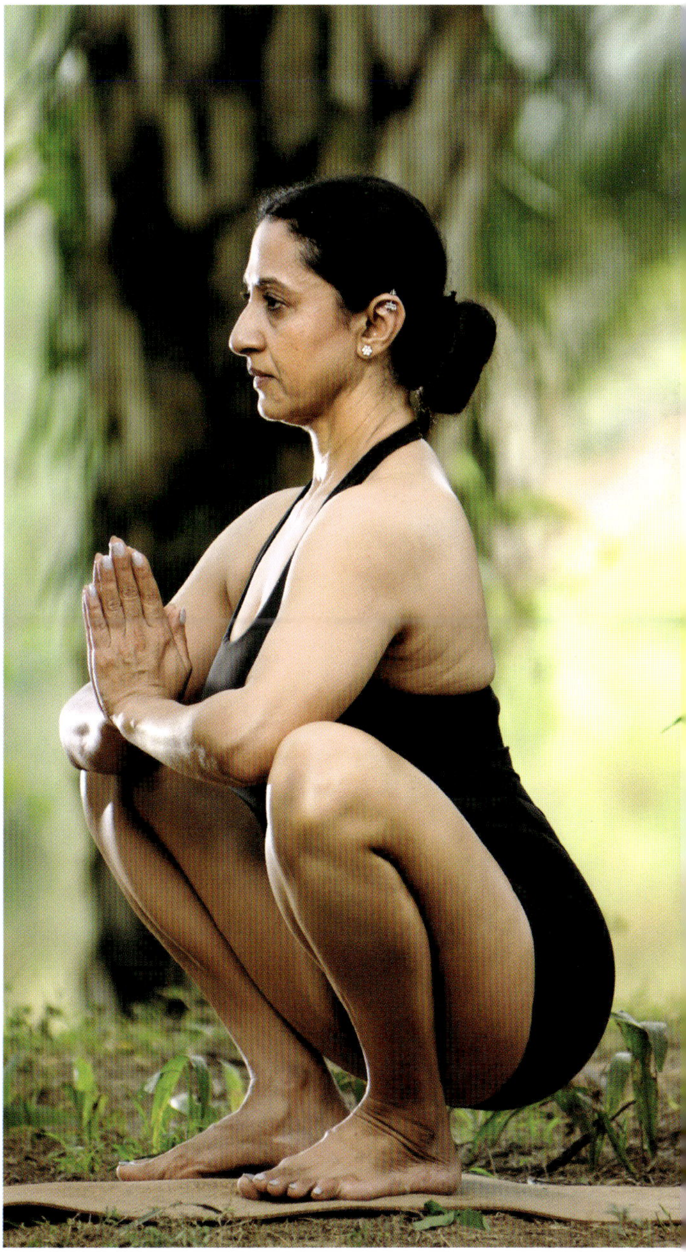

Shani (Slowing Down)

In yogic and spiritual philosophy, *shani* symbolizes patience, discipline and the power of slowing down. Derived from the Sanskrit word *shan*, meaning 'slow' or 'gradual', it represents the idea that true transformation happens over time, not instantly.

On the other hand, instinctive behaviours enable negative samskaras. This needs to be curtailed with a careful study, greater focus, stronger refection and then correct action. The process of setting this change from a negative samskara to a positive one is a slow and gradual process, which needs to be monitored at every stage.

Vidya (Awareness)

The root of negative samskara lies in *avidya* (ignorance). Once the root cause is identified, clarity sets in. This is *vidya*, or knowledge. It is important to have knowledge of the samskara that requires change. This awareness helps identify thoughts and behaviour patterns leading to the cause of the particular samskara. However, just identifying the pattern is not enough. Guidance from a guru to help understand the pattern of change and also monitor the process of change can prove to be very helpful. It should be understood that despite the intention to change the samskara being strong, certain unseen forces can cause obstacle in the path of change.

Abhaya(Fearlessness and Confidence)

Samskaras are powerful and deeply ingrained, making them alluring even as they bind us to repetitive patterns. When the desire to clear a samskara is strong, it must be accompanied by *abhaya* (fearlessness), as breaking an old samskara may bring discomfort or uncertainty. The key to liberation lies in moving forward without fear, unattached to the results—only then can one truly disconnect from the endless cycle of patterns and their consequences.

Darshana (Vision or an Insight)

A vision for change is important. Having this insight is an energy force by itself, capable of destroying the old patterns. To create new memories and release deeply buried emotions, one must be guided by a clear vision for a new and a healthier pattern.

Abhyas (Practice)

Practising a new routine with consistency will create a new pattern. With practice, the new samskara starts gaining power and strength. The stronger it gets, the lesser there is a chance of a relapse of an old samskara.

There is often resistance to change a samskara, for the fear of losing a major part of one's identity. It is important to understand what the trigger of a samskara is, so that it will be easy to monitor and avoid its relapse. Sometimes, samskaras can also be rooted in the mystery of karma which cannot be changed. But working on creating a positive karma can help change the samskara.

AUTHOR'S NOTE

Creating a new samskara is an organic pattern. The change starts from a decision. This decision is like a seed sown in the fertile mind field that has to be nurtured and facilitated enough for the process to take place. It should be remembered that all samskaras, whether positive or negative, has an inbuilt pre-existing pattern. Change can be brought in with patience and practice.

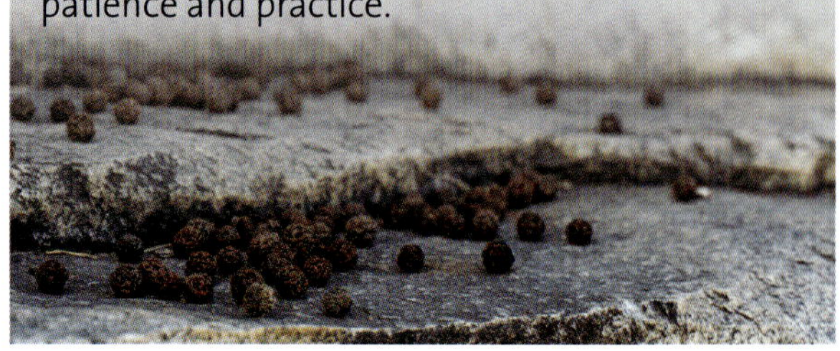

ASHTANGA PRINCIPLES FROM PATANJALI'S YOGA SUTRAS

Yoga Sutra is a valuable compilation by the great sage Patanjali who set up a systematized practice guide. The points mentioned in the *Yoga Sutra* are codified findings of a number of sages who documented their understanding. This was compiled by Sage Patanjali. The sutras serve as a comprehensive manual and guide for yoga practitioners. This is a master text that explains the afflictions of the mind and has a systematic and holistic approach recommended to resolve those afflictions.

The *Yoga Sutra* outline eight steps, known as ashtanga, to master the mind and free it from distractions, leading to inner peace and self-realization. Sutra 2.29 of Patanjali's *Yoga Sutra* defines the Ashtanga Yoga:

YAMA

Yama is the first limb of Patanjali's Ashtanga Yoga, guiding ethical and moral conduct in our interactions with the world. It is important to keep the mind pure and free of conflict.

It requires strong restraint over the mind to overcome any possible affliction. The sutra lists five main enemies in the path of spiritual growth.

- *Ahimsa*: It encourages not to cause physical or mental harm to any living being. It extends beyond actions to include words and thoughts too.
- *Satya*: It encourages to be truthful and honest, focusing on integrity and transparency.
- *Asteya*: It encourages honesty, contentment and respect for what belongs to others.
- *Brahmacharya*: Excessive indulgence in sensual pleasures can distract one from achieveing life's higher purpose. Brahmacharya encourages moderation, self-discipline and mindful use of energy to cultivate inner balance and spiritual growth.
- *Aparigraha*: Aparigraha teaches freedom from greed and attachment, discouraging the desire to accumulate more than what is necessary. It promotes contentment, simplicity and a mindful approach to material and emotional possessions.

NIYAMA

In this limb of Ashtanga Yoga, the focus is on cultivating dharmic virtues. *Niyama* translates to 'guidelines for self-discipline', fostering responsible behaviour, a loving attitude and harmonious relationships—with both people and nature. It is the foundation for inner growth and spiritual refinement. It consists of five key principles:

- *Shaucha*: Purity of the body and mind
- *Santosha*: Being grateful
- *Tapas*: Exercising the body and mind, fasting, learning art and skills to enhance knowledge
- *Svadhyaya*: Periodical reflection into one's personality is the key to progress to be even better than today
- *Ishwara Pranidhana*: The belief and trust on some power beyond human are the essence of this limb. Complete surrender to this higher power to keep the mind away from the fear of the unknown is the essence of this limb

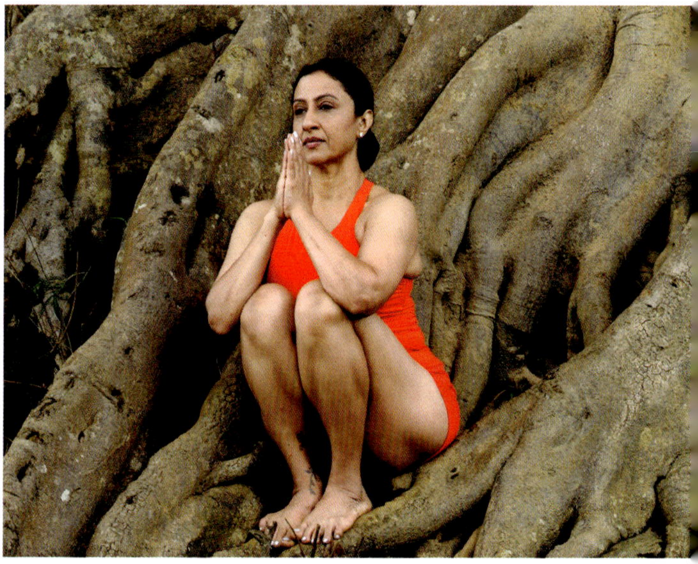

AUTHOR'S NOTE

Peace and harmony arise from the power of being truthful to oneself. Through dedicated practice of niyama, a practitioner cultivates an aura of serene strength, unwavering in the face of external disturbances. Yoga Sutra 2.35 states that even wild animals can recognize and respond to the presence of one who embodies yama and niyama with deep sincerity.

ASANA

A healthy body is important for a healthy mind. Asanas help prepare body and mind for meditation. Amongst the 196 sutras, asana practice has one dedicated sutra. The essence of this sutra centres around learning how to sit for meditation for a long period of time, without getting uncomfortable and constantly adjusting and readjusting the position.

The practice of asanas/postures is most popular these days. Even complex asanas are taught and practised with great enthusiasm in modern yoga studios. Unfortunately, the essence of getting the body to stay stable and still is not a priority.

PRANAYAMA

Breathing exercises also help prepare the body and mind to practise meditation. The ancient yogis discovered a physiological principle, which is well known to modern science, and it is that breath and the nervous system are closely connected. This limb focuses on breathing techniques involving inhalation, exhalation and breath retention. Practising pranayama techniques has great benefits for the mind as well as the body.

When faced with stress, the breathing naturally becomes rapid and shallow. When there is calmness, breathing slows down and deepens. A disturbed nervous system affects breathing, and in the same way breathing affects the nervous system. Rapid shallow breathing stimulates the system while slow deep and steady breathing calms it. Pranayama is a fundamental practice that prepares the mind and body for meditation and other spiritual pursuits.

PRATYAHARA

Pratyahara is the practice of withdrawing the mind from external disturbances and mastering one's reactions. It cultivates the ability to disengage the senses, allowing the mind to remain undistracted, much like when fully absorbed in something captivating. This practice fosters inner focus and mental clarity.

DHARANA

The practice of pratyahara leads to dharana, the cultivation of one-pointed focus. There are many dharana techniques offered in the scriptures. The main purpose of practising dharana is to find the object of concentration—which is a personal choice. Some choose to focus on the sound of 'Om', some a sacred image, lamp or chanting of a mantra. When the practice of dharana matures mind becomes absolutely one-pointed, completely free from distraction, and focused on the object of meditation.

DHYANA

Dhyana is the next stage once the object of meditation is set. It is a state of an uninterrupted flow of identical thoughts. The final state of meditation is achieved once the flow of thoughts gets uniform. Even though the mind is active, this uninterrupted flow of identical thoughts will result in deep stillness.

During dhyana in the beginning, the object of meditation is separate from the meditator. As the meditation deepens, the sense of distance between the meditator and the object of meditation becomes less. Then it gradually diminishes until finally, there is no distance left, and the object of meditation and the meditator becomes one. This is the state of total absorption or samadhi.

SAMADHI

Samadhi is not a state of thoughtlessness but an unchanging and unwavering thought.

It is referred to as the highest state of consciousness one achieves after dhyana. This is the state where the mind and the object of meditation merge.

Samadhi can be understood as a state of mind initially because when the meditator stops focusing on dhyana, they will come back to the original state. The ultimate goal of a spiritual seeker cannot be transient. Proper planning and the help of a guru can be the next steps towards one's journey to samadhi.

PRACTICAL TECHNIQUES FOR TRANSFORMATION

The scriptures clearly mention that human beings are endowed with immense potential to change or transform their life as and when they decide. However, right knowledge, correct planning and execution, and a sustained effort or consistency is very important. Before taking any major step towards transformation, it is important to make a complete assessment of the self (svadhyaya). Based on the finding, the next stage would be to determine the scope and intensity of the desire to transform. In the process, it is vital to recognize personal strength and weakness.

SETTING UP A GOAL

- Set the process of transformation with a clear goal in mind.
- Deal with resistance to change.
- Change is challenging and uncomfortable. Get used to the discomfort.
- Explore the true nature of your personality—journaling can aid in this process. Consider how you respond to adversity.
- Examine the present moment and how it may shape future outcomes.
- Acknowledge the present and recognize any feelings of gratitude for life's natural gifts.
- Contemplate whether you could depart from the world with grace and dignity.

Such reflection will help find a path and a purpose. Acting on it will pave the way for ultimate freedom.

SURRENDER

Surrender might sound like a negative moment and inaction. But the scriptures treat this as a very active stage, one that requires thorough monitoring. Surrender in the true sense is winning over oneself. Dropping the negativity and moving courageously towards positivity is the essence of true surrender. A guru plays a vital role in the process.

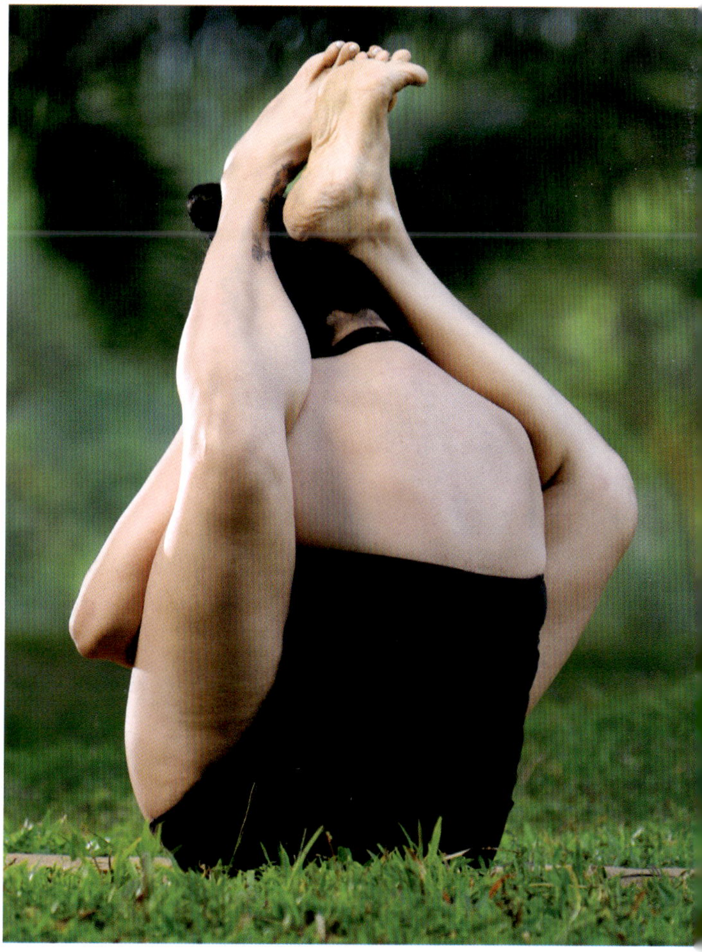

BHAKTI

Unshakeable faith is another approach for bringing about transformation in life. Infusing every action with devotion, faith and love towards the ultimate reality is a crucial step. Bhakti, or complete devotion, is about dedicating all efforts with a sense of offering, free from personal attachment.

In the *Yoga Sutra*, bhakti is referred to as 'Ishwara Pranidhana'. Sage Patanjali explains that true bhakti is not about acting with personal intent but realizing that we are mere instruments of a greater purpose, surrendering completely to the universe.

THE POWER OF MEDITATION

Meditation has been a sacred practice of sages and scholars since ancient times, though its exact origins remain unknown. Ancient scriptures describe its profound effects on the mind and body. Over time, diverse meditation techniques have emerged, each evolving to meet specific needs and cultivate unique potentials. In recent years, new methods have been developed, incorporating systematic relaxation, visualization, breathwork and simple concentration techniques—accessible approaches for beginners to start their practice.

BREATHING

Simple breathing techniques are best to begin with. It helps release the tension in the body and gently build up concentration. This is a good way to train the mind without imposing upon it.

- Sit comfortably with your head, neck and hips aligned, allowing your body to relax completely.
- Keep your gaze soft and neutral while looking straight ahead.
- Gently roll your eyes upwards and close them lightly.
- Focus on your breath as it flows in and out through your nostrils.

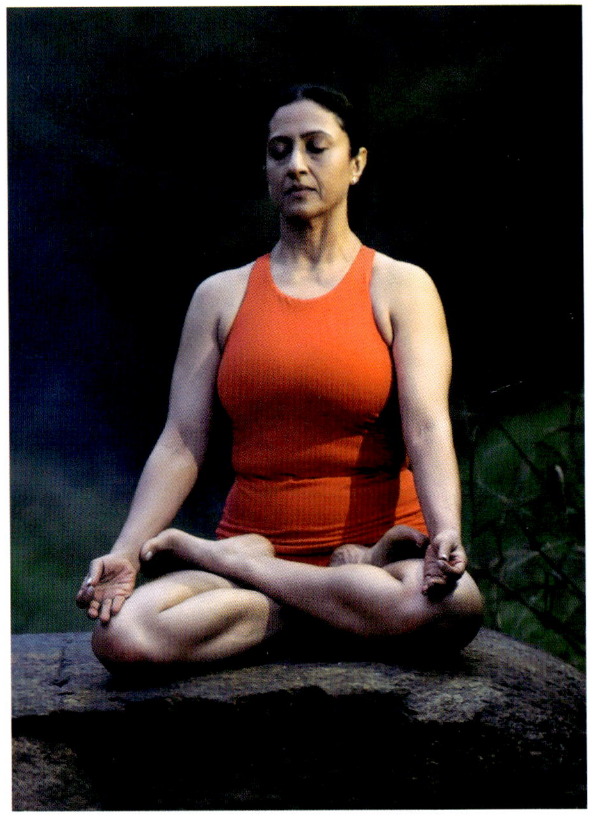

- Notice the coolness of the air as you inhale and the warmth as you exhale.
- Maintain a calm, even breath without force—this helps still the mind and enhances focus.
- Experimenting with slight variations in breathing rhythm can aid concentration.

Samavritti Breathing

Also known as 'equal breath', this breathing technique is used to balance the breath and calm the mind, especially during times of stress. The practice involves creating a rhythm where the length of the inhalation and exhalation are equal.

- Sit in a comfortable, upright posture, ensuring your spine is aligned. Close your eyes gently and begin to bring your awareness to your breath.
- Make a slow, deep inhalation through your nose, filling your lungs completely.
- Aim for a steady and smooth inhalation without rushing. Begin by counting, for example, to four,

ensuring the inhalation is steady and even. This is the first step in making the inhalation equal in length to the exhalation.

- Exhale slowly and completely through your nose, releasing the breath smoothly and evenly, for the same count as the inhalation (e.g., to a count of four). The key is to ensure the exhalation is just as controlled and gentle as the inhalation.
- Continue inhaling and exhaling in an equal ratio (for example, a four-count inhalation and a four-count exhalation).
- With each cycle, focus on maintaining smooth, even and controlled breathing, without force or strain.

As you practise, you can gradually extend the length of both the inhalation and exhalation, but the important part is that they remain equal.

Vishamavritti Breathing

Vishamavritti breathing involves uneven or 'irregular' breathing patterns. Unlike *samavritti*, where the inhalation and exhalation are of the same length, vishamavritti focuses on creating an unequal ratio between the inhalation and exhalation. This practice helps to balance the mind and body by promoting focus, relaxation and energy.

- Sit in a comfortable, upright position. Keep your spine straight, shoulders relaxed, and close your eyes gently.
- Begin to tune into your breath, noticing its natural flow.
- Inhale slowly but deeply through your nose, making the inhalation longer than the exhalation. For example, you can inhale for a count of four, six, or eight (or longer, depending on your comfort level).
- Focus on filling your lungs completely, but do not force the breath.
- Exhale through your nose for a shorter duration than the inhalation. For example, you might exhale for a count of two, four, or six (again, depending on your level of comfort).
- Make sure the exhalation is controlled and smooth, but it should not be rushed.
- Repeat the cycle of inhaling longer than the exhalation, maintaining the uneven pattern (e.g., inhale for six counts, exhale for four counts).
- As you continue, try to keep the breath smooth and relaxed, even though it is uneven. Focus on the sensation of breathing and the feeling of balance this pattern creates.

Practise the two breathing techniques over a period of time (six months or more to build up the focus). Focus on at least two rounds of samavritti breathing and two rounds of vishamavritti breathing. Notice the benefits—of a relaxed and refreshed feeling.

MOVING MEDITATION (AS AND WHEN POSSIBLE)

This meditation can be practised in both indoor or outdoor settings. With five minutes of focus, it can help improve breathing and cardiovascular health, stabilize mood, relax the nervous system, boost energy and, most importantly, quieten the mental chatter. This method has three components: breathing, movement and a steady slow stride. It can be divided into six stages.

- Stand with your feet together, distributing the body weight on both feet.
- Fixing the gaze straight, walk 30 steps forward and 30 steps backward in a comfortable stride and pace.
- Observe the breathing and heartbeat, and change the rhytm of the stride accordingly.
- For every inhalation and exhalation, walk four steps each.
- Walk for about two minutes monitoring the movement and breathing.
- Stop after two minutes, close your eyes, and observe your breath and your bodily response with full awareness, being as relaxed as you can possibly be.

- Complete the exercise by repeatedly making the 'soo' sound as you breathe in and 'hum' sound as you breathe out. Keep your feet together in a comfortable position, eyes closed, and breathe naturally. The breathing should be comfortable and not too strong.

This technique can be practised whenever time allows, as it helps cultivate awareness and keeps the mind focused and alert.

STILLNESS MEDITATION

1. Start by finding a quiet place and a comfortable seated position. It is important to keep the spine erect with pelvis, chest and head in a straight line to ensure smooth flow of breath.
   - Sitting on a chair is a good idea if the back is not strong.
   - Sitting on the floor gives more focus. To protect the lower back from getting tired, a blanket or a cushion may be placed under the hips.
2. Visualizing a circle of light around the circumference of the body creates a sense of boundary—like sitting within a protective shell of light, distinct yet at peace with your surroundings.
3. With practice and patience, unnecessary tension can be released from the mind and body. The best and the only way to deal with distraction is by becoming aware of the breath and strengthening that awareness. Do not feel pressured into practising deep breathing or rhythmic breathing.
4. As the attention to breath establishes, follow the breath as it reaches to different areas of the body. Observe the air filling into the chest, expanding it and moving along right shoulder to left shoulder, below the chest and belly, towards the lower belly and the lower back, and then down towards the legs.
5. Focus on the breath as it flows around the nostrils for a while, then gently shift your attention to the centre of the eyebrows. To deepen your focus, silently repeat 'soo' with each inhale and 'hum' with each exhale—allowing the rhythm to guide you into complete stillness.
6. To end the meditation, shift the attention from the centre of the brow to the whole body. Return to visualizing the wheel of light surrounding you, then gradually expand your awareness beyond its boundary.
7. It is important to rest the body in Shavasana for at least 10 minutes. Sit upright and briskly rub your palms together for 30 seconds. Then, gently sweep your hands from the top of your head down along the length of your body, releasing energy outward through your feet.

MEDITATION TO SUSTAIN A YOGA LIFESTYLE

Meditation provides a sense of stability in the ever-changing world. Meditation should be a consistent practice, like a daily ritual with dedication and reverence. Ideally, a space and a time to be fixed for meditation will help initiate a regular practice. Early morning hours are the best time suited for meditation.

The body and the mind are in a constant state of change, influenced by circumstances, environment, diet, and even the nature of our thoughts. Meditation helps to be kind to the mind and self, which in turn helps the mind to rest, reflect and renew.

Meditation is the key to cultivating a yoga-inspired lifestyle, enhancing not only external achievements but also fostering deep self-awareness. It encourages healthy self-reflection and personal growth. The fundamental meditation techniques outlined in this book hold immense potential to help overcome limitations and unlock the subtle power within. As we deepen our awareness, we become more creative and dynamic. Meditation helps bring hidden thoughts and lingering emotions to light, allowing us to release what no longer serves us. Each day, waves of thoughts will rise, seeking resolution. This is a natural process, and the key is to remain steadfast—continuing the practice without giving in to doubt or distraction.

MEDITATION BENEFITS

1. Meditation is the most certain path to discovering our true identity. As the scriptures teach, 'the world within is more important than the external world'. Through meditation, we turn inward, uncovering the deeper essence of who we truly are.
2. Meditation has the power to restore inner strength, which often becomes depleted by uncontrollable external circumstances.
3. It helps mind remain focused which is very important to reach one's destination.
4. Meditation will help realize that true joy doesn't come from external world but comes from within, in the form of inner joy.

YOGA SEQUENCE BEFORE MEDITATION

Meditation requires focused attention, a relaxed body and a peaceful mind. Establishing a consistent routine, a dedicated time and a serene space can enhance the practice. A well-structured asana and pranayama routine helps prepare the body, allowing for stillness and comfort during meditation.

Standing Asanas

SURYA NAMASKARA A (FOR REFERENCE, SEE PP. 4–5)

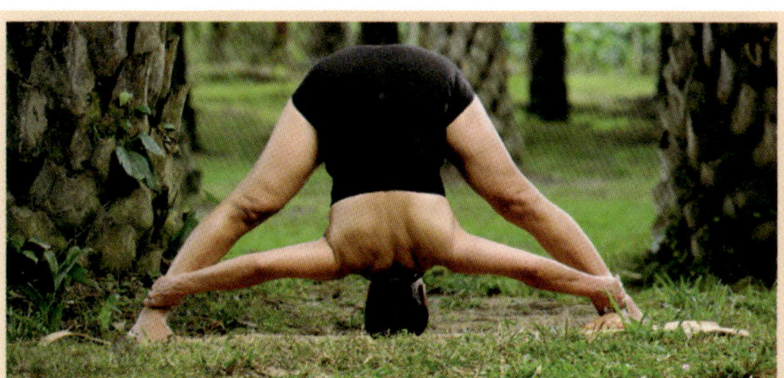

PRASARITA PADOTTANASANA

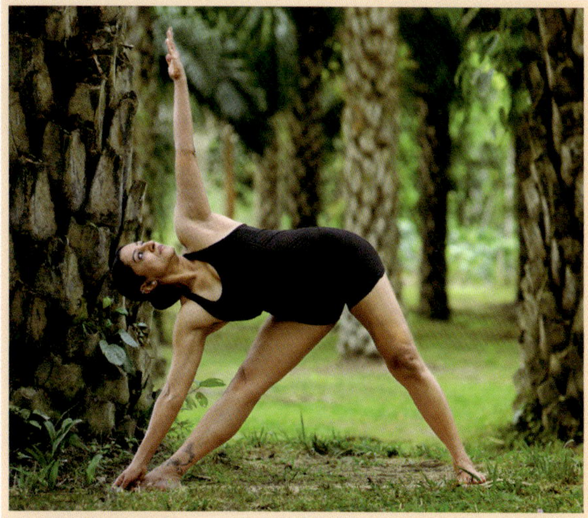

TRIKONASANA

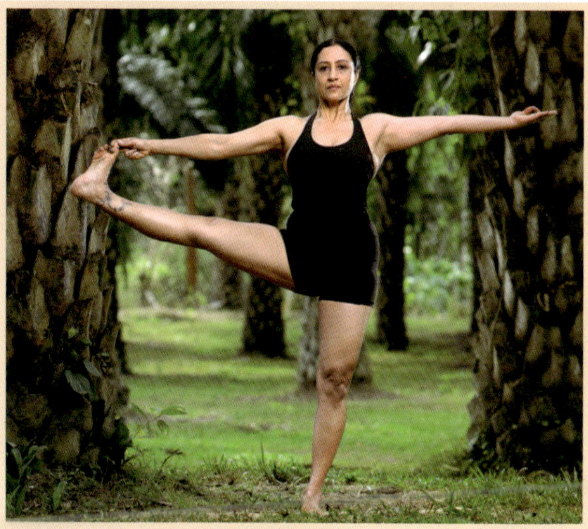

HASTA PADANGUSHTHASANA

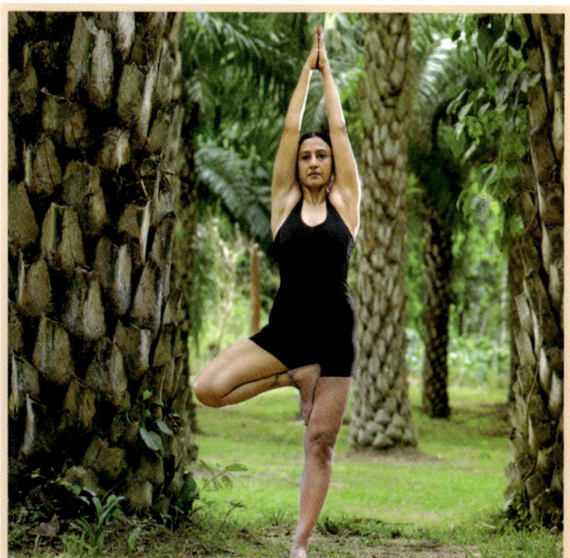

VRIKSHASANA

Floor Asanas

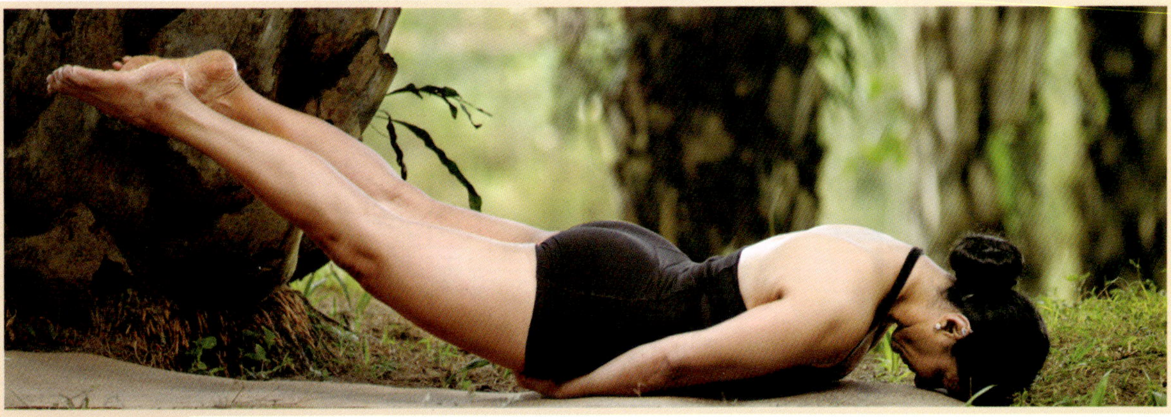

SHALABHASANA

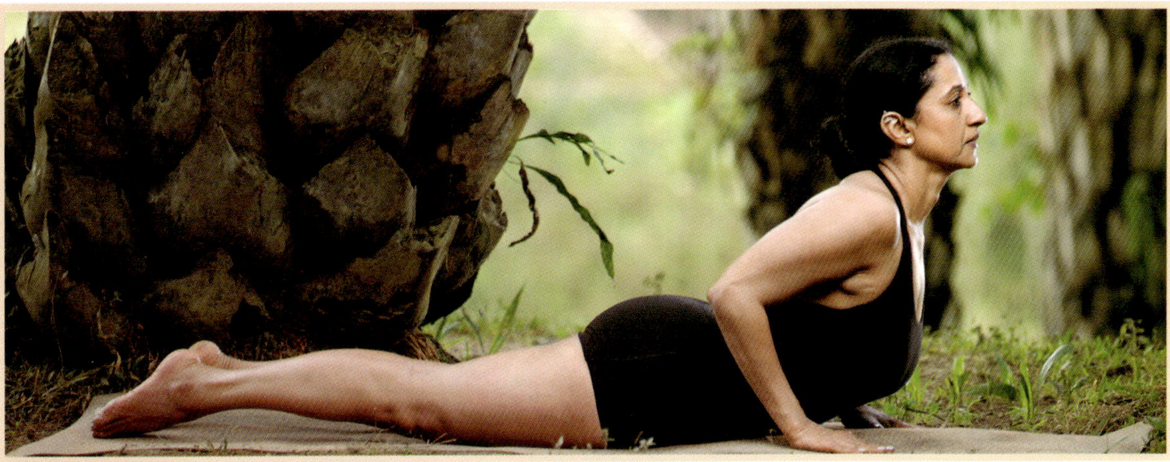

BHUJANGASANA

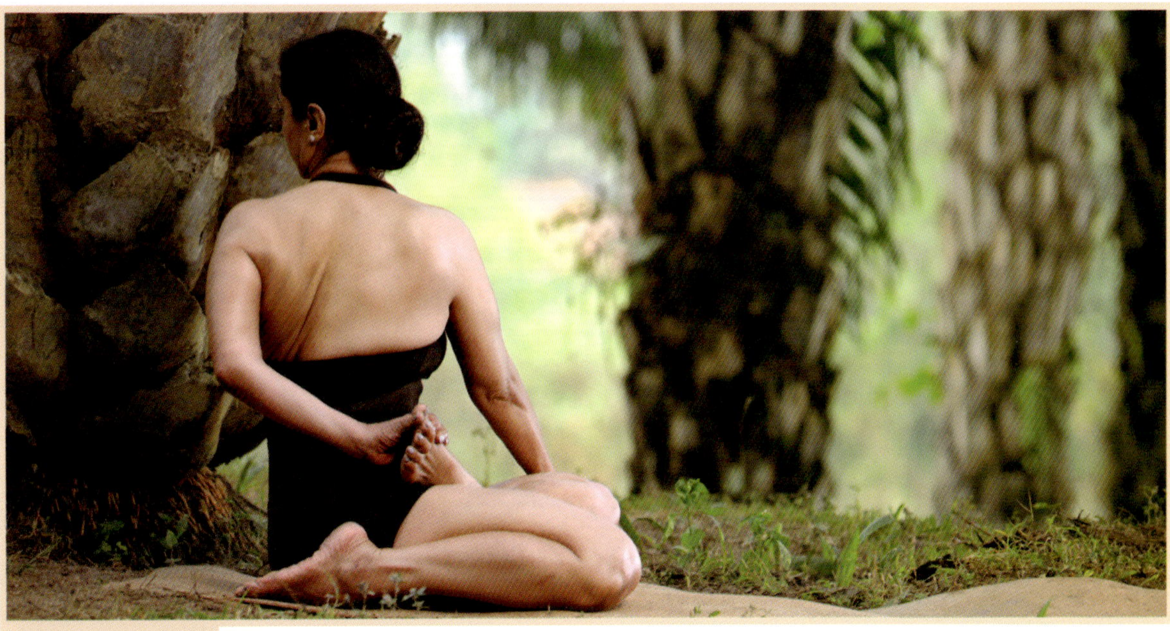

BHARADWAJASANA

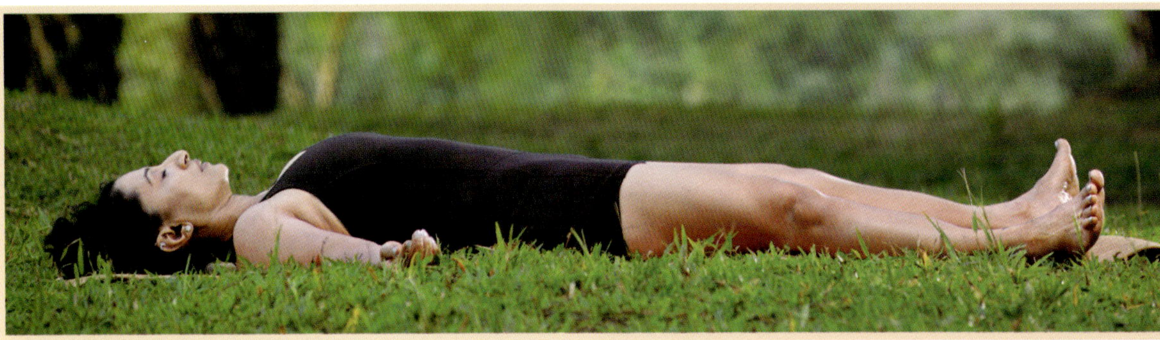

SHAVASANA (FOR 5 MINUTES)

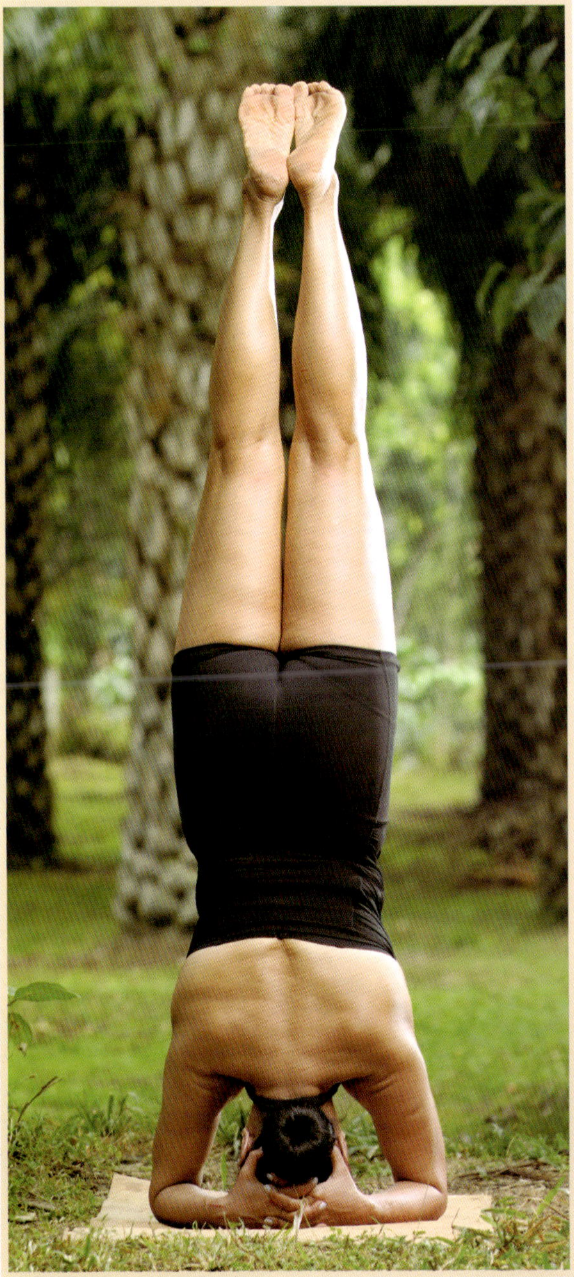

SHIRASANA (OPTIONAL)

Pranayama

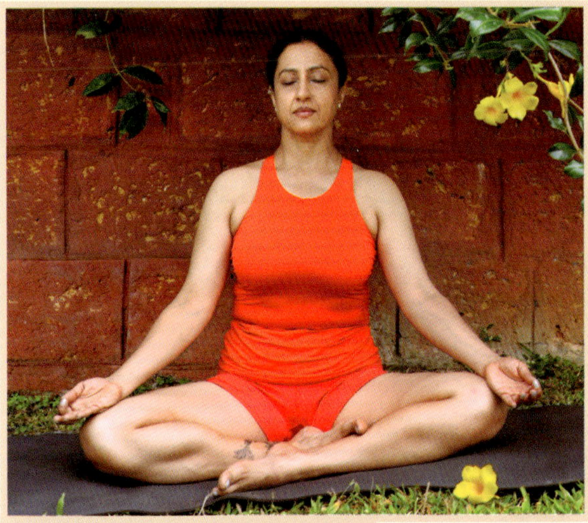

UJJAYI (WITH ANTAR KUMBHAKA)

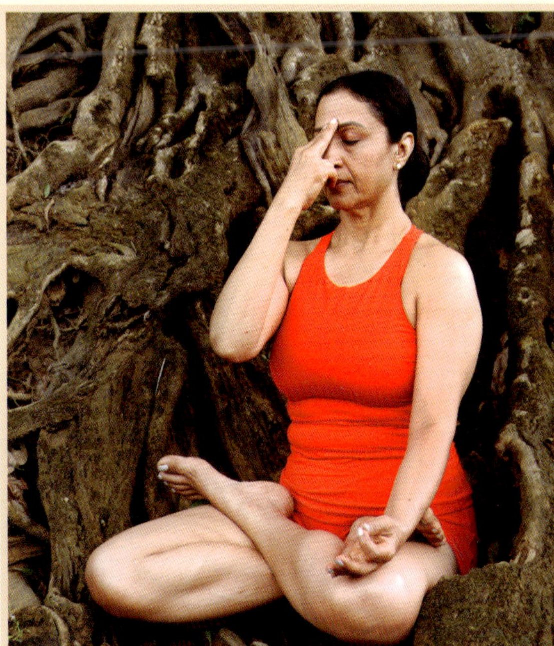

ANULOM VILOM (WITH ANTAR KUMBHAKA)

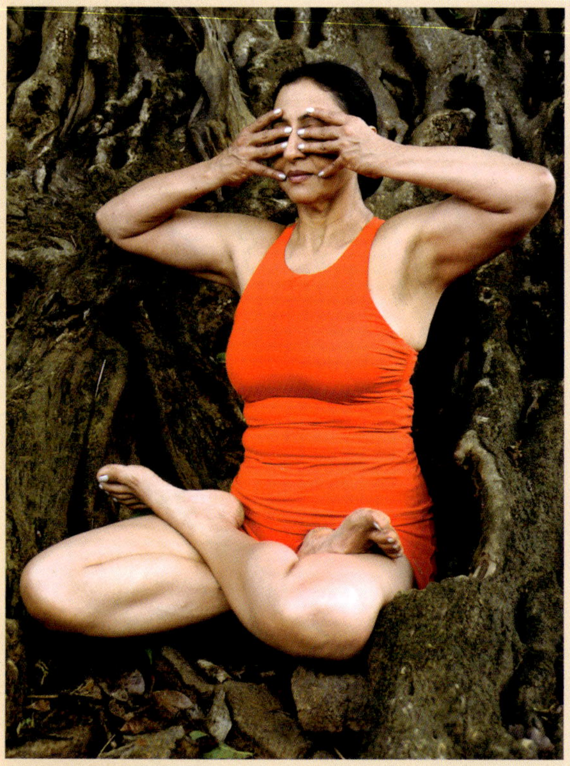

BHRAMARI

GENERAL TIPS TO SIT STILL

- In the early stages of meditation, the body may present obstacles such as restlessness, muscle twitches, slight tremors, itching or swaying. These sensations are natural and will gradually subside with time, patience and consistent practice.
- It is important not to heed to the obstacles surfacing in the mind and body. The mind will get very busy and distractive as the body gets still, casuing pain and discomfort.
- A healthy body lays the foundation for a strong meditation practice. Regular breathing exercises cultivate a steady, calm breath, which in turn nurtures a peaceful mind. Focusing on the breath is one of the most effective ways to quiet—mental turbulence. By simply observing the breath, the mind becomes steady, enhancing focus and inner stability.

GENERAL TIPS FOR STEADYING THOUGHTS

- The main focus here is paying attention to the breath. Initially, it may shift between regular and irregular, especially as thoughts flood the mind. It is important to remain patient.
- Another effective way to stabilize the mind is by choosing an auspicious object or symbol as a point of focus, helping to anchor awareness and cultivate inner stillness.
- Chanting affirmation or mantras initiated by a guru can also help initiate the process of meditation.
- There is always going to be a flow of worldly activities which is bound to disturb the mind. Observing thoughts without responding to it is an effective way of steadying thoughts.
- The process demands patience and consistency. This is something which can be done through one's own effort, with trial and error. The most important thing is to not to give up.

MANTRA

A mantra is usually given by a teacher to a student. It is usually given after an assessment of the student, wherein the teacher evaluates and prescribes a mantra best suited for the student according to their attitude, emotions, desire and habits.

A mantra has four koshas:

- It begins as a word.
- It deepens with meaning.
- It is enriched by feeling.
- It dissolves into silence.

Reaching the fourth kosha, the meditator gets deeper into practice and a constant awareness of mantra sets in.

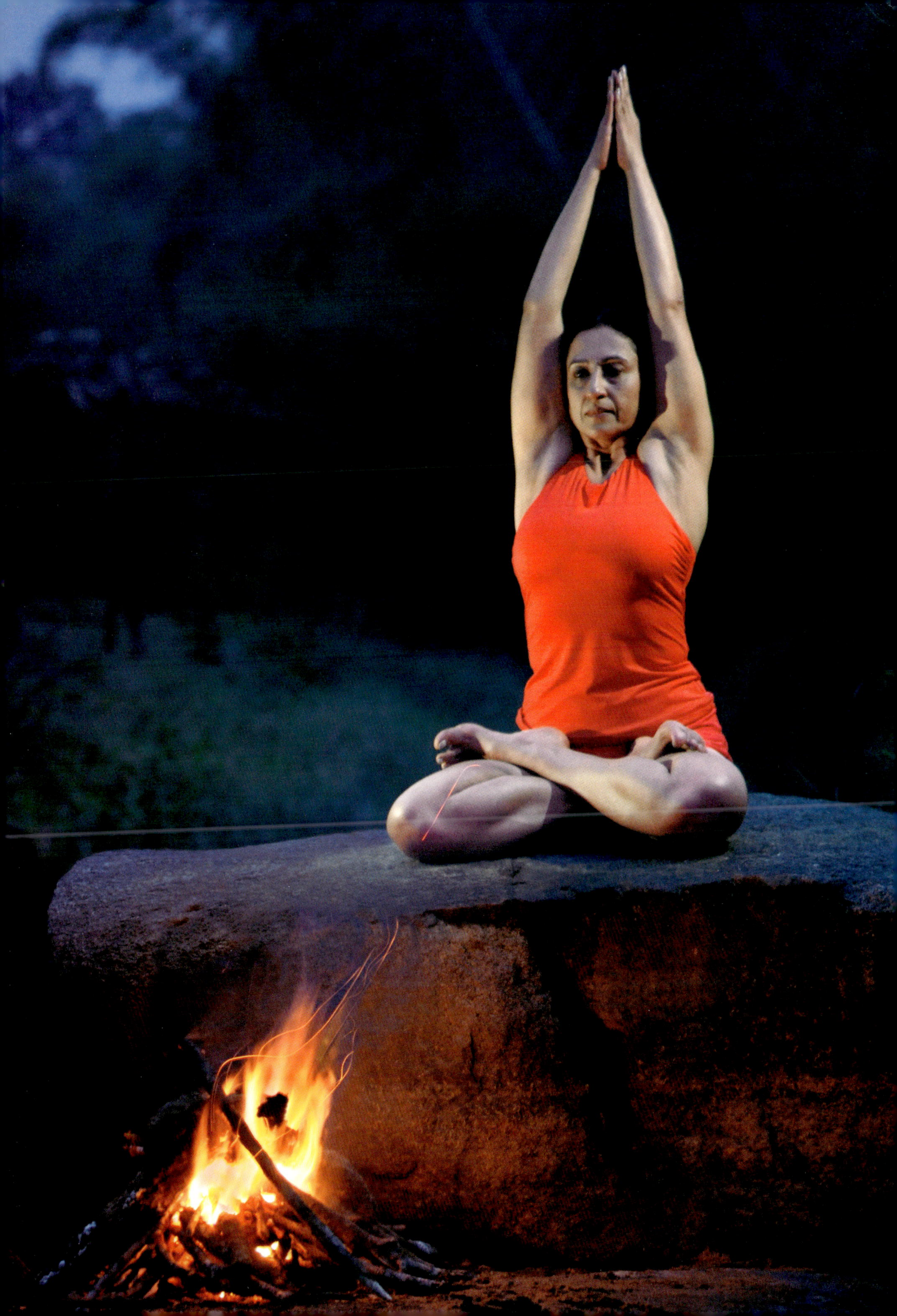

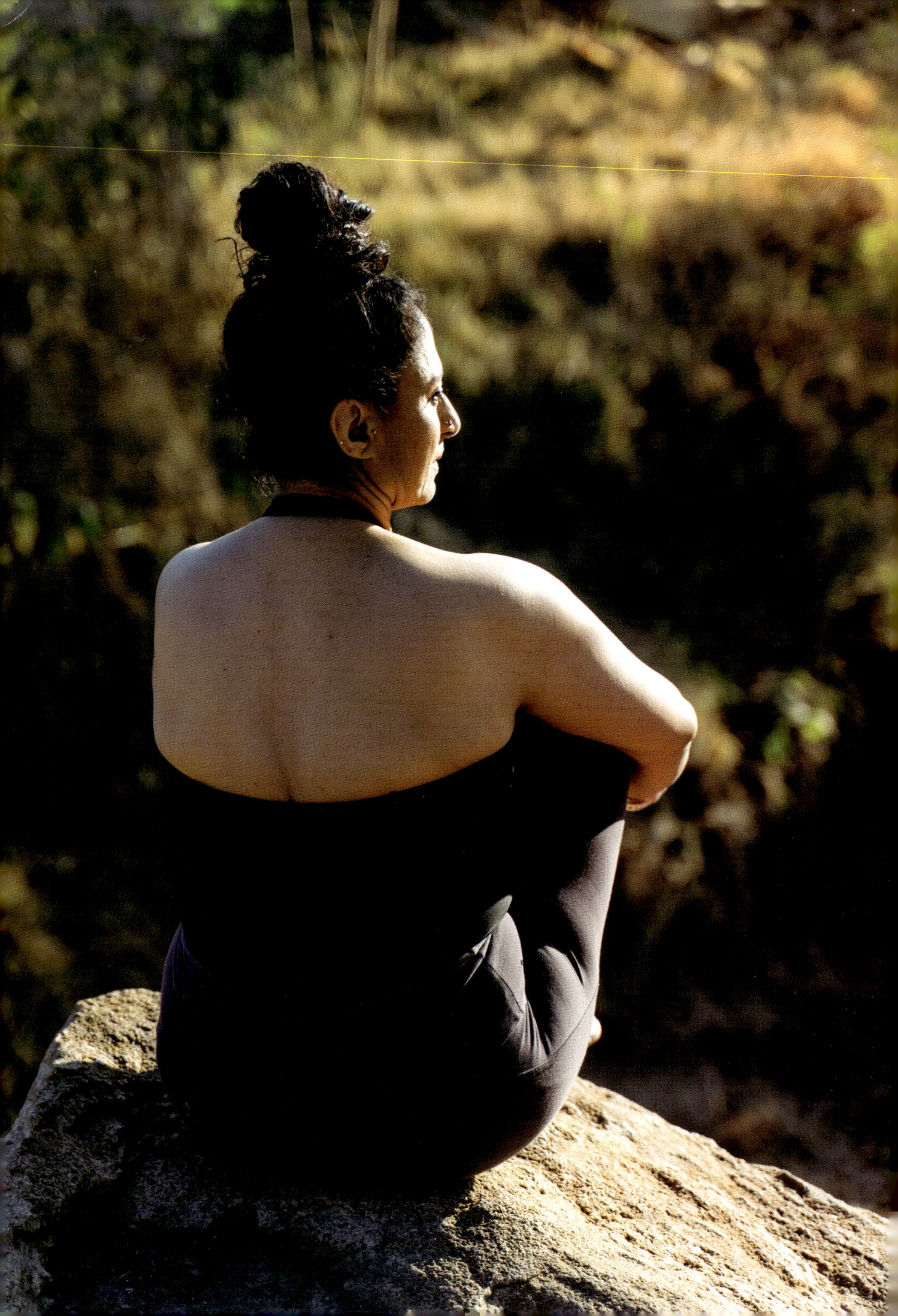

AFTERWORD

Study and practice of yoga are incomplete without understanding the essence of the practice. It is also important that we understand the context in which the practice of yoga took its origin and why it has such a profound influence on the culture of ancient India.

Yoga in the recent times has often been dismantled and practised as a set of physical routine to get flexible and strong, while some others regard it as a discipline for enhancing mental well-being, and many others consider it as an esoteric practice for mystical experiences. This book is about an integrated practice of yoga for an all-round benefit.

This book provides essential knowledge for yoga practitioners seeking to move beyond the physical aspects of practice and explore the deeper dimensions of yoga. It offers valuable insights into the intricate layers of human existence, as described in ancient texts and scriptures.

Understanding this wisdom enables self-reflection, helping individuals navigate life's challenges with clarity and ease, reducing the strain of ignorance. Our ancient masters, through intense penance and dedicated practice, have left behind profound teachings—timeless and invaluable guidelines that continue to serve as a gift to humanity for generations to come.

This book is an attempt to simplify this vast knowledge system which has taken a back seat in this modern time and age. It is like a preparation to transform from a level of yoga asana practice and move towards the other limbs of yoga system.

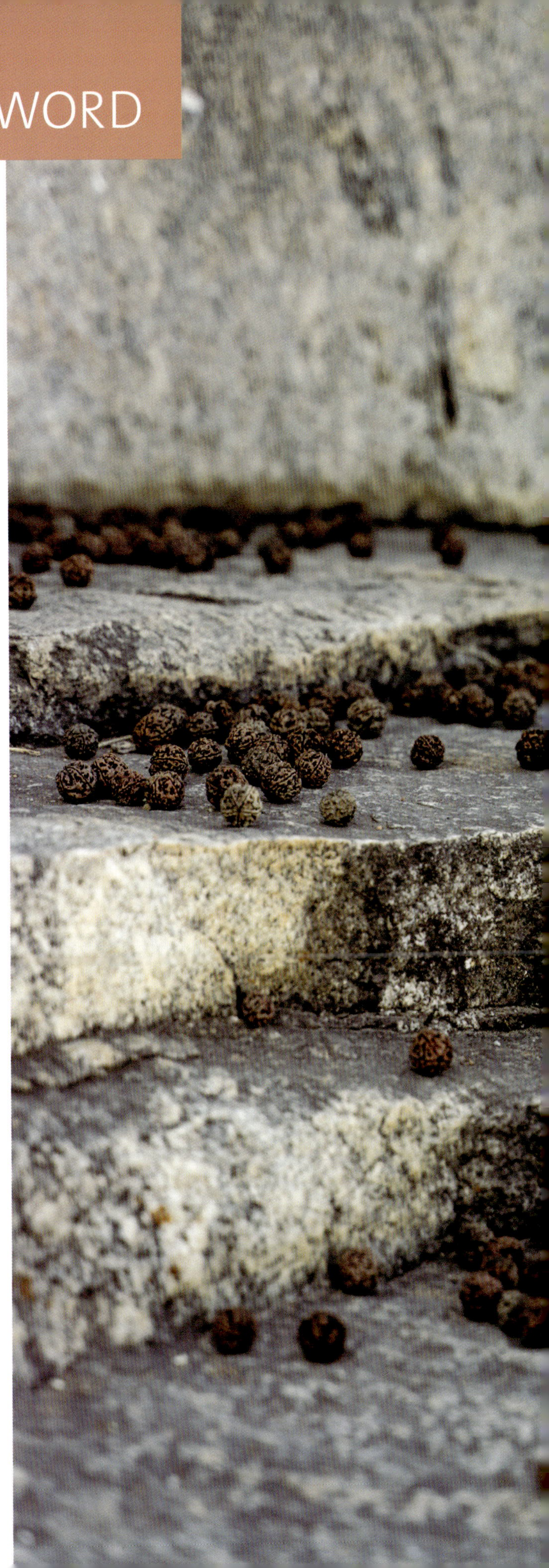

GLOSSARY

Abhaya - Fearlessness
Abhyas - Practice
Agni - Fire
Ahimsa - Non-violence
Akasha - Sky/ether
Anand - Highest state of happiness
Anubhava - Experience
Aparigraha - Non-possessiveness
Asana - Posture
Ashtanga - Eight limbs
Asteya - Non-stealing/non-covetousness
Asthi - Bone tissue
Atma - Eternal radiant self
Bhakti - Faith and devotion
Brahmacharya - Self-control
Buddhi - Intellect
Chakshu - Eye
Chitta - Storehouse of impressions in the mind
Darshana - Auspicious sight
Dharana - Mental concentration on an object or idea
Dharma - A code of proper conduct conforming to one's duty and nature
Dhyana - Profound meditation
Drishti - Sight
Gandha - Smell
Guna - Attribute
Guru - One who guides from darkness to light
Hasta Mudra - Hand gestures
Ishwara Pranidhana - Surrender to the Divine
Jal - Water
Jihva - Tongue
Jnanendriyas - Five sensory organs
Kaivalya - Final liberation
Kapha - One of the three doshas, representing the element of water
Karmendriyas - Five organs of action (mouth, hands, feet, excretory organ and genitals)
Karna - Ear
Kriya - Action
Kosha - Five layers of existence
Kumbhaka - Breath retention
Majja - Bone marrow
Mamsa - Muscle tissue
Manas - Mental faculty or mind
Meda - Fat tissue
Moksha - Release from cycle of rebirth
Mudra - Hand gestures
Mutra - Urine
Nabi - Navel
Nasika - Nose
Nirodha - Restraint
Niyama - Observing discipline
Pancha Bhootas - Five elements of nature
Pitta - One of the three doshas, representing the element of fire
Prajna - Insight
Prakriti - Material existence
Prana - Life force
Pranayama - Breathing exercises
Pratyahara - Turning mind inwards for self-introspection
Prithvi - Earth
Puraka - Inhalation
Purisha - Faeces
Purushartha - Purpose of human life
Rakta - Blood
Rasa - Plasma/lymph
Rasana - Taste organ
Rechaka - Exhalation
Rupa - Form
Samadhi - Spiritual enlightenment/ culmination of meditation
Samskara - Deep-seated mental imprints/impressions

Sankalpa	-	Strong intention or a solemn vow
Santosh	-	Contentment
Satya	-	Truth
Seva	-	Selfless service
Shabda	-	Sound
Shani	-	Slow mover
Sharira	-	Physical body
Sharira traya	-	Yogic model of human existence comprising the gross, subtle and causal bodies
Shaucha	-	Cleanliness
Shukra	-	Reproductive tissue
Sthula	-	The gross or physical body (comprising earth, water, fire air and ether or space)
Sparsha	-	Touch
Sukshma	-	The subtle body comprising mind and life energy
Sutra	-	Aphorism in Sanskrit literature prepared for memorization
Svadhyaya	-	Self-study
Sweda	-	Sweat
Tapas	-	Austere spiritual meditation
Twak	-	Skin
Upadesha	-	Spiritual guidance
Vasana	-	Behavioural pattern
Vata	-	One of the three doshas, representing the elements of air and ether (space).
Vayu	-	Wind/Air
Vidya	-	Knowledge
Vinyasa	-	Yoga postures accompanied by regulated breathing
Vrata	-	Religious observance
Vritti	-	Waves created in the mind by ever-changing thoughts
Yama	-	Ethics

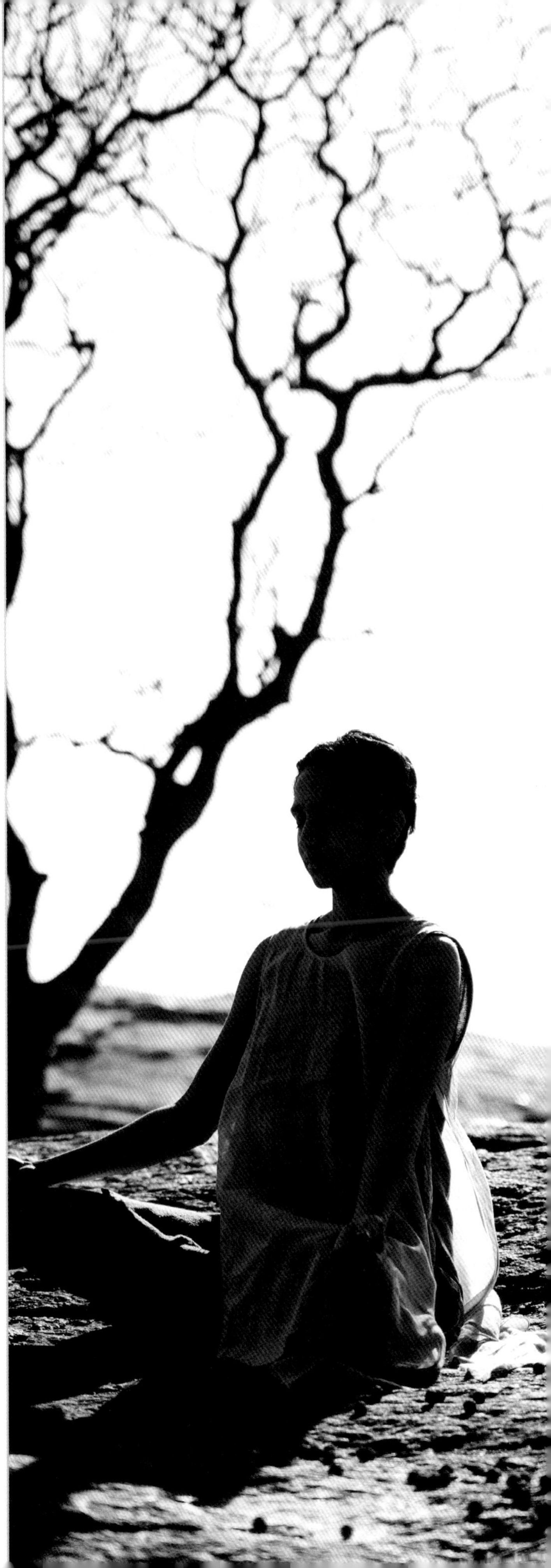

INDEX

Y

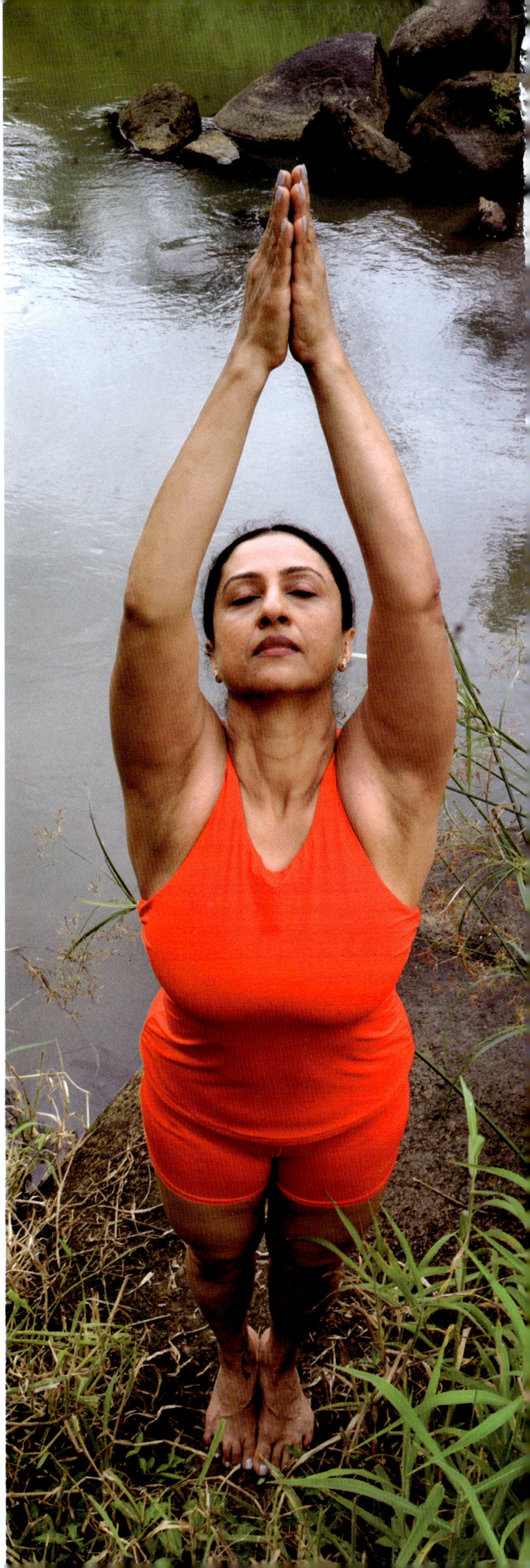